PRAISE FOR THE CARNIVORE CODE

"Dr. Paul Saladino is driving an incredibly compelling carnivore diet movement, with a thoughtful and measured presentation that compels everyone to pay close attention. With Paul's broad experience in both traditional and functional medicine, he is able to embrace the big picture of healing and achieve breakthrough results."

Mark Sisson
NYT Bestselling Author of *The Primal Blueprint* and *The Keto Reset Diet*, Founder of MarksDailyApple.com

"Paul Saladino is, by far, one of the most brilliant new minds in the health and nutrition sector. This guy is the real deal. He is well researched, practices what he preaches, and has a passion for digging for the ultimate truth. I can't recommend him or his work highly enough."

Ben Greenfield
NYT Bestselling Author, Voted America's Top Personal Trainer

"Paul is an extraordinary out-of-the-box thinker. He has deeply researched the science and provides some compelling arguments that challenge conventional nutritional wisdom regarding the need for eating plants to achieve optimal health."

Dr. Mercola
Multiple Time NYT Bestselling Author, Founder of Mercola.com

"Paul extols the benefits of carnivorous eating and backs it up fully with science. He's done the hard work and fact-finding so you don't have to. As a functional medicine physician, he looks at human health from all angles. He's got this one covered in *The Carnivore Code: Unlocking the Secrets to Optimal Health by Returning to Our Ancestral Diet*."

Dave Asprey
CEO of Bulletproof, Leading Biohacker

"Paul Saladino is a bright thinker who has a unique ability to present the complex science surrounding diet and nutrition in an understandable way. In *The Carnivore Code* and his work, he does just that, showing us the compelling research supporting the many benefits of a carnivore diet. If you are looking to optimize your health, you need to read this book. You won't be disappointed!"

Robb Wolf
Two-Times NYT Bestselling Author of *The Paleo Solution* and *Wired to Eat*

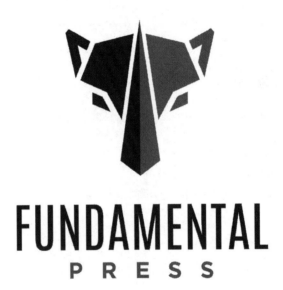

FUNDAMENTAL

PRESS

THE

CARNIVORE CODE

PAUL SALADINO, M.D.

FOREWORD BY MARK SISSON

The Carnivore Code

© 2020 by Paul Saladino
Published by Fundamental Press

Edited by Jackson Haynes, Tim Neller, and Shawn Mihalik
Interior design by Nikkita Kent
Illustrations by Judy Cho

Printed in the United States of America
ISBN: 978-1-7346407-0-0

First edition

Disclaimer: None of the information contained in this book should be construed as medical advice. If you have questions about anything mentioned or recommended in this book, please consult your personal physician.

*To my mother, father, and sister. You have shown me unwavering
love and support throughout all of my adventures.
I owe the best parts of who I am to you all.*

*And to my patients, you are my inspiration and my greatest
teachers. I am so much richer from hearing your stories,
and what you have taught me is immeasurable.*

CONTENTS

SECTION III

The Myth of the Blue Zones
Won't I Get Scurvy Eating Only Animal Foods?
Summing It Up

CHAPTER ELEVEN: MYTH IV—RED MEAT CAUSES THE HEART TO EXPLODE

The Basics of Lipoproteins and Cholesterol
The Vital Role of LDL in Our Body
Could More LDL Be Protective?
LDL in Heart Disease: Criminal or Firefighter?
Atherosclerosis—It's All About the Stickiness!
Further down the LDL Rabbit Hole
The Skinny (and Not So Skinny) on Insulin Resistance
Other Causes of Insulin Resistance
Why Does LDL Rise on a Ketogenic Diet?
Should You Take a Statin for an Elevated LDL?
TMAO: The Sheep in Wolf's Clothing
Saturated Fat: Why Vegetable Oil Companies Say It's Bad
The Edge of Zion

SECTION IV

CHAPTER TWELVE: WHAT TO EAT ON A NOSE-TO-TAIL CARNIVORE DIET

Is It Ethical to Eat Animals?
How to Eat a Nose-to-Tail Carnivore Diet
Tier 1: The Carnivore-*ish* Diet
Artificial Sweeteners and Spices
Didn't Our Ancestors Eat Fruit?
Tubers and Berries
What About Fungi?
What to Drink on a Carnivore Diet
What About Alcohol?
When to Eat on a Carnivore Diet
Tier 2: The Meat and Water Carnivore Diet
Tier 3: The Freshman Carnivore Diet
What About Seafood on a Carnivore Diet?
What About Chicken, Turkey, and Other Birds?
What About Pork?
Tier 4: The Junior Varsity Carnivore Diet
Liver Magic
Is It Possible to Eat Too Much Liver?

FOREWORD

The carnivore diet has suddenly arrived into a prominent position in the world of ancestral health. Over the years, I've come across the occasional fringe character touting a carnivore-style diet and never paid it a second thought. Back in the 1970s, Venice Beach bodybuilders were known to eat only steak and eggs for a few weeks to get cut up for contests. In 2017, when fitness expert Danny Vega told me that his prolonged carnivore experiment generated dramatic improvements in blood values, as well as increased energy and peak performance, I shrugged off the story because it didn't align with my personal belief system. As a guy who prides himself on being able to think critically, remain open-minded, and always willing to revise his positions when new information arises, I humbly apologize for my resistance.

In recent years, the carnivore message has evolved from fringe to legit. In 2019, when Dr. Paul started making the rounds of podcast interviews, his carnivore message caught my attention and held it. Truth be told, I was captivated by the way Dr. Paul gracefully addressed the most controversial aspects of carnivore with reasonable, precise, and scientifically validated responses. For example, we know that most plants, including the vegetables beloved by all the diet experts, contain anti-nutrients that are difficult to digest and even toxic. That's why we must elaborately soak, sprout, ferment, and cook our plant foods to render them edible. Even then, many of us experience side effects like gas, bloating, and digestive pain that are so commonplace we have come to view them as normal. As Paul will detail in this book, it's not normal to suffer when consuming meals that are supposed to be healthy!

Carnivore is an area where I am doing some deep thinking, research, and personal experimentation. Placing sustainably raised nose-to-tail animal foods at the center of your diet and minimizing exposure to inflammatory foods (not just grains, but even vegetables in sensitive people) is simply too compelling to ignore or dismiss with a stylized reaction. Carnivore seems extreme at first glance, but researchers confirm that human evolution was driven by a nutrient-dense diet where calories came predominantly from nose-to-tail animals and secondarily from the plant kingdom. We most certainly evolved as omnivores—don't let any whole food, plant-based zealot or carnivore stalwart tell you differently—but when Dr. Paul proposes that plants were merely the "survival foods" of evolution, we must carefully consider this premise. After all, as you will learn in the book, our ancestors' increasing consumption of nutrient-rich animal foods was strongly correlated with an increase in brain size. This was the primary catalyst for us to branch away from our leaf-chewing ape cousins and ascend to the top of the food chain.

Granted, the carnivore argument advanced so clearly and comprehensively in this book is just one point of view. Today, there are many loud and passionate voices in the health and diet scene dispensing so much information that it's easy to get overwhelmed, confused, and frustrated. What I appreciate about Paul's message is his measured and respectful tone and his ability to thoughtfully weigh opposing points of view. That said, Paul wastes no time and pulls no punches in attacking what he believes to be misinformation, flawed science, or conventional wisdom propaganda. When even my beloved Bigass Salad is taken to task, it leaves a lasting impression. I'm confident that this book will do the same, and I encourage you to absorb the information in the same good spirit with which Paul wrote it: with an open mind, a willingness to learn and grow, and a desire to discover the most satisfying and nutritionally optimal diet for you.

Mark Sisson
October, 2019
Miami Beach, FL

INTRODUCTION

I like puzzles, and the puzzle of what humans should eat in order to kick as much butt as possible is absolutely the most fascinating one I've ever found.

If you were going to construct the ideal diet for humans, what sort of metrics would you use to define this selection of foods? I would want this diet to include (1) all of the nutrients that we need to function optimally (2) in the most bio-available forms (3) with the smallest amount of toxins. It should have all of the vitamins, minerals, amino acids, and other building blocks we need to thrive but none of the stuff that messes up our biochemistry or causes inflammation and cellular damage. Sounds reasonable, right? I call this the **optimal diet riddle**. It's really the holy grail of nutrition and medicine, and I believe that a nose-to-tail carnivore diet is the best solution to it. But don't just take my word for it; that's what this book is all about. It's my shot at convincing you that animal foods are the best foods on the planet and that plant foods are sub-optimal, containing smaller amounts of nutrients that are much less bio-available and a myriad of toxins that do nothing but harm us.

This book is going to ruffle some feathers. It's going to be controversial, it's going to have a lot of critics, and it's going to challenge many long-held beliefs that have wrongly been accepted as canon. But I'm okay with the push-back, because it's also going to help a whole lot of people.

So now I ask you, *Do you want to be radically healthy?* Do you want to have endless energy, mental clarity, a rocking libido, a sexy physique, and emotional resilience? Of course you do. We all want to be the best versions of ourselves and show up as powerfully as we can.

This book is the story of how we can all reach our radical potential. These goals are attainable for every single one of us, and I believe that the biggest factor in achieving them is what we consume in our diet. The food we eat is the key determinant in whether we take the path towards obesity, brain fog, and fatigue, or the path towards optimization.

There's just one tiny problem … we've forgotten *what* we are supposed to be eating. Okay, let's be honest, this is actually a really big problem, and it shows! As a whole, our health today as humans is pretty abysmal, and it's not getting any better. Estimates are that an overwhelming 87.8 percent of Western populations have some degree of insulin resistance and metabolic dysfunction. Let's let that sink in for a second … 87.8 percent! That's a staggeringly large number and a vicious indictment of how unhealthy we are today.

As a physician, I have seen the evidence of this firsthand, and it's not pretty. So many people that I have encountered during my medical career have suffered with illness that Western medicine was powerless to correct. Sure, we could offer medications that might ameliorate symptoms for a short amount of time, but often, the side effects of these are worse than the diseases that are being treated. Inevitably, the underlying inflammation also continues undetected and ultimately leads to even more issues down the road.

Throughout my medical training and practice within mainstream allopathic medicine, I've come to one very disappointing conclusion: the system that I was trained in isn't helping people lead better lives. Sure, it can correct acute problems like a ruptured appendix or a broken leg, but when it comes to chronic disease and correcting the root cause of illness, it's failing miserably.

This isn't a book about what's wrong with the medical system, however. Those books have been written, and that's not my goal here. This is a book about how to take back your own health with careful attention to what you are eating and, in the process, manifesting your inner superhero who can kick more butt than you've ever thought possible. All I will say about the current medical system is that it will never be able to treat the root cause of illness until the fundamental paradigm of treating disease changes. Physicians need to realize and accept that food has everything to do with whether we become deeply sick or vitally healthy.

The Lost User Manual

If you're still reading this book and you think there's some truth to what I've said thus far, you are almost certainly asking a very important question: how do we figure out what we should eat? Which foods will make us into the demigods we all deserve to be and which will only serve as roadblocks on this quest? I've been obsessed with this question for the better part of two decades, and the pages you are holding are the result of my own personal quest to find the answer.

I believe that the solution to the riddle of what we should be eating lies in our "user manual," the template that we should follow for proper fuel and nutrition. Sadly, this user manual isn't an actual book that is delivered to our ecstatic families along with our slippery bodies when we enter the world. That would be amazing and would make this question a lot easier to answer. Alas, the universe doesn't work this way. Our user manual is really a code written into our genes. It's in our DNA and it's been there since we became "human" about 3–4 million years ago.

So how are we supposed to rediscover this code in order to become the superhuman beings we are meant to be? We've clearly lost the user manual somewhere along the way, as our previously discussed declining health would indicate, and we are now suffering the consequences. Growing up, whenever I would lose my Transformers or GI Joes, my mom would always ask me where I last saw them. There's a lot of wisdom in this. I think we should begin our search for the user manual where we last saw it. Our ancestors knew the answer to this puzzle, and this special set of knowledge was passed down between generations, woven into our being from before we were even born.

Ultimately, this book is an adventure story. It's the narrative of my own personal search to rediscover the code that will allow all of us to thrive in ways few of us thought possible. I've been looking for this piece of treasure for many years, and I think I've finally found it. It's been an incredible experience that I can't wait to share with you, but before we dive in, I think it's important to display a bit of my past and where I've been on my own personal journey.

BEGINNINGS

My father is a physician and my mother is a nurse practitioner, so I was exposed to medicine a lot while growing up. Dinner table conversations were about things like atrial fibrillation, hypertension, and cholesterol. When I would go with my dad to the hospital, I saw illness firsthand at a young age, and this created a fascination within me. I wanted to know what was wrong with my father's patients and how they could return to health. I had to know why a patient suffered from heart failure or a stroke, why they struggled to breathe, or why their bones had become so brittle. I wanted to know why certain people were healthy with bodies that functioned well and why others experienced sickness and disease.

The underlying factors causing these disparate outcomes have always been fascinating to me.

Even though my parents were healthcare professionals, there wasn't much emphasis on healthy eating in our home. We ate a pretty standard American diet that included TV dinners, fast food, bread, pasta, and processed carbohydrates. I also grew up in a time period when fat was the enemy, having been wrongly demonized by the cereal and processed food industries since the 1950s. After school I remember ravenously devouring multiple bowls of cereal, never feeling full. I also experienced irritability, childhood obesity, asthma, and eczema. I was a child of the low-fat era, and it showed.

My health got a little better in college, but it certainly wasn't ideal. I studied chemistry at the College of William and Mary with the original intention of going to medical school. During my four years of college, I had numerous severe eczema flares and often required oral steroids like prednisone. Those drugs quelled the raging auto-immune process that was going on, but they also caused horrible insomnia, mood swings, and weight gain. Things were still way out of balance, but I had no idea that these symptoms could be caused by the foods I was eating. That notion wasn't even on my radar, because it's not something that is taught in pre-medical courses nor in the formal medical training of my family or any of the doctors I saw. I studied really hard in high school and college, and by the end of my time at William and Mary, I was a bit burned out. I'd been successful at gathering a number of accolades while there, graduating *suma cum laude* and being elected to Phi Beta Kappa, but I knew that medical school wasn't the right next step.

Instead, I became a vagabond and had a fantastic time doing it. At that time in my life, I had no idea how long my gallivanting would last, but the freedom was intoxicating. I spent a summer in Maine teaching outdoor education to middle school students and then headed West to the wilderness lands I had seen only on calendars. Many adventures followed: a thru hike of the 2,700-mile Pacific Crest Trail, multiple explorations of the New Zealand backcountry (highlights included swimming a flooded river and nearly falling off a mountain while lost), and years as a ski bum in such hallowed locales as Telluride, Alta, and Jackson Hole.

After six years of personal exploration and adventuring around the American West, my scientific curiosity was reawakened, and I again began to crave academic learning. The thought of medical school crossed my mind at that time, but I was dissuaded by the brutal lifestyle I had seen my father assume as an internist. I opted instead to become a physician assistant (PA) and hoped that this would provide me with some balance between seeing patients and maintaining a healthy personal life outside of work.

Working as a PA in cardiology provided me with my first real taste of what being in the trenches of Western medicine was like. It stunk. I was immediately disillusioned and disappointed with what I encountered, but this wasn't due to lack of intelligent or kind and well-intentioned physicians. I was fortunate to have the opportunity to be mentored by many incredibly talented individuals who taught me a lot about how medicine is practiced. My greatest disappointment was in the overall medical paradigm and the medical system itself. Neither in the hospital nor in the clinic were patients getting better, and the progression toward worsening disease was constant. At times, their decline was slowed by medications, but the march toward morbidity was relentless.

I began to question my role in all of this. Was I really helping people lead fuller, higher quality lives with statins, blood pressure medications, insulin, and blood thinners, or was I just delaying the inevitable? Was there really no way to reverse conditions like heart disease, high blood pressure, or diabetes by addressing them at their root? Did our ancestors suffer the same cruel chronic illnesses that we face today? Or had there been some sort of fundamental shift in the way that we are living that could be behind these observed departures from mental clarity, strength, healthy body composition, and vitality?

I didn't have the answers to these questions at that time, but I knew in my core that these were the questions I should be asking. I realized that seeking these answers would be a worthwhile endeavor and perhaps the most worthwhile venture that I could possibly embark on. After spending a few years as a PA, I realized that I couldn't go on working within a system that I didn't believe in when such fundamental questions as these remained unanswered.

THE SECOND TIME AROUND

Not many people get to go to medical school twice, but in many ways, I did. During my four years of medical school at the University of Arizona and my following four years of residency in psychiatry at the University of Washington, I saw everything from a different perspective than during PA school. The six years I had already spent in medicine (two in PA school and four practicing as a PA in cardiology) allowed me to have a different approach the second time around. I asked a lot of questions. I think I pissed off more than a few professors, attending physicians, and residents with my incessant entreaties for deeper knowledge regarding the cause behind diseases we encountered. The same was true in residency. Since the days of following my father in the hospital, I always wanted to know "why," and I hoped these would be my opportunities.

You can probably guess what I'm going to say next—they weren't. There were a few glimmers of hope and "ah-ha!" moments during those eight years, but for the most part it was more of the same. As my good friend Dr. Ken Berry likes to say, medical school and residency are about teaching you which pill to give. They are not about understanding what is causing illness. So I did what I was supposed to and learned over and over again which pill to give. I crushed my board exams at the end of it all but still didn't feel like I knew how to help my patients get well, and that was profoundly disappointing. I had studied as hard as I possibly could and learned all the answers to the standard questions, but still my patients were suffering. It wasn't supposed to be that way.

To add insult to injury, I also hadn't been able to heal myself. During my time as a physician assistant, I had discovered the paleo diet and the concept resonated with me. For the decade that followed, I shunned grains, beans, and dairy and ate a strictly organic diet based around animal and plant foods. With this change, I definitely noticed some improvements in body composition and mental clarity, but my stubborn eczema persisted and became very severe at times. During medical school, I began learning Jiu-Jitsu, and practicing this marital art humbled me in ways I had not experienced previously in my life. It proved to be both the source of great suffering and deep satisfaction. Unfortunately, all of the time on the mats with elbows and knees exposed caused my eczema to flare severely, and eventually it became infected with a strain of Streptococcal bacteria. As a result, I developed impetigo, followed by cellulitis, and then an episode of sepsis. I was plagued with fever and chills and had to get IV antibiotics. It was not exactly the ideal scenario for a third-year medical student in the midst of the most grueling portion of his education.

Somehow, I survived. Trust me, it wasn't the salads that got me through, but we'll get to that soon enough. In residency, the ezcema continued to flare intermittently, and at times, it was so severe that most of my lower back was a weeping, infected, mess. By this point, I knew that food was a huge factor in health and disease. I had tried cutting out things in the past: high histamine foods, high oxalate foods, high lectin foods, nuts, seeds, and chocolate. Eventually, I tried cutting out everything I could think of for several months. I was basically eating avocados, salads, and grass-fed meat, along with a few supplements that I thought

I needed based on my genetics. Still, my body attacked itself and the eczema continued to besiege me.

I'll never forget the day I was listening to Jordan Peterson on Joe Rogan's podcast while driving to the Washington coast to go surfing. I'm sure the weather was rainy and cold and the waves were mediocre, but that trip was entirely worth it. At the end of the podcast, I heard Jordan talk about his meat-based diet. He related how it had helped his daughter, Mikhaila, overcome a lifetime of severe autoimmune disease and how it had helped him lose weight and resolve his own sleep apnea and similar autoimmune issues. Suddenly, I had a paradigm-shifting thought that changed the course of my life from that moment forward. *What if my own autoimmune issues and so many of the inflammatory problems we see manifested as chronic disease today could be triggered by the plants we are eating?*

Immediately, I dismissed the idea, burying it beneath a mountain of decades of indoctrination that plants, fiber, and phytonutrients were essential for human health. How would I poop without fiber? What about all the benefits of these so called *polyphenolic* compounds? What about my microbiome? Wouldn't all the good bugs living in my gut starve without pre-biotic starches? All of the Jiu-Jitsu I had studied during medical school could not prepare me for the grappling match between everything I had been taught and this new, radical notion that was about to take root in my brain. A royal rumble of epic proportions did indeed occur, but after months of studying the literature and a careful consideration of the ideas behind the carnivore diet, I decided to give it a try. I knew that if I didn't change something, my eczema wasn't likely to get any better, and I wasn't satisfied with using medication to treat it long term.

Within the first three days, I knew there was something special about this way of eating. I began to feel a level of emotional calm and an increasingly positive outlook on life unlike anything I had experienced before. I wasn't expecting this feeling, but it was a pleasant surprise. It felt like some sort of sand paper had been wrapped around my brain but was slowly being removed. Suddenly, things were softer and smoother in my psyche. I now believe that this was due to gradual resolution of low-level inflammation in my body that began in my gut and was translated to my brain. Some have described similar improvements in mental clarity with states of ketosis, and this no doubt played a role later in my carnivore journey, but when I first began to explore this way of eating, I included honey in my diet and was getting plenty of glucose. It was the removal of plants that had resulted in this profound change in my experience of life, and I was deeply intrigued at what other benefits a carnivore diet might have.

Since then, I have been eating only animal foods and am thriving like never before. My outlook on life remains extremely positive, my emotions are stable, my sleep is restful, and my body is strong. My energy is full, my libido robust, and yes, I poop every day and it is beautiful.

Bloodwork, you ask? Remember that I am a physician obsessed with understanding how all of these things work. I've literally done hundreds of assays on myself, all of which have looked great. *My kidneys and liver are healthy*, and I definitely don't have scurvy. Nor do I have indications of inflammation or insulin resistance. In fact, *my inflammatory markers are nearly undetectable* and my *blood sugars are in the ideal range throughout the day* without any significant change after I eat. What about my autoimmune disease? *Since going carnivore, I haven't had a single eczema flare.* Prior to making this change, I had been suffering from eczema every month with many periods of persistent rash and itching.

My story is not unique. There are now thousands of people with experiences similar to mine demonstrating improvement and resolution of a variety of diseases such as ulcerative colitis, Crohn's, lupus, thyroid disease, psoriasis, multiple sclerosis, rheumatoid arthritis, and psychiatric illnesses like depression, bipolar, and anxiety. This is in addition to the thousands of others who have used the carnivore diet to lose weight, reverse diabetes and insulin resistance, or to improve libido and mental performance. Many of their incredible stories are catalogued at the website MeatHeals.com, which is indexed by condition.

Sound too good to be true? It did to me, too! It sounded totally crazy when I first heard about it, so if you are having those thoughts, you are in good company. The experience that I had with this way of eating was so impactful that I dove head first deeper into the research in an effort to understand the benefits, the mechanisms behind the benefits, and the potential pitfalls. This book is the story of what I learned along the way and how I came to believe that so many of our long-held nutritional beliefs are flat out wrong and often prevent us from achieving our true potential. The majority of the disease and illness we experience today is autoimmune and inflammatory in nature, and I believe that by focusing on nutrient-rich animal foods while avoiding the toxins found in plants that trigger these processes, we will swiftly return to our ancestral birthright of radical health and vitality.

THE GOAL OF THIS BOOK

My goal is to share with you why I thoroughly believe in the carnivore diet, and why it makes sense from an evolutionary, medical, nutritional, and biochemical perspective.

In **Section I**, we will begin at the beginning, a time when we knew how to eat, and a time when we thrived as humans because we were hunting and eating animals ... lots of them! We'll then talk about the time in human history when I believe we lost the user manual. Seduced by "the cult of the seed," we stopped hunting and began farming. As you'll see, the resulting impact on our health was strikingly detrimental.

In **Section II**, we will explore why our decision to increase the consumption of plants was a bad idea. Ultimately, neither plants nor animals want to get eaten. But while animals have their legs, fins, teeth, and horns as defense mechanisms, plants are stuck in the ground and have been for 450 million years. During this time, in order to survive, they had to evolve complex chemical defense mechanisms that can wreak havoc in our bodies if we don't pay attention to them.

In **Section III,** we will compare the nutritional quality of animal foods to plants and will illustrate how animal foods are the clear winner in this duel. One of the things I find most egregious is when animal foods are unjustly vilified, so we'll then debunk many of the myths we've been told about animal foods, including notions that meat will cause cancer and heart disease or shorten our lives.

Section IV is devoted to the nuts and bolts of how to eat a nose-to-tail carnivore diet. I'll break it all down for you in great detail and will do my best to leave no question unanswered. We'll cover several areas of the carnivore diet: what to eat, different styles of eating carnivore, and how to include organ meats. Based on your goals, we will also include when to eat and how much should be eaten.

If you are most interested in learning about how to construct a carnivore diet and want to jump into this way of life ASAP, you may want to skip to this final section of the book and read Chapters Twelve and Thirteen first. In Chapter Twelve, you'll also find some personal stories shared by others in the carnivore community who have found incredible improvements with this way eating.

We're almost ready to jump into the "meat" of it all, but before we do, I want to talk about one more key concept that will help frame all of our further discussions of the carnivore way of life.

THE QUALITY OF LIFE EQUATION

I'm well aware that many of the concepts I'll talk about in this book depart abruptly from societal norms and that many of you may be asking yourselves, "Is he really suggesting that I should only eat meat for the rest of my life? I could never do that!"

This book isn't meant to limit but, rather, to empower you with knowledge to make choices that will positively affect your quality of life. It is also intended to help you along your own personal journey to have the most optimal experience of life each and every day. Ultimately, this is YOUR adventure. By sharing with you what I've learned, I hope to give you the tools needed to embark on your own quest, rather than to simply mimic mine.

One of these tools is the **Quality of Life** equation. Simply put, when following this equation, the goal is to always solve for your highest quality of life, and in order to do this, we'll need to know what our goals are. Each person has unique experiences and different goals depending on where they currently are in their journey, and these factors will translate into a different highest quality of life for each person at any given moment. For some, the highest quality of life will always be optimal performance, both mentally and physically. In this situation, deviating from an intentional way of eating, be it carnivore, keto, or paleo, would result in a lower quality of life because their performance might decline. I myself fall into this category. The good news is that this book isn't written only for people like me, but also for the men and women who are better at moderation than I am.

I know that for the majority of these individuals, performance is the main goal most of the time. At other times, community or relaxation takes priority and participating in activities aimed at fostering these needs leads to the highest quality of life. This is totally okay. It's okay not to want to be a carnivore or even carnivore-*ish* all of the time. As long as we are solving for the highest quality of life as much as possible, we'll be living amazing lives, full of rich experiences, personal growth, and profound health.

Let's consider an example to illustrate how the quality of life equation works. Meet Joe, a forty-five-year-old man who's happily married with two healthy and energetic children. Joe has noticed that he's gained about 20 pounds over the last few years, feels less energetic, has a waning libido, and some aching joints. A friend told Joe about this crazy "carnivore diet" that he's been on for the last few months and delights in sharing with him tales of weight loss, improved sleep, increased energy and sex-drive, a better mood, and less joint pain. Joe's friend hands him a copy of this very book and encourages him to read it. Intrigued by the idea, Joe reads the book intently and decides to give the carnivore diet a try.

This is where the quality of life equation comes into play. Joe decides that his main goal is improving his health and gaining improvements in many of the things that have been nagging him recently. If I could give Joe advice, here's what I would say to him:

"High five, Joe! I really think you are going to feel amazing on this diet. It's going to be a change from what you are used to, but in exchange for the hard work of making this lifestyle change, I'm willing to bet more than a few ribeyes that many of the things you've noticed becoming sub-optimal over the last few years will quickly begin to improve. It's not going to happen over night. Give it at least a month or two, but by the end of those thirty to sixty days, you're going to feel amazing. Here's one more thing to think about as well: the closer you can adhere to the diet, the better your results will be, but if you slip up, it's definitely not the end of the world. There are also likely going to be special occasions when your highest quality of life is not performance and optimizing your health, and that's totally okay. If you want to have a dessert with your wife on your anniversary or a bite of cake on your son's birthday because that shared experience is meaningful, realize that may be your highest quality of life in the moment. You're not going to torpedo the whole endeavor when you do something like that from time to time. Do these things intentionally and then return to your original goals by again asking yourself what your highest quality of life is. It will probably be back to optimizing your own health, and with that shift, you can return to a focused effort on the carnivore diet. Always seek your highest quality of life."

The quality of life equation isn't meant to be a "get-out-of-jail-free card" or an excuse to eat cake. It's a gentle nudge to always be aware of what nourishes your soul most in the moment. It gives you the freedom to pause any effort to change your lifestyle if your highest quality of life temporarily changes. As I mentioned earlier, for some people, the highest quality of life will always be improving their personal health. Those with autoimmune disease or significant evidence of inflammation might fall into this category. For those who are generally well and looking to optimize, however, there might be a bit more flexibility.

This is *your* life. This is *your* adventure. You decide what *your* goals are. I'm just here to share with you the amazing things I've discovered so that you can go on your own Rambo adventure mission. With that said, the time has now come, brave adventurers! Let's begin our quest to find the lost user manual, crack the code, and become radically healthy humans!

SECTION I

CHAPTER ONE

OUR BEGINNINGS

I still remember my mom's recommendation when I lost my GI Joes and Transformers. She was spot on with her suggestion to look for them where I last saw them, and I think we should do the same in our search for the lost user manual. So where did we last see the precious tome that holds the key to our optimal health and performance? *Within our history.*

There is a caveat along any theoretical journey back in time: anthropology isn't perfect, and we don't have a time machine to go back and witness past events. I'm working on building one, but I'm having trouble finding a source of the 1.21 gigawatts needed to power it. Until I figure that puzzle out, we can use the evidence that *is* available to reconstruct our history as best we can—and that's what we'll do in this chapter. Onward! An incredible adventure awaits us!

INDIANA JONES STUFF

Eating animals has been an integral part of our existence as humans and pre-humans for a very long time, probably for at least 5–6 million years. Primate evolution preceded ours by about 60 million years, and during that time period, the size of the primate brain stayed essentially constant at around 350 cubic centimeters (cc), with some variation among species depending on body size. This research means that 60 million years of eating fruit and leaves didn't result in a bigger brain for our primate predecessors.

It is thought that the hominid lineage diverged from chimpanzees about 6 million years ago when our distant ancestors came down from the trees and entered the open grasslands of North Eastern Africa after the shifting of tectonic plates caused changes to their environment. The oldest fossils from our lineage are dated to about 4.2 million years ago and were discovered in Northern Kenya. This genus, known as *Australopithecus*, includes fossilized female remains affectionately named "Lucy" after the well-known Beatles song that was played nightly in camp during the arduous process of excavation. Lucy appears to have walked upright, like a human, but the size of her brain is estimated to be only slightly larger than her chimpanzee ancestors. By looking at skeletons like Lucy's and others from more recent times, we are able to track the brain size of our distant relatives along the timeline of our history and see a fascinating story unfold.

The size of our predecessors' brains gradually increased after Lucy's time, and then, about 2 million years ago, something incredible happened: they suddenly began to grow much more rapidly. They continued to increase in size, attaining an apex volume of 1600cc about 40,000 years ago. This increase in brain size correlated with a growing complexity in the neocortex (the outer portion of our brains) and upgraded intelligence—both of which allowed for better communication and more sophisticated group behaviors, like organized hunting. Bigger brains equaled smarter people and smarter people figured out how to hunt animals in groups more successfully.

This dramatic change in brain size raises a foundational question: what was the magical event that occurred 2 million years ago that allowed our brains to grow and our ancestors to become more intelligent? No one knows for sure, but there are a couple of key clues in the archeological record. 2.5 million years ago, with the appearance of *Homo habilis,* is also when we begin to see the first evidence of stone tools and the hunting of animals. Fossilized animal skeletons from this time period show damage from weapons and cut marks on bones from the earliest butchering practices.[1,2,3] There's evidence that our ancestors were eating some animal foods prior to this point in history during Lucy's time, 4–5 million years ago, but 2 million years ago, we appear to have evolved from scavengers to hunters.

As scavengers, we could access only a few parts of the animal, like bone marrow and brain, that were encased by skeletal tissue other animals couldn't break through.[4,5] However, when we could hunt animals in organized groups with stone tools, we suddenly had first dibs on all parts of our kill. That meant we had access to the visceral (abdominal) organs and fat as well as the muscle meat. I believe it was the eating of these parts of the animal, with all of their unique micronutrients and caloric abundance, that allowed our brains to grow beyond the initial increase in *Homo habilis* and made us into the humans we are today. *Eating animals nose to tail is what made us human!* Transitioning from scavengers to hunters appears to have been the defining moment in our evolution as humans.

Some would argue that it was cooking that resulted in the sudden increase in the size of the human brain, but many scientists agree that our torrid love affair with fire did not begin until about 500,000 years ago, 1.5 million years after our brains began to grow exponentially.[6]

In the following graphic, you'll see a representation of the size of our ancestors' brains over millions of years. At approximately 4 million years ago, you'll see Lucy and her *Australopithecus* lineage. Her brain was the size of a small grapefruit. Between Lucy and *Homo habilis*, however, the brain increased to the size of a medium grapefruit: about 500cc. Then, 2.5 million years ago, with the advent of stone tools and hunting, our ancestors' brains began to grow even more rapidly. In fact, they doubled in size over the next 1 million years. Based on the fossil record, it appears we reached a maximum brain size of 1600cc about 40,000 years ago, and that our brains have shrunk slightly since then. The takeaway message from this graphic is that a significant change in the rate of growth of our ancestors' brains coincided with stone tools and hunting. *We are the humans we are today because we began eating animals.*

HUMAN EVOLUTION INCREASE IN BRAIN SIZE

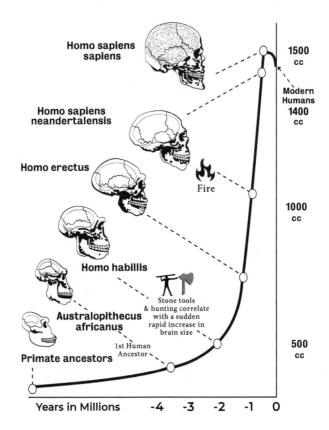

As we'll see in the next chapter, there was a colossal shift in the way we ate that coincided with a gradual shrinking of our brains. It was when we began eating less animals and more plants. Clearly, eating animal foods has been a vital part of our evolution from the beginning. Katherine Milton, a researcher from UC Berkeley, came to the same conclusion in her paper "The Critical Role Played by Animal Source Foods in Human Evolution," which states:

> *"**Without routine access to animal source foods, it is highly unlikely that evolving humans could have achieved their unusually large and complex brain** while simultaneously continuing their evolutionary trajectory as large, active and highly social primates. As human evolution progressed, young children in particular, with their rapidly expanding large brain and high metabolic and nutritional demands relative*

to adults would have benefited from volumetrically concentrated, high quality foods such as meat."[7]

How Much Meat Were We Eating?

But weren't our ancestors eating both plants and animals? Weren't we gatherers as well as hunters? Great question! As I began digging into the anthropological literature, I asked myself the same thing. Thankfully, we do have a sort of "time machine" here that helps us answer this question.

In order to determine the proportion of animal foods in the diets of our predecessors, we can examine the amount of δ15 nitrogen in their fossilized bones. By looking at levels of this isotope, researchers are able to infer where in the food chain animals reside by identifying their protein sources. Herbivores generally have δ15N levels of 3–7 percent, carnivores show levels of 6–12 percent, and omnivores display levels between these two. When samples from Neanderthal and early modern humans were analyzed, they demonstrated levels of 12 percent and 13.5 percent, respectively, even higher than that of other known carnivorous animals like hyena and wolves.

What can we make of this? These extremely high levels of δ15N isotopes suggest that 40,000 years ago, *Homo sapiens* and concurrent Neanderthal were high-level trophic *carnivores*. They were consuming the vast majority of their protein from large mammals like mammoths rather than from plant sources. Who wants to share a woolly mammoth ribeye with me?

Similar patterns are seen further back in the fossil record as well. At the time of *Australopithecus,* there appears to have been a separation into two different lineages of hominids, one of which became *Homo habilis* and the other, known as *Paranthropus*, which went extinct.

Like δ15N in bones, levels of strontium, barium, and calcium in fossilized teeth can also be used to indicate the dietary patterns of our ancestors. Studies comparing ratios of these elements suggest that while *Australopithecus* ate a mix of plants and animal foods, the diet of *Homo habilis* consisted of significantly more animal foods,[8] a shift that coincides with the rapid growth of the brain observed at this time in our history. *Paranthropus*, on the other hand, appears to have relied more heavily on plant foods, a preference that was likely its undoing.

HUMANS AS FAT-HUNTERS

The data here is very clear and has been replicated repeatedly when looking at nitrogen levels in preserved fossils. And from an energy efficiency standpoint, hunting large animals makes more sense. Gathering plants and stalking small animals deliver much less of a caloric and nutrient bounty relative to the energy that is invested. Across more recently studied indigenous peoples, we observe a similar pattern that clearly indicates preference for animals over plant food.[9,10] For example, in his studies of the Eskimo, Vilhjalmur Stefansson writes:

> *"The Eskimo situation varies from ours still more when it comes to vegetables. In the Mackenzie district these were eaten under three conditions:* **The chief occasion for vegetables here, as with most Eskimos, was famine...**"[11]

But our ancestors weren't just looking for any animals. They were looking for the animals with the most fat on them. Larger animals have more fat by weight, and fat appears to be the macronutrient we sought most for survival. There are many sources of protein in the animal world, but the sources of fat are more scarce.

Many anthropologists studying disparate indigenous peoples have noted a predilection for fat and fattier animals. In his book, *The Paleoanthropology of and Archaeology of Big Game Hunting*, Speth states:

> *"...fat, not protein, seemed to play a very prominent role in the hunters' decisions about what animals (male vs. female) to kill and which body parts to discard or take away."*[12]

In the !Kung of the Kalahari:

> *"Fat animals are keenly desired, and all !Kung express a constant craving for animal fat."*[13]

And of the James Bay Cree, it is stated:

> *"The Cree considered fat the most important part of any animal. One reason they valued bears above other animals was because of their body fat."*[14]

Among the Yolngu of Arnhem, Australia, a similar sentiment is noted:

> *"Animals without fat may indeed be rejected as food."*[15]

Why were our ancestors and more recent indigenous peoples so intent on finding fat? At a very basic level, it was probably about sheer calories. By weight, fat provides more than twice as many calories than do protein or carbohydrates. In addition, the human metabolism makes fat a uniquely valuable and necessary food. If we think of ourselves as automobiles that need fuel for our metabolic engines, we shouldn't put protein into our gas tank. For best results, our metabolic engine runs more efficiently on fat or carbohydrates, and our bodies seek to use protein first for building blocks rather than for energy. Although we can use protein for energy in a pinch through a process called gluconeogenesis, it doesn't work well as our primary energy source.

Historical accounts of arctic explorers tell us of the dangers of "rabbit starvation," a condition that occurs when we eat too much lean protein without carbohydrates or fat.[16] Our liver has a limited capacity to turn the nitrogen from amino acids into urea, a water soluble compound that we excrete in our urine.[17] Once the liver's capacity to turn the nitrogen from protein into urea is exceeded, the excess can cause ammonia levels to increase, leading to all sorts stress on the body. You may have seen the term "BUN" on your labs. This stands for blood urea nitrogen, and is an indication of how much nitrogen you are converting into urea before it is filtered out in the urine through your kidneys.

The upper limit for protein in our diets seems to be about 40 percent of our total calorie intake, beyond which point we might exceed the liver's ability to process this macronutrient. This means that 60 percent of our caloric needs must be met by either fat or carbohydrates. Have you ever tried to look for digestible carbohydrates in the wilderness? They are pretty darn rare! Depending on the latitude, fruit might be available a few times a year for a very short period of time, but we also would have to compete with other animals, insects, and mold. In addition, although some plants have root portions that might be edible and contain some carbohydrates, they are rare, and many are toxic. As we shall see in future chapters, aside from occasional fruit and tubers, the stems and leaves of plants don't contain much in the way of carbohydrates, and they are often riddled with plant-defense chemicals as well. The vast array of carbohydrate-rich plant foods we see in grocery stores today is *nothing* like the selection of plants in the wilderness or the plants our ancestors would have had to choose from.

Let's pretend I did get the time machine working and we were able to go back in time. Set the dial to 50,000 years ago and off we go for a ride to the period when both *Homo sapiens* (our relatives) and Neanderthals were around. I hope you brought your loin cloth so we don't stick out too much, and I hope you know how to make a spear because pretty soon, we are going to get hungry. Should we set off in search of some bitter leaves that will probably give us diarrhea, or would you prefer to dig up some roots that are incredibly fibrous and taste horrible? On the other hand, how about hunting for some big game? It will give us a lot more energy as well as provide us with food that will last for the next several days or even weeks.

This choice seems like a no brainer, and it would have been for our ancestors as well. Forget the leaves and fibrous tubers, we're going hunting! And we're going to feast on mammoth or buffalo for days when we get one. As we saw from the stable isotope studies, this approach appears to be *exactly* what our ancestors did. I'm glad they chose wisely and figured this out, because I don't think humans would have survived as a species if they hadn't.

At this point in the book, I want to share with you my **Carnivore Code Hypothesis**: *I believe that throughout our evolution, our ancestors have hunted animals preferentially, and have eaten plant foods only during times of scarcity or starvation.* I base my hypothesis on the following factors:

1. Anthropological data including brain size, stable isotope data from bones and teeth, and examples from indigenous peoples as we have just discussed.

2. The significantly higher availability of energy from animals relative to plant foods per energy invested.

3. The vastly superior nutrient content of animal foods (we'll talk all about this later in the book, Chapter Eight)

I'm not suggesting that our ancestors never ate plant foods but that they favored animal foods based on caloric and nutritional superiority. If we couldn't find animal foods, we might have eaten plants as a backup plan, but they do not appear to have composed any significant part of our ancestors' diets.

Take a moment to let the notions I am advancing in the last paragraph sink in. It's basically canon at this point to consider humans as omnivores, but what does this really mean? If we dig into this characterization a bit and examine ourselves in comparison to other omnivorous and carnivorous animals, some enlightening realizations will occur.

EVOLUTIONARY ADAPTATIONS TO EATING MEAT

Since we're about to chow down on woolly mammoth, let's start with the digestive system and begin in the mouth. Critics of the carnivore diet love to point out that our teeth don't look like the teeth of other carnivores like lions or tigers. However, this isn't really a fair comparison, because our evolutionary lineage is completely separate from felids and appears to have diverged about 90 million years ago. Our primate ancestors ate mostly plant foods, so it makes sense that we have molars for chewing these foods. On the other hand, it's interesting to note that our molars are ridged like a dog's rather than flat like a sheep's or other strict herbivore's. From an evolutionary perspective, even though we have been eating mostly meat, it probably benefited us to retain molars for times of starvation when we might have chewed more fibrous plant material.

In addition to molars, human smiles quickly reveal the incisors and canine teeth best suited for biting into animal flesh—an indication that we have been eating meat for some time. It's also interesting to note that humans have jaws that are better adapted for vertical rather than rotary chewing, an adaptation that likely assisted us in gnawing on sinewy animal tissues. Thus, depending on the availability of food sources, our mouths appear to be adapted to eating both plant and animal foods. As we move down the digestive tract, however, we begin to see stronger inclinations toward eating animal foods.

THE CAULDRON OF FIRE IN YOUR BELLY

As you take that first bite of mammoth meat and it passes to your stomach, let's pause and notice something very striking about this upper region of the human digestive tract. Our stomachs are basically cauldrons of acid, eagerly waiting for food to arrive from the esophagus to then digest it into more basic components. It is in the stomach that we break down the complex protein, fats, and carbohydrates that compose our food. By the time that bite of mammoth steak leaves your stomach, it looks nothing like it did going down the hatch. The pH of a healthy human stomach is around 1.5, which is very acidic on the pH scale that spans from 0 to 14 (lower is more acidic and higher is more alkaline). If your stomach contents with a pH of 1.5 were to leak out into the rest of your abdomen, you would literally melt yourself from the inside out.

So how does the human stomach's acidity compare to the chimpanzee's? Our distant primate ancestors have a stomach pH of 4–5, which is much less acidic.[18] pH is a logarithmic scale, and every increase of 1 translates to a 10x less acidic solution. Our stomachs are about 1000x more acidic than a chimpanzee's. 1000x is no joke, and it certainly wasn't an accident. Our stomach became much more acidic because 3–4 million years ago, our diets changed from predominantly plant foods to including many animal foods—and then 2 million years ago to mostly animal foods.

Remember Lucy and her brain size? The first "pre-humans" (generally considered to be *Australopithecus*) are thought to have been primarily scavengers, going after meat that was less than fresh. An extremely acidic stomach would have been very helpful for such an endeavor. Even today, the low pH in our stomach protects us from pathogens in the environment and breaks down food so intensely that it's not seen as foreign by the immune system that resides in the walls of our intestinal tract. Pharmaceutical medications like proton pump inhibitors raise pH levels and thereby increase the risk of contracting pneumonia, infections, and numerous allergies.[19,20] In addition, with less acidity in the stomach, undigested food particles could pass into the small intestine and interact with the armies of immune cells that reside a single cell layer away from the lumen in the gut wall. Clearly, maintaining a low stomach pH was, and continues to be, critical for optimal human health. The fact that it's much lower than our primate ancestors' is no accident. It points directly to a radical change in diet early in our evolution as hominids and indicates selective pressures for those best adapted to eating fresh and not-so-fresh animal meats.

EXPENSIVE TISSUE

Once that amazing bite of mammoth steak has been partially digested in the stomach, it passes into the duodenum, the first portion of the small intestine. It is here that the stomach contents mix with bile from the gallbladder and digestive enzymes from the pancreas before they embark on a serpentine journey through the remainder of the small intestine and then into the colon. Comparing the structure of our digestive tract to a primate's reveals significant divergence, likely driven by shifting dietary preferences 2–3 million years ago. We possess a small intestine of much greater length, while our colons have shrunk substantially.

Primates must spend the majority of their days chewing on leaves and other vegetable matter to obtain enough calories, mostly in the form of plant-based carbohydrates. These pass through their shorter small intestines quickly before arriving at a voluminous cecum (the first portion of the large bowel) and colon. In primates, plant matter hangs out in the massive large bowel where it undergoes fermentation and results in the production of large amounts of short-chain fatty acids, which are then used as the main source of their calories. Even though primates are eating mountains of carbohydrate-based plant matter, they are actually running on fat! They need such large colons to house the bacteria that ferment all of the plant fiber they eat into these fats for energy. If you've seen monkeys or apes, you'll notice that their rib cage angles outward with protuberant bellies to accommodate their commodious colons.

Beginning with Lucy and progressing to *Homo erectus* and beyond, the layout of our guts began to change as we ate more and more animal foods. Remember how our brains were beginning to grow during this time as well? A compelling theory called the "expensive tissue hypothesis" elegantly ties all of this together.[21] Both brain and intestine are very metabolically active tissues that require a lot of energy to function properly relative to their mass. A gram of brain tissue requires 22 times the amount of energy to function as a gram of muscle tissue. Our intestines are similarly greedy.

According to the expensive tissue hypothesis, in order for our brains to grow in size without significantly increasing our overall caloric needs (increasing caloric needs would have been highly selected against in the evolutionary context), another tissue in the body would have needed to shrink in size and energy demands. Disparate organ systems needed to make an energetic trade off, and this is exactly what appears to have happened with the brain and the intestines. It appears that our small intestine expanded slightly to be able to better absorb the new protein and fats in our animal-based diets, allowing the colon and the overall size of the gastrointestinal tract to shrink substantially. As the gut shrank in size and in energy needs, the brain was free to gradually expand over generations into the stellar instrument we possess today. With shrinking guts also came straighter rib cages and flatter bellies. Not only can you thank the animal foods our ancestors ate for your big brain, you owe your six pack abs to them too! If you've lost your six-pack, I promise you that a carnivore diet will be an amazing first step to getting it back.

CHANGE IN HUMAN GUT SIZE AND THORACIC STRUCTURE WITH INCREASED RELIANCE ON ANIMAL FOODS

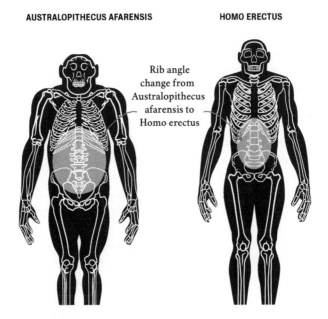

AUSTRALOPITHECUS AFARENSIS   HOMO ERECTUS

Rib angle change from Australopithecus afarensis to Homo erectus

AMYLASE GENE DUPLICATIONS

Some have argued that the striking increase in brain size observed in our ancestors might have been due to heavy consumption of starch-rich tubers, but there are two major problems with this theory. The first of these is that our ancestors don't appear to have begun using fire until 1.5 million years after the sharp change in cranial vault size, and in order for tubers to provide accessible carbohydrates and calories, they must be cooked. The timing here appears to be off.

The second major problem with the notion that humans have been eating significant amounts of tubers throughout our evolution comes from evidence regarding observed duplications of the salivary amylase gene. This gene codes for an enzyme present in our saliva that helps break down complex carbohydrates in the mouth, beginning the process of digestion before they reach the stomach and making the calories within them more accessible. It's widely accepted that these duplications likely occurred as an adaptation in response to increased consumption of starchy foods. Multiple copies of the salivary amylase gene are found in

99 percent of living humans today, suggesting that we are all descendants of a population that was eating tubers.

What's most interesting about this story, however, is the fact that Neanderthals and Denisovans do *not* possess amylase gene duplications like our *Homo sapien* ancestors did.[22,23] These separate lineages of humans are believed to have branched off from our common ancestor, *Homo heidelbergensis*, approximately 600,000 years ago.[24] At that time, some early humans are believed to have left Africa and migrated into Europe and Asia, resulting in the Neanderthal and Denisovan lineages, respectively. Members of the *Homo heidelbergensis* species that stayed in Africa appear to have evolved into our direct predecessors, *Homo sapiens*, who left Africa much later, around 70,000 years ago.

We don't know why our more recent *Homo sapien* ancestors left Africa at this time, but upon arriving in Northern Europe, they encountered Neanderthals—and stable isotope levels found in the bones of both of these species suggest that the majority of their diet consisted of animal products, as we've discussed previously. We also don't know exactly when the amylase gene duplication phenomenon occurred in our history, but the fact that neither Neanderthal nor Denisovans possess these duplications strongly suggests that up until at least 600,000 years ago, our ancestors were probably *not* eating many starchy foods. If they had been, we would likely have observed this gene duplication much earlier in human history.

Thus, for the *majority* of our evolution as humans, we were probably not eating many starchy foods like tubers, and the consumption of these types of foods is likely a recent adaptation due to the shifting of food availability. Many have hypothesized that our migration out of Africa 80,000 years ago was related to declining populations of megafaunal animals due to overhunting,[25] a predicament that certainly could have spurred our ancestors to obtain more calories from starchy foods and favored duplications of the amylase gene.

With what we've learned so far, we can now add to my earlier premise: eating animals made us human by providing higher quality, nutrient-rich foods. Those foods required less of an energy-intensive, fermentation-focused digestive tract and, as a result, opened the energetic gates for an increase in brain size and complexity. Furthermore, access to nutrients like omega-3 fatty acids in highly bio-available forms probably played a role here as well. We know from studies of developing infant brains that *a lot* of DHA and EPA are needed to make a human brain.[26,27] The more of these nutrients that pregnant mothers and infants can get, the better. Indeed, DHA has been said to have a "unique and indispensable role in the neural signaling essential for higher intelligence."[28] We'll talk much more about DHA in future chapters, but here's a bit of foreshadowing: DHA *doesn't* occur in plants, and humans are horrible at converting the precursor form of omega-3 into this precious brain-building block.

Intriguingly, the expensive tissue hypothesis appears to be valid for animals other than humans. There's a critter known as the elephantnose fish that inhabits African freshwater streams and displays features suggesting similar trade-offs between the brain and the intestines. These nasally robust fish have the largest ratio of brain-to-body oxygen use of all known vertebrates. Relative to the size of its body, the brain of an elephantnose fish is three times the size of other fish brains and uses 60 percent of its total body oxygen consumption.

Where's the tradeoff? Just like we have seen in humans, it appears that in order for elephantnose fish to get such big brains, their guts had to shrink. They have a very small gut compared to other fish and they are *carnivorous*. It appears to be a dietary strategy that has allowed this trade off to occur. Across the species, we observe that consuming foods with higher nutrient quality allow for smaller intestines, ultimately freeing the brain to grow in an energetic trade-off throughout evolution. Pretty cool, right? If I can get that time machine working, I'm also going to use it to go forward in time to check in on this little guy's evolutionary progress. With that big brain, I wouldn't be surprised if he's evolved into some sort of super-fish in a few million years.

THE APEX PREDATOR

"Wow, that chimpanzee has a wicked fastball!" Said no one ever!

Have you ever seen a chimpanzee throw a rock? How about a spear? I didn't think so. Another significant difference between humans and our distant primate relatives is the design of our shoulder joint.[29] It's truly a masterpiece of evolution. The human shoulder allows us to throw objects like baseballs, rocks, or stone-tipped spears at speeds high enough to kill the targeted animal. No other species on the planet can do this, and we certainly don't need to throw rocks at plants to harvest them. Our shoulders evolved this way as a *hunting* adaptation, and a darn good one at that. Being able to kill at a distance allowed groups of our ancestors to hunt larger and more dangerous animals that provided them with richer sources of nutrients and calories necessary for fertility and survival.

During our evolutionary journey from Lucy to *Homo habilis* and then to *Homo sapiens*, we also developed changes in our pelvis that resulted in bipedalism,[30] a fancy term describing the structure that allows us to walk in a more upright position and makes us especially well-suited for distance running. Relative to other animals, humans aren't great at sprinting, but we are very good at the walking and running of long distances that would have been needed to track down and hunt animals.

Our feet also changed during this time to assist in long distance running and walking.[31] The big toe became more aligned with the rest of the foot, and our heel pad grew to provide cushion as we walked more upright. There were also changes in our knees and spine to optimize posture and upright mobility. Taken together, all of these skeletal changes allowed our ancestors to move and interact with their environment in new ways that facilitated our growing ability to procure animals as food, a key turning point in our evolutionary past. Running upright and hurling spears and rocks at prey, our ancestors quickly became the apex predator on the ancient landscape and eventually expanded across the globe, dominating every species they encountered.

Another human adaptation to hunting is found in our eyes. Humans have a white portion of the eye outside of the iris, known as the sclera, but primates' sclera are darkly colored to help disguise the direction they are looking. Primate society is intrinsically competitive, and chimpanzees battle each other for food and other resources. Within such a culture, it's advantageous for animals to disguise the direction they are looking—be it at food, a potential mate, or the direction of a planned escape/attack. But somewhere along our evolutionary journey, these patterns shifted, and our ancestors realized they were better off cooperating in endeavors like hunting or fighting off attackers. In these situations, knowing where our compatriots were looking was a very good thing. The whites of our eyes are thus believed to have been one of the key adaptations that evolved over the last 6 million years and that allowed us to communicate with tribe members in silence. By showing them where our attention was directed without speaking aloud, we could communicate more quickly and with greater stealth.[32] This enhanced communication allowed groups of ancestral humans to hunt together with greater success and cooperate more efficiently in communal projects. At our core, we are cooperative beings, and shifting to this type of interaction was a key part in our evolution as humans.

OUR DESTINY

Lest you think my claim of humans as the ultimate hunters is far fetched, or that lions and tigers might take this crown rather than us, I'll ask you:

What other animal on the planet is capable of hunting as many species as us? What else can hunt whales, seals, mammoths, buffalo, birds, and a host of other potential food sources? Sure, lions and tiger are well adapted to chasing down a gazelle or wildebeest on the open plains, but they are specialized for only that type of prey. On the other hand, over the last five million years, humans have evolved to acquire elegant shoulder joints, upright postures, and pelvic girdles that have allowed more fluid running, as well as more acidic stomachs, smaller guts, white sclera, and bigger brains. These adaptations have all propelled our species toward one destiny: becoming the best hunters this planet has ever seen.

We didn't evolve to be the best gatherers or the best farmers—we evolved to be the best hunters. And it was this hunting that provided us with the best food available: animal foods. Having access to animals meant receiving more calories with less energetic input, in addition to providing a complete array of nutrients. Not only did hunting and eating animals make us human, it also allowed us to thrive as a species. In essence, that is *the* reason that we are who we are today. To reflect how important this concept is, I'll note that the title for this book was almost "Apex Predator."

"But wait!" you ask, "what about agriculture? Isn't that why we are who we are today?" As we'll see in the next chapter, the advent of agriculture happened only about 12,000 years ago. This is the blink of an eye in evolutionary terms, and as I'll describe, our health as a human species took a nose-dive with that change. I'd say that's exactly where we lost the user manual, foolishly discarding it for the empty promises of farming and a non-nomadic existence—a move some have called "the worst mistake in human history."

CHAPTER TWO

OUR WORST MISTAKE

I know what you're thinking right now: *isn't that statement about farming being "the worst mistake in human history" a bit of a hyperbole?* To be certain, it's a neck-and-neck race between farming, the mullet, and pop-tarts, but the way I see it, farming is the leading contender for this dubious honor right now. Let me explain why.

I'll begin by asking you a question. What is the most valuable thing you possess? Some people might think of their home or their car. Others might think of their families. But I'd be willing to bet that after some careful consideration, most of you will come to the same conclusion that I have: the most value thing that each of us posses is our health. When we are well, we don't think about how incredibly lucky we are to possess health and are easily preoccupied with the day-to-day stressors in our lives. This is normal, and it's a trap I fall into as well. It is only when we suddenly lose our health that its value becomes clear. When that happens, we recognize that nothing matters more than regaining and recovering our vitality. It is only then that we will be able to resume our lives and enjoy the natural world around us as we care for our families and share our time with others.

My own personal experience has taught me this lesson. When I was in medical school, my eczema flared to such an extent that I was hospitalized and eventually developed cellulitis (an infection of the deeper layers of the skin). Right in the middle of the most grueling time of my medical education, I was sidelined with fevers, fatigue, and an aggressive skin infection. I couldn't sleep, my energy was gone, and it was hard to think clearly because my body was so inflamed. As a result, instead of thinking about my current internal medicine rotation, my upcoming exam, my patients, and what I was going to do that weekend, all I could think about was how to get rid of my current illness. I became solely focused on how to get well. More importantly, I wanted to know what was causing my eczema in the first place. The *only* thing that mattered to me at that point was being healthy and being able to do all of the cool stuff I was previously doing in my life. What if I were to tell you that at one point in our evolutionary history, our health went from appearing pretty good to being basically abysmal almost overnight? Well, this is exactly what happened about 12,000 years ago during the Neolithic Revolution when we began farming and joined "the cult of the seed." This colorful moniker was given to the advent of agriculture by Jared Diamond, author of numerous works examining our human journey through time. He stated:

> "*Archaeology is demolishing another sacred belief: that human history over the past million years has been a long tale of progress. In particular, recent discoveries suggest that the adoption of agriculture, supposedly our most decisive step toward a better life, **was in many ways a catastrophe from which we have never recovered.** With agriculture came the gross social and sexual inequality, the disease and despotism, that curse our existence.*"[1]

He goes on to note that this revisionist interpretation may strike some as incongruous. After all, aren't we better off now than our Paleolithic ancestors were? These sorts of arguments quickly lead us into speculative quagmires often riddled with inaccurate comparisons. Although we live longer today than at any other point in our past, our overall health is inferior, and chronic disease is rampant despite the mountain of technology and other "advancements" we've created. Claiming that the advent of agriculture is responsible for many of the pleasantries we enjoy today is an overly bold intellectual leap reliant on many unexamined assumptions.

How Healthy Are We Really Today?

Perhaps the most prominent of these assumptions is the notion that prior to farming, our lives were nasty, brutish, and short. The way of life observed in current indigenous groups indicates otherwise. Hunter-gatherers of today, like the previously mentioned !Kung, Hadza, Inuit, and Maasai, enjoy profound vigor late into their lives and are generally free from the chronic disease epidemics that now plague modern Western society.

Haven't we been told that the life expectancy of these groups is pale in comparison to ours? It is important to note that this statement fails to mention the mortality hazard factor in hunter-gatherer societies. During the first fifteen years of their lives, they are seventy-five to one hundred and ninety times more likely to die than individuals in Western societies.[2] That is, from birth to age fifteen, you'd be much more likely to die as a hunter-gatherer than as a Westerner. The factors that contribute to this mortality hazard include less access to clean water, lack of sanitary waste facilities, infectious illnesses, and traumatic wounds.

Comparisons of life expectancy between these groups are confounded by these inflated childhood mortality rates. When we compare the health, vitality, and quality of life in elderly indigenous groups to that of Westerners, the former are clearly superior in all aspects.

I imagine that you're thinking, *Isn't sanitation the result of our progression from farming?* Kudos to you, astute reader—this is a great question. My point with this portion of the book is not to say that our societal progression away from our previous days as hunter-gatherers (emphasis on *hunter*) has been *all* bad, but rather, to point out that while some beneficial things have been gained along this journey, many negative things, like rampant chronic disease, have as well.[3] Current estimates indicate that 88 percent of the westernized population have some form of metabolic disease, pre-diabetes, and insulin resistance. I'll discuss insulin resistance much more in Chapter Eleven, but for now, suffice it to say that this condition is behind the majority of chronic illnesses that cripple our society today, including diabetes, heart disease, hypertension, and infertility.

In today's mental health sphere, depression and anxiety affect a combined 600 million people worldwide and have increased 17 percent in the last ten years. Depression also takes the dubious honor of being the number one cause of disability in the world.[4] Dementia affects 50 million people in the westernized world today and is expected to triple by 2050. Sure, we've had some brilliant minds in Western society, but as a whole, hunter-gatherers have healthier brains and bodies. Despite our apparent longer life expectancies, we are sadly a very *unhealthy* population. Don't be fooled by estimates of life expectancy that are confounded by childhood mortality rates. Hunter-gatherers demonstrate superhuman health and vitality compared to us, and the aforementioned chronic illnesses of insulin resistance, depression, and dementia are virtually unheard of in these groups.

HUNTER-GATHERER LIFE

What were our day-to-day lives like before the advent of agriculture (also known as the Neolithic Revolution)? No one knows for sure, but we take some indication from the study of present-day hunter-gatherers. Diamond notes:

> *"Scattered throughout the world, several dozen groups of so-called primitive people, like the Kalahari bushmen, continue to support themselves that way.* **It turns out that these people have plenty of leisure time, sleep a good deal, and work less hard than their farming neighbors.** *For instance, the average time devoted each week to obtaining food is only 12 to 19 hours for one group of Bushmen, and 14 hours or less for the Hadza nomads of Tanzania."*[1]

Does this sound "nasty and brutish" to you? I wouldn't mind only working fourteen hours a week, especially if I had the rest of the time to do self-care, catch up on sleep, spend time in the ocean chasing waves, and be with friends and family.

Studies of present-day hunter-gatherer tribes invariably reveal robust health and freedom from chronic disease like diabetes, depression, and dementia.[5,6,7,8] But what do we know about the health of our more distant pre and post Neolithic Revolution ancestors? Once I get the time machine fully operational, we'll be able to answer these questions. Until then, we again must rely on fossil records, which in this case suggests some pretty striking contrasts between these two groups.

THE RETURN OF INDIANA JONES

In western Illinois, perched atop a bluff near the confluence of the Spoon River and Illinois River, lie thirteen earthen mounds that hold treasure. It is not the type of golden treasure our good friend Indy would have been after, but *historical treasure*. These are burial mounds that provide evidence of the lifestyle of the hunter-gatherers who lived in this area from around 950 AD to 1200 AD—a time period in which a very interesting thing happened. For reasons unknown, the population appears to have undergone a massive shift in the way that they were eating. They went from a hunter-gatherer lifestyle to a lifestyle based primarily on maize (ancient corn) agriculture. Multiple theories exist as to why this may have happened. It may have been out of necessity due to increasing population numbers or perhaps the development of a new technology that allowed tilling of the soil. Other possible reasons include overhunting and the decline of large animal populations. There are still others who point to the hypothetical Younger Dryas meteor impact that caused climate changes and mass faunal extinctions.

For whatever reason, these groups shifted their practices, and the population increased ten times in the span of the 250 years after they adopted agriculture. But there was a dark side to this growth. Comparison of bones from these pre- and post-agriculture groups reveal striking differences indicative of a marked decline in health with the introduction of agriculture.[9,10] Dickson Mounds researchers noted a clear decrease in both femur length and tibia diameter in children from the post agricultural period. Adult skeletons from this area displayed the same pattern as well as a significant reduction in stature after farming was introduced.

Similar discrepancies in height have been found in other ancient civilizations. Skeletons from Greece and Turkey reveal that 12,000 years ago, the average height of hunter-gatherers was five feet, nine inches for men and five feet, five inches for women. But with the adoption of agriculture, adult height plummeted—dashing any hopes these poor pastoralists would have had of dunking a basketball or playing competitive volleyball, if those sports had existed at the time. By 3,000 BC, men in this region of the world stood only five feet, three inches tall, and women a diminutive five feet, reflecting a massive decline in their overall nutritional status. Many studies across varied populations show a strong correlation between adult height and nutritional quality. One study looking at male height across 105 countries came to the following conclusion:

> *"In taller nations…the consumption of plant proteins markedly decreases at the expense of animal proteins, especially those from dairy.* Their highest consumption rates can be found in Northern and Central Europe, with the global peak of male height in the Netherlands (184 cm)."[11]

In this large study of nutritional quality, it is intriguing to note that the intake of *animal* foods directly correlated with greater height in males. The authors point out that even under conditions of caloric equivalency in plant-heavy versus animal-heavy cultures, height levels were higher in the latter societies. Other studies have come to similar conclusions regarding the key role that nutritional quality plays in determining adult height:

> *"Evidence across studies indicates that short adult height (reflecting growth retardation) in low- and middle-income countries is driven by environmental conditions, **especially net nutrition during early years**... This review suggests that adult height is a useful marker of variation in cumulative net nutrition, biological deprivation, and standard of living between and within populations and should be routinely measured."*[12]

In addition to declining height, there is also evidence that the Native Americans buried at the Dickson Mounds suffered increased bacterial infections. Such infections leave marks on the outer surface of the bone, known as the periosteum, with the tibia being especially susceptible to such damage due to its limited blood flow. Examination of tibias from skeletons found in the mounds shows that post agriculture, the number of such periosteal lesions increased threefold, with a whopping eighty-four percent of bones from this period demonstrating this pathology. The lesions also tended to be more severe and to show up earlier in life in the bones from the post agriculture peoples.

Another type of bone lesion, known as porotic hyperostosis, occurs in the skull and thinner bones of the body and is suggestive of nutrient deficiencies such as zinc and iron. These striking lesions cause the thin bones to have a "spongiform" appearance as the marrow expands and the other layers erode. At the Dickson Mounds, eye sockets and skulls demonstrated porotic hyperostosis, again with markings that display an increase in occurrence and severity after hunting practices were deemphasized in favor of farming. The incidence of joint and spine arthritic degeneration also appears to have doubled between these two periods. Defects in tooth enamel, suggestive of inadequate intake of the fat soluble vitamins unique to animal foods, increased across this time span as well. Clearly, eating less animals and more farmed plants was a disaster for the health of these peoples. Despite an increase in the population, their overall health took a serious nose dive.

DECLINE IN HUMAN HEALTH DURING NEOLITHIC REVOLUTION

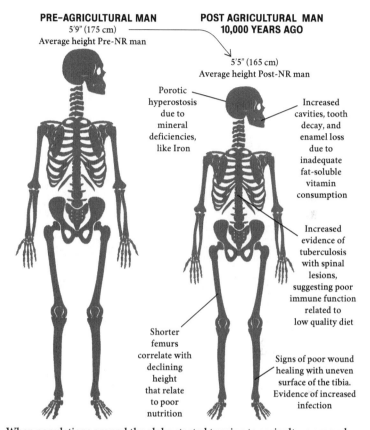

When populations around the globe started turning to agriculture around 10,000 years ago, regardless of their locations and type of crops, a similar trend occurred: the height and health of the people declined. Skeletal analysis suggests that these Neolithic peoples experienced "greater physiological stress due to under nutrition and infectious disease." Ulijaszek, Stanley J., et al., 1991 Human Dietary Change. Philosophical Transactions: Biological Sciences, 334 (1270): 271-279.

These types of negative health shifts weren't occurring only among the hunter-gatherers of Illinois, however. In *Paleopathology at the Origins of Agriculture*, the authors describe this trend in nineteen out of twenty-one cultures undergoing the agricultural transformation.[13] Similarly, in *Nutrition and Physical Degeneration*, Weston A. Price observed a stark contrast in the physical and dental health of populations around the globe when they were eating traditional diets versus processed westernized food.[14] Price observed that animal foods were favored above plants among people living traditional lifestyles, and further, that animal foods *always* constituted a significant portion of the diet, with special emphasis on organ meats and fat.

Good old Weston was way ahead of his time. He traveled all over the world to study these indigenous groups at the edge of civilization, learning from peoples as disparate as Northern European, Swiss, Gaelic, Polynesian islanders, African tribes, and Australian Aborigines. What did he learn from all of this adventuring? Dr. Price noticed a number of trends, including the fact that not *one culture* was thriving eating a plant-based diet.

> *"It is significant that I have as yet found no group that was building and maintaining good bodies exclusively on plant foods."*[14]

He also observed that in similar regions of Africa, tribes consuming more animal foods were healthier and dominant over the tribes that relied more heavily on plants. Comparing the Maasai, who eat an almost entirely animal-based diet, to the Kikuyu with their agricultural emphasis, he stated:

> *"In the Maasai tribe, a study of 2,516 teeth in eighty-eight individuals…showed only four individuals with caries. These had a total of ten carious teeth, or only 0.4 percent of the teeth attacked by tooth decay… In contrast with the Maasai, the Kikuyu tribe are characterized by being primarily agricultural people. Their chief articles of diet are sweet potatoes, corn, beans and some bananas, millet, and Kafir corn, a variety of indian millet…* **The Kikuyus are not as tall as the Maasai and physically they are much less rugged***…A Study of 1,041 teeth in thirty-three individuals showed fifty-seven teeth with caries, or 5.5 percent. These were 36.4 percent of the individuals affected."*[14]

This is a huge difference in dental health with noted inferior height and robustness in the agricultural Kikuyu, and it mimics the contrasts we've seen between hunter-gatherers and farming peoples at the Dickson Mounds and other locations throughout the world.

In addition to the Maasai, Eskimos demonstrate exemplary overall health and pristine dentition with an almost entirely animal-based diet. Price was particularly impressed with this group of people, stating:

> *"The Eskimo race has remained true to ancestral type to give us a living demonstration of what Nature can do in the building of a race compe-*

tent to withstand for thousands of years the rigors of an Arctic climate. **Like the Indian, the Eskimo thrived as long as he was not blighted by the touch of modern civilization, but with it, like all primitives, he withers and dies.** *In his primitive state he has provided an example of physical excellence and dental perfection such as has seldom been excelled by any race in the past or present."* [14]

Our other explorer friend, Vilhjalmur Stefansson, left his position as an anthropologist at Harvard to live with the Eskimo people of northern Alaska, whom he noted ate an almost entirely animal-based diet for much of the year. He remarked on the profound health that resulted from such a diet:

> *"***It seemed to me that, mentally and physically, I had never been in better health in my life***....During the first few months of my first year in the Arctic, I acquired...the munitions of fact and experience which have within my own mind defeated those views of dietetics reviewed at the beginning of this article. I could be healthy on a diet of fish and water. The longer I followed it the better I liked it, which meant, at least inferentially and provisionally, that you never become tired of your food if you have only one thing to eat. I did not get scurvy on the fish diet nor learn that any of my fish-eating friends ever had it...There were certainly no signs of hardening of the arteries and high blood pressure, of breakdown of the kidneys or of rheumatism...These months on fish were the beginning of several years during which I lived on an exclusive meat diet...***To the best of my estimate then, I have lived in the Arctic for more than five years exclusively on meat and water.***"* [15]

When Stefansson returned from his time with the hunters of the great white North, he made bold claims like these and described his findings to physicians of the 1900s—but they were certain he was off his rocker. Vilhjalmur was determined, however, to prove that a meat based diet was not only safe, but health promoting. In what became one of the most amazing studies of human nutrition, he spent the next *year* cloistered in Bellevue Hospital in New York City eating an entirely animal-based diet under the close scrutiny of skeptical physicians.

> *"The broad results of the experiment were...so far as the supervising physicians could tell,* ***that we were in at least as good average health during the year [eating a meat-only diet] as we had been during the three mixed-diet weeks at the start.*** *We*

*thought our health had been a little better than average. We enjoyed and
prospered as well on the meat in midsummer as in midwinter, and felt
no more discomfort from the heat than our fellow New Yorkers did."* [15]

I can only imagine the cognitive dissonance the previously skeptical
physicians must have had when they observed these results. We'll talk all
about how eating a carnivore diet won't lead to scurvy or other nutritional deficiencies in later chapters, but Vilhjalmur displayed this conclusion over ninety years ago.

HUNTER-GATHERERS OR JUST HUNTERS?

I know what you might be thinking at this point. The Native Americans
of the Dickson Mounds and many of the other peoples studied by
Weston Price were both hunters and gatherers. This is true. In fact, most
recently studied indigenous populations are observed to consume both
animals and plants. However, it is important to remember the *carnivore
code hypothesis* here and to think about the animals that are available for
more modern hunter-gatherers to hunt versus the animals that were
available to our more distant ancestors 70 thousand years ago or even 2
million years ago. Based on energetic and nutrient superiority, our ancestors have always favored animal foods over plant foods *when animal foods
were available.* Current estimates of the plant-to-animal consumption ratio
in present-day hunter-gatherers suggest an approximate fifty-fifty split.[5]
But, as many have pointed out, these populations no longer have access
to large game and are forced to adapt to their changing environment by
gathering more plant foods. Thus, currently living populations of hunter-gatherers are a poor indication of the relative amounts of animal and
plant foods consumed by more distant predecessors.

The groups studied by Weston Price were trying to survive, just like
today's indigenous cultures are trying to survive. But we are trying to
thrive. Calories are no longer a limiting factor as they have been throughout much of human history. None of the 87.8 percent of our population who are metabolically broken are suffering from a caloric deficiency.
As the apex predators on this planet, we can now access the most optimal foods for humans all of the time. Whether or not we should do
this becomes an ethical and environmental question that I will address in
Chapter Fourteen, but here's a hint that may surprise you: properly raised
ruminant animals are actually *good* for the environment.

We know that our predecessors ate some plant foods, but these
were eaten as survival foods rather than as components of the diet that
provided unique nutrients. It's also revealing to discover that indigenous

groups have unique ways of preparing many plant foods to help render them less toxic, like fermentation. Oh yes, plants are full of toxins! They are cunning little critters that have co-evolved with insects and animals that want nothing more than to munch on them, so they had to adapt— and they found some ingenious ways to do so. In the next few chapters, we'll dive into all of these phenomena as we talk about the chemical weapons that plants have been developing for the last 400 million years. It's scary stuff!

SECTION II

CHAPTER THREE

CHEMICAL WARFARE

Remember when your siblings buried you in the sand at the beach with only your head sticking out? Imagine that happening to you again, except this time you are buried so well that you can't escape. *You are stuck in the ground and can't run away.* Now we're going to paint your face like a soccer ball as the entire six-year-old pee-wee soccer team arrives at the beach full of energy. How are you going to feel? **Vulnerable**! You are going to hope and pray that there are some adults around so these irascible six year olds don't decide to start playing soccer with your head. That would really stink.

Welcome to the world of plants. When insects and animals decide to go munching on our green neighbors, plants can't run away, bite, or verbally threaten them to defend themselves. Just like you would be defenseless against the inclinations of the pee-wee soccer team players, so too are plants vulnerable to the appetite-driven whims of everything around them. They have faced this quandary since the beginning of their evolutionary history, about 470 million years ago, and over that time span, they've come up with a solution: creating extensive defense mechanisms, both physically and chemically.

Turns out, plants are pretty darn crafty. For a long time, they've been in a constant "arms race" with everything that wants to eat them.

In order to protect themselves, they have managed to produce a variety of defense mechanisms as they evolved—many of which we are familiar with. Ever go hiking in the desert and accidentally bump into a cactus? Ever play in the woods and stumble into a patch of brambles? Ouch and double ouch! We are much less aware of the molecular mechanisms plants have evolved to defend themselves, however, and these chemical "spikes" can cause just as much harm as the spines on a cactus or the thorns on a rosebush.

A CASE OF MISTAKEN IDENTITY

I'm not exactly sure why we've come to believe that plants are fundamentally benevolent and that anything that comes from a plant should be good for us. Maybe it's because there are a lot of beautiful plants out there, full of colors and smells, that delight the senses and curry romantic favor on anniversaries, holidays, and birthdays. On the surface, most plants look friendly enough, but if we look closer—it's an entirely different story. Most of the compounds we think of as "phytonutrients" are in fact "phytoweapons," meticulously designed by plants to discourage insects, animals, and fungi from consuming them for breakfast. Plants do *not* want to be eaten (sure, fruit is a different story and we'll talk about that later, but it's still not that good for you). They have the same agenda as the rest of the living things on this planet: to proliferate and pass their DNA on to future generations. Being chewed up by a moose doesn't exactly make it onto a plant's to-do list.

I have some heartbreaking news to tell you, but I'm your friend and know you need to hear this. Kale doesn't love you back. Broccoli is just not that into you. Spinach isn't a real friend. Feel free to break out the tissues if you need to wipe the tears from your eyes. Trust me, you're better off without these bad relationships in your life—they are only going to break your heart in the end.

The statement "plants don't want to be eaten" is often countered with the assertion that animals don't want to be eaten either, and I couldn't agree with this more. However, remember that animals have evolved different sorts of defense mechanisms to combat predators. Usually, this is simply getting the heck out of Dodge when a hungry predator shows up and bears its sharp teeth. Other times, when push comes to shove, prey animals fight back with talons, claws, and teeth of their own. This isn't the case with plants, and as we vividly displayed earlier, they're rooted in the ground, so the arms race between plants and animals continues. Let's examine the various types of weapons plants have devised and what we know about them.

SWORDS, SPEARS, AND AXES

The plant armamentarium is vast, like James Bond's weapon collection on steroids. There are literally hundreds of thousands of chemicals produced in the plant kingdom that can harm us. Broadly speaking, we can divide these toxic compounds into a few categories. The largest category is the phytoalexins—chemicals directly produced by plants to ward off attack from insects, fungi, and animals. This category includes many of the compounds that we have been told are good for us, including glucosinolates and many polyphenols. Glucosinolates might sound like an alien term, but you're likely familiar with one of the by-products of this family of compounds called sulforaphane, which is formed in large amounts when we eat broccoli sprouts. In the next chapter, we'll go into great detail about why this compound is not all it's cracked up to be, and how it could actually be harming you in many ways.

The colloquial term "polyphenol" has been used to refer to many plant compounds, though technically it identifies a family of carbon-based organic plant molecules with multiple phenol-like rings. Some well-known examples are pictured below. These compounds are often also formed as phytoalexins or as plant pigments. The most well-known polyphenols are probably resveratrol and curcumin, and if you believe the hype, by taking these you'll live forever, cleanse yourself of inflammation, and maybe even grow wings. In Chapter Five, I'll debunk the many myths surrounding the purported benefits of polyphenols and show you evidence that polyphenols are potentially damaging our bodies.

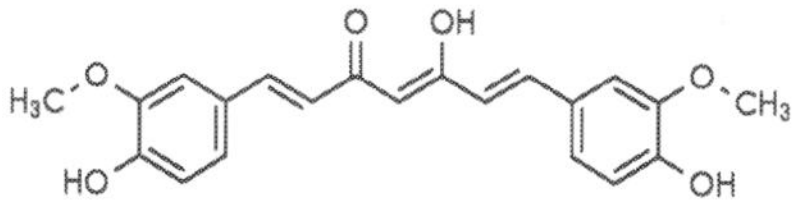

curcumin

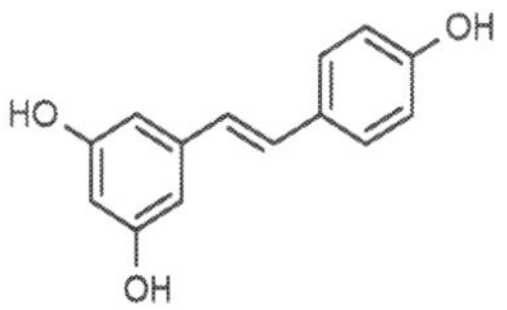

resveratrol

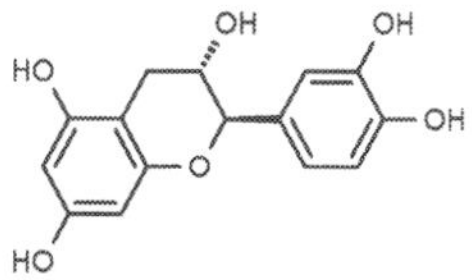

catechin

Does it sound like I'm going to turn mainstream nutritional ideas on their head? Good, because that's exactly what this book is intended to do. As I said in the introduction, I'm not here to parrot nutritional dogma that has been accepted as canon for decades. In reality, it has always been based on shaky science. I'm here to ruffle some feathers, kick a whole lot of butt, and take names along the way, while challenging you to think outside of the box.

PLANT PESTICIDES

Phytoalexins can also be thought of as plant pesticides, but not the type of pesticides we are used to thinking about that are sprayed on plants, like Roundup (glyphosate). The plant pesticides I am speaking about here are produced *by the plants* as defense chemicals.[1] In his comprehensive scientific article titled "Dietary Pesticides: 99.9% All Natural," researcher Bruce Ames highlights the fact that humans consume 99.99 percent of their pesticide load from plants themselves and only 0.1 percent as pesticides sprayed on food. Glyphosate and other synthetic pesticides are certainly harming people, but the amount of these consumed pales in comparison to the quantity of plant-produced pesticides in our diet. Ames states:

> *"We estimate that Americans eat about 1.5 g of natural pesticides per person per day, which is about 10,000 times more than they eat of synthetic pesticide residues… there is a very large literature on natural toxins in plants and their role in plant defenses.* **The human intake of these toxins varies markedly with diet and would be higher in vegetarians.** *Our estimate of 1.5 g of natural pesticides per person per day is based on the content of toxins in the major plant foods."[2]*

Ames goes on to note that plant pesticides are pervasive, with at least forty-two compounds known to occur in a seemingly benign food such as cabbage. Furthermore, many of these compounds have been shown to be damaging to DNA in humans and animals, a process known as clastogenesis.

> *"Thus, it is probable that almost every fruit and vegetable in the supermarket contains natural plant pesticides that are rodent carcinogens."*

We'll talk much more about this concept in Chapter Four and Chapter Five. Brace yourself!

The butt-kicking doesn't stop with polyphenols. Lectins are another category of toxic substances in plants that you need to know about and avoid if you're in search of optimal health. Dr. Steven Gundry has raised awareness of these carbohydrate-binding proteins with his book, *The Plant Paradox,* which many of you may be familiar with. In Chapter Seven, I'll talk about lectins and build on many of the ideas he has advanced in order to demonstrate how these pervasive molecules in plants may damage our gut and lead to autoimmunity and inflammation.

Oxalates are another chemical spike found in plants. Plants use these organic molecules to bind minerals in their own unique biochemistry. But oxalates aren't used in human biochemistry and instead are a by-product that results when the human body metabolizes amino acids. This small amount of oxalates is treated as a waste product and is excreted daily in the urine. In plants, however, very large amounts of these compounds occur and are known to contribute to significant pathology in humans. Calcium oxalate kidney stones are a well-known effect of oxalate consumption, and in Chapter Six, we'll dive into research suggesting that breast cancer, thyroid disease, vulvodynia (pelvic pain in women), and skin rashes are also connected with oxalates in our diet. Don't believe me? When you see the picture of the vicious microscopic needles, called raphides, that oxalate crystals form, you might never look at spinach or sweet potatoes the same way again. All I can say is, ouchie!

DISPARATE OPERATING SYSTEMS

Before we dive headlong into the tumultuous sea of plant toxins, there's a key concept I'd like to introduce. As we sail across the rough waters ahead, it will become very clear that plant molecules don't work very well with our biochemistry and usually just end up throwing a big fat monkey wrench into the elegant workings of the human machine. This shouldn't come across as a surprise, however. It's believed that plants and animals diverged from a single-celled precursor more than 1.5 *billion* years ago, and in that time, these two disparate kingdoms of life have evolved in very unique ways.

Let's try to place the overall timeline of life on earth into context here. The earth is thought to be about 4.5 billion years old, and the first evidence of life dates back to around 3.5 billion years ago. Some scientists say life may have originated even earlier than this, but we can't say for sure. We're not sure exactly how life started, but most hypothesize that it began with the coalescence of atoms into more complex molecules, and then into structures resembling DNA, before the first single-celled organisms arose.[3,4]

For now, I'll focus on the split between plants, animals, and fungi, which happened 1.5 billion years ago. At that time, we looked like a blob, a single-celled blob to be more exact. We were nothing like the animals, plants, or fungi that appear today. Since that fateful day *billions* of years ago, these three main lineages of life have been humming along doing their own things in very different ways. Each kingdom has evolved its own ways of getting nutrients from the environment and transforming them into the energy needed to power their internal "engines."

We might think of these families of life as three different "operating systems," like Mac, Android, and Linux. Because I'm partial to Macs, I think of humans as these, with plants as Android, and fungi as Linux. Each operating system has been programmed in a different code and has different internal processes that allow it to run smoothly. If you try to take a program from Android and run it on your iPhone or your MacBook, it's not going to work, and it might even cause other programs to crash. You're going to need special software to convert the program to an operable format, and in reality it's best to just run Mac programs on a Mac because they were specifically designed for that operating system.

You might also think of the three different kingdoms of life as three different types of cars, let's say Tesla, Ferrari, and Porsche. You're not going to be able to use Tesla parts in your Ferrari or your Porsche. If you want your car to perform the way it's supposed to, it's wisest to use parts that were specifically designed for it.

Plant molecules like phytoalexins, polyphenols, oxalates, and lectins are like computer programs from a different operating system than ours. They are Android and we are Mac; the programs are not very compatible. When we try to use plant programs in our human operating system, they generally just mess things up, sometimes causing massive problems akin to the "blue screen of death" on your computer. Plants have evolved these molecules for their own personal biochemistry and metabolism, not for ours!

Those Porsche parts don't work in your Tesla. Contrary to popular belief, plant molecules do not play a role in human biochemistry or metabolism. As you'll see in future chapters, so called "antioxidants" from plants don't directly serve an antioxidant role in your body. In fact, they are often doing the opposite—acting as "pro-oxidants." Our body has its own intrinsic antioxidants, like glutathione, that are part of *our* programming and that manage the balance of oxidation and reduction just fine on their own. In fact, multiple studies have shown that supplementation with plant "antioxidant" molecules do nothing to improve antioxidant status in humans and are often associated with worse outcomes.[5,6,7-10]

When we eat animal foods, we are eating foods from the same operating system as humans. The biochemistry and metabolism of animals look a whole lot more like ours than those of plants or fungi. Plants use photosynthesis to generate energy as they inhale carbon dioxide and expire oxygen. Animals do the opposite, breathing in oxygen and producing carbon dioxide as a by-product of cellular respiration. Similarly, the plant-based forms of many vitamins and nutrients look very differently from the corresponding animal-based forms. Beta-carotene vs. retinol (vitamin A), alpha-linolenic acid (ALA) vs. DHA (omega-3 fatty acids), and vitamins K1 vs. K2 are all examples of this and will be discussed in much greater detail in Chapter Eight. In that chapter, we'll also discuss the many nutrients key to optimal human function that don't occur in appreciable amounts in plants or fungi, like vitamin B_{12}, choline, taurine, carnitine, carnosine, vitamin K2, and others.

The "operating systems" concept is meant to serve as a framework for many of the discussions that will follow in this book. We'll see that when humans consume plants and fungi, problems result because their foreign molecular programs often aren't compatible with our physiology. In the following chapters, I'll discuss the many types of plant toxins in detail. I'll also explain the inferior ability of plants to provide us with vitamins and minerals due to their less usable forms and their decreased bioavailability. Animals, on the other hand, provide a much more compatible framework for human nutrition based on their similar design.

BRACE YOURSELF FOR A CHEMISTRY LESSON

The concepts of antioxidants, oxidation, and reduction are going to be spoken about frequently in this book, and I want to make sure that we have some sense of what these really mean. At a biochemical level, life can be distilled to the exchange of electrons between molecules and the harvesting of energy stored in bonds between atoms. We eat food in order to gather energy stored in the bonds of its molecules, translating this energy through the movement of electrons into other storage forms of energy, namely into a molecule called ATP, or adenosine triphosphate. Oxidation and reduction refer to the molecular loss and gain of electrons, respectively. When a molecule is oxidized, it loses an electron to another molecule, which is simultaneously reduced as it gains that electron. When I was in college studying chemistry, we used the mnemonic "LEO the lion says GER" to remember that Loss of Electrons is Oxidation (LEO), and Gain of Electrons represents Reduction (GER).

Free radicals are molecules with an unpaired electron, and they are an unruly sort of character. They are highly reactive and have a predilection for stealing electrons from proteins, lipids, and nucleic acids—which results in oxidation of these molecules. Free radicals aren't entirely bad, however, and they do serve important signaling roles in the human body—but if overproduced, they can cause oxidative stress, a condition in which the delicate balance of oxidation and reduction is thrown off, resulting in cellular damage and aging.[11] However, our body has an amazing system to manage this balance that generally works pretty well as long as we are providing the nutrients needed for it to function. Minerals like zinc, copper, selenium, and magnesium help power the reactions that keep our redox system in balance, and the amino acids glycine, cysteine, and glutamine form glutathione, which is part of our body's major antioxidant police force. What are the best sources of these nutrients? Without a doubt, animal foods provide the richest array of bioavailable vitamins and minerals used in our biochemistry. We don't need plant molecules to achieve optimal redox balance or overall function. On the contrary, optimal redox balance *can* be achieved by consuming just the nutrient-rich animal foods that our ancestors favored for millions of years.

ANIMALS EATING PLANTS

If animals and plants are from different operating systems, how do herbivorous animals eat plants and thrive? The answer hearkens back to the disparate paths that humans and herbivores have traveled in their respective co-evolutions with plants. As we discussed in the first two chapters of this book, it appears that when we broke away from our plant-focused ancestors in the evolutionary chain, the source of our food changed dramatically. This allowed for much bigger brains and fundamental changes in many aspects of our bodies, like a more acidic stomach, a smaller GI tract, and structural changes of feet, pelvis, shoulder, and jaw.

In other words, our environment changed dramatically and we evolved with it, becoming well adapted to eating animal foods. The evolution of herbivorous animals parallels ours, but with plants as the main dietary driving factor. Just as we adapted to eating an animal-based diet, herbivores similarly adapted to consuming plants in high quantities while mitigating the plant defense molecules that come with this way of eating. With our shifting dietary preferences and needs, we didn't evolve the same adaptations, however. We can detoxify some of the harmful chemicals in plants, but herbivores are much more suited to this. While humans have been feasting primarily on animal foods for the last 2 million years, similar selective pressures from plant toxins have not been present for us, and we appear to be much less adapted to eating significant amounts of plants for long periods of time.

Moose and many other grazing animals have evolved proteins in their saliva to deactivate tannins present in leaves, which act as digestive enzyme inhibitors.[12] Ruminants also possess multiple stomachs, which accomplish the task of digesting plants and breaking down plant toxins much differently than monogastric (single stomach) animals like humans do. Rabbits and other small animals often chew plants like sage brush excessively, allowing for many of the volatile plant toxins to be off gassed in the process.[13,14,15,16] In what is thought to be a detoxification behavior, herbivores have also been observed eating clay or dirt along with more toxic plants when these are all that is available.

Herbivores aren't often considered the brainiacs of the animal world, but examination of their grazing practices reveals a keen sense of the relative toxicity of various plants.[17,18] They appear to know how much of any particular plant they can eat without it making them sick, and then they move on to selectively eat other plants before over-consuming any one source of a particular toxin. When populations of herbivorous animals like deer and buffalo are overcrowded and forced to abandon their innate feedings and grazing patterns, mass deaths occur as a result of over-consumption of only a small variety of plants. If cows could laugh, they would surely have a good chuckle at our expense if they saw us shoveling loads of kale, spinach, and other toxin-ladened leafy greens into a blender, imagining that this was good for us without any regard to the boatloads of plant toxins contained within them.

In the next chapter, we'll begin our deeper examinations of the multiple types of plant toxins as we explore the broad family of isothiocyanates, like sulforaphane. I hope the concept of disparate operating systems will help you understand why these molecules aren't actually beneficial for humans at all. They're produced by plants for their own cellular processes, not other animals'. Like programs from a foreign operating system that aren't compatible with ours, they don't help us, and often they get in the way of optimal functionality. As we'll see in the case of isothiocyanates, this involves interfering with proper thyroid functionality and damaging our DNA. The next few chapters are definitely a journey through some rugged territory, so lace up your boots, and let's continue our adventure.

CHAPTER FOUR

BROCCOLI—SUPERHERO OR SUPERVILLAIN?

Perhaps more than any other single plant food, broccoli has been uniquely hailed as a magical vegetable. Is there any truth behind this praise or was George H. W. Bush right when he famously declared in 1990, "I've never liked it. I'm the President of the United States, and I'm not going to eat my broccoli!"?

As the subject of our detective work, broccoli belongs to the *Brassica* family of vegetables, all of which are derived from an ancient type of mustard plant. The many faces of this family, also known as crucifers, include kale, collard greens, Brussels sprouts, cabbage, kohlrabi, horseradish, wasabi, Swiss chard, cauliflower, rutabaga, bok choy, watercress, radishes, mustard, and turnip. A unique feature of this family is the presence of the sulfur-containing compounds known as glucosinolates—which are transformed into isothiocyanates and related compounds when acted on by the enzyme myrosinase.

I know I'm handing you a lot of esoteric chemical names, but bear with me. I'm going to break it all down and it's important to understand this for the broader discussion. Perhaps you've heard of the compound sulforaphane associated with all sorts of fancy health claims from "cancer fighter" to "antioxidant hero." This molecule is an isothiocyanate derived from the glucosinolate molecule, glucoraphanin. In this case, sulforaphane is formed when myrosinase does its enzymatic work on glucoraphanin, and out of this process come magical rainbow unicorns. While that's the popular narrative that supplement manufacturers and many in the health space want you to believe, I'm not buying it and you shouldn't either. Allow me to show you the dark side of sulforaphane and the whole family of these isothiocyanate molecules.

Although it is true that when myrosinase acts on glucoraphanin the end result is sulforaphane, this happens *only* when plants are under attack and are being chewed to pieces by predatory insects and animals. Sulforaphane does not exist in a healthy, living broccoli plant. It only shows up as a defense chemical in response to damage being done to the plant cell walls. When everything is hunky-dory in broccoli's world, glucoraphanin and myrosinase never get together to make sulforaphane. They are separated into different cellular compartments that mix only when the plant's cell walls are destroyed as Bambi eats it for breakfast. Sulforaphane is a plant weapon. It's a phytoalexin, a plant toxin that does not play a role in plant biochemistry, and is only employed to do its dirty work when helpless broccoli is being turned into a snack. Like a booby trap waiting to be sprung, or a highly dangerous covert operative, it's deployed only when things get really bad. Sulforaphane is so toxic that it can't be present in a healthy broccoli plant, or it would cause massive damage due to it's strong capacity as a pro-oxidant.

sulforaphane

So how does sulforaphane do its dirty work? In animals, including humans, it has two main mechanisms of toxicity, a slow one and a fast one. The fast mechanism of harm is accomplished by acting as a vicious pro-oxidant, causing the formation of free radicals that damage the delicate lipids in cell membranes, proteins, and DNA. In human cell culture, sulforaphane and many other related isothiocyanates have been shown to damage DNA in the process of clastogenesis, causing chromosomal breaks.[1,2,3-5] Trust me, damaging these cellular components is not a good thing.

DAMAGING DNA

In mouse trials for toxicity, sulforaphane has been found to cause sedation, hypothermia, loss of motor coordination, leukopenia (low white blood cell count), and even death.[6] It's important to note that animal studies aren't always a great proxy for human effects and that doses used in this study were high, but there are also multiple animal studies that demonstrate toxicity of broccoli and broccoli extracts in animals at much lower doses. Research has shown that feeding good old broccoli to mice and rats resulted in DNA damage, and the same results occurred when raw broccoli was fed to pigs and freeze-dried broccoli extract was given to fruit flies.[7,8,9-11] Though no one has looked at the potential for this to occur in vivo in humans (in the body), isothiocyanates have repeatedly been shown to have these adverse effects in human cell culture. Damaging DNA can lead to a number of problems in our body and is generally accepted as the main precursor event in most types of cancers.[12] To make matters worse, sulforaphane is only one of seventeen isothiocyanate compounds known to be present in broccoli. Other cruciferous vegetables have even more. Cabbage, for instance, demonstrates forty-two known plant toxins.

SLOW DAMAGE

Acting as a pro-oxidant and causing damage to DNA, membranes, and proteins through the formation of free radicals is just the "fast" way that sulforaphane and this family of compounds seek to fight back against the animals eating *Brassica* plants.[13] There's also a "slow" mechanism, which earns this family of plants the ignominious moniker of "goitrogens," signifying their ability to produce enlargement of the thyroid gland known as goiter. If you've seen photos of people with very large necks related to iodine deficiency, you'll be familiar with what this condition looks like. These extreme examples are from regions of the world where iodine-rich foods are often scarce and people eat many goitrogenic foods like cassava and cruciferous plants out of necessity, but similar mechanisms are at work whenever we consume isothiocyanates.

When we eat broccoli, or any plant from the *Brassica* family, some of the absorbed sulforaphane is immediately detoxified because our body knows it's a toxin and doesn't want it. Whatever is not broken down circulates in the bloodstream and competes with iodine for absorption at the thyroid—preventing this gland from getting one of the minerals it needs to make thyroid hormones. Cases of hypothyroidism induced by over-consumption of crucifers have been reported even in westernized populations but are extremely common in underdeveloped regions of the world.[14,15,16,17] Consumption of cruciferous vegetables has also been linked to increased rates of thyroid cancer in Melanesian women who had low intakes of iodine.[18] Does that broccoli-sprout-and-kale smoothie still seem like a good idea? As we'll see in the next chapter, many polyphenols, such as green tea catechins, have also been shown to interfere with proper thyroid function.[19,20]

Within the plant kingdom, there are multiple examples of this type of chemical booby trap system whereby toxins are released only upon the mechanical destruction of cell walls by predators. Cassava is a plant native to South America, the roots of which are widely consumed as a source of carbohydrates in poor regions of the continent where there is limited access to more nutrient-rich food. In all parts of the plant, but concentrated in the roots, is the molecule linamarin, which is a cyanogenic glycoside.[21,22] These compounds are also found in the pits of stone fruits like peaches, apricots, and plums, and they are highly toxic. Linamarin itself isn't toxic, but when combined with the enzyme linamarase, it's broken down into hydrocyanic acid,[23] which is exactly as toxic as it sounds.

When ingested, hydrocyanic acid quickly breaks down into cyanide—an extremely potent mitochondrial poison. This is the stuff of real secret agents and even small quantities can be a swift path to the grave. Cyanogenic glycosides in other foods, like the aforementioned pits of stone fruits, can similarly break down into cyanide, and poisonings have been reported with overconsumption. In order to be eaten, cassava must either be fermented for three days or ground up and left to dry in the sun while the majority of the hydrocyanic acid is released into the air. As if this wasn't bad enough, cassava also contains isothiocyanates, just like the *Brassica* vegetables, and has been associated with the development of endemic goiter.[24,25,26]

HOW WE'VE BEEN LED ASTRAY

With all of these strikes against broccoli and its cousins, why would anyone want to consume these foods? Surely, there must be another side to this story. There definitely is, and we'll explore that before I share with you why I think the purported benefits of these foods are overblown and myopic.

Many of the laurels thrown toward sulforaphane come from researchers touting its potential as a cancer chemoprotective agent and claiming that it acts as an antioxidant.[27,28] I'm all for plant compounds as potential therapeutic agents in cancer, and many of the chemotherapies we use in medicine today are derived from plants. But just because a compound has shown benefits against cancer does not mean it's good for the general population.

Would you take chemotherapy like a multivitamin every day? Of course not! Chemotherapy agents are vicious chemicals that kill both cancer and native cells, often leading cancer patients to the brink of death. Sulforaphane has been shown to have potential benefit in cancer-fighting models *because it damages cells* and can induce programmed cell death, or apoptosis. But when introduced into our bodies, it's going to target our healthy cells too. In studies with human tissue, sulforaphane has been shown to alter the way genes are turned on and off in both cancerous and healthy cells.[29] No chemotherapy yet developed can perfectly target cancer cells while leaving the rest of our body unscathed. We're getting closer to this with some targeted cancer therapeutics, but we're still not perfect. A molecule like sulforaphane is certainly not going to be specific, and as you'll see in the next chapter, neither are many of the touted polyphenolic molecules, like curcumin, that have also been shown to be toxic to both cancerous and native human tissues.[30]

Remember when I said earlier that sulforaphane had a fast mechanism of toxicity? This is part of the chemical karate it uses to attack cancer cells, but it also harms our healthy cells in the process. Sulforaphane can create so many reactive oxygen species in both cancerous and non-cancerous cells that programmed cell death is initiated.[31] In this process of oxidative-stress-induced apoptosis, the hyperdrive engines in our cellular spaceships become overloaded and can explode, potentially damaging many surrounding healthy cells. In a valiant act of selflessness, our cells sense this happening and initiate a controlled self-destruct sequence so as not to harm other cells around them.

The study of plant molecules as possible cancer chemotherapies can reveal valuable adjunctive treatments for this tragic set of ailments, but the ability of a molecule to harm malignant cells reveals very little about its usefulness for a healthy population. Chemotherapeutic compounds do not work well as chemopreventive agents. They're just too toxic. If we are interested in preventing the genesis of cancer within our bodies, the answer isn't to take toxic plant molecules like sulforaphane. On the contrary, our goal is to live in as healthful a manner as possible and allow our immune system's natural surveillance mechanisms to act as they are designed. I believe we can best achieve this through our diet, and in the next chapter, I'll go into detail about the other health behaviors that can complement our food choices and enable us to truly reclaim our health, all of which contribute to what I call "living a radical life."

HORMESIS RE-EXAMINED

The other claim about potential benefits of sulforaphane champion its role as an antioxidant. Throughout this chapter, I've repeatedly stated that these isothiocyanate molecules act as pro-oxidants. Am I lying to you? No way! We've been badly misled on this point. Let's take a very close look at what happens when sulforaphane or other isothiocyanates are ingested to clear up this confusion.

When we eat cruciferous vegetables, glucosinolates like glucoraphanin combine with myrosinase during the chewing process, forming isothiocyanates like sulforaphane. This is the booby trap pattern of plant toxins we discussed earlier. A small fraction of this sulforaphane is absorbed and rapidly detoxified in the liver through a process of conjugation to glutathione. It is then excreted in the urine.

We will see this same pattern with all of the plant compounds examined in this book: *our body does not want these foreign molecules*. They are not actively absorbed, and the small fraction that makes it into our body is rapidly detoxified in the liver before being excreted in the urine and the stool. This process can be contrasted with the active absorption and biochemical utilization of the vitamins and minerals found in our food. Plant compounds like glucosinolates and polyphenols do not participate directly in our biochemistry. Instead, they often trigger defensive reactions in our body.

Due to its pro-oxidant tendencies, sulforaphane triggers a cellular cascade designed to sense oxidative stress. One of the key components of this system is a transcription factor known as NRF2. Let's pause for one moment and describe what a transcription factor is. In molecular biology terms, when genes encoded in DNA are turned on, they are *transcribed* into RNA, which is then *translated* into that gene's protein product. In a simplistic model, your genetic code is written in the alphabet of DNA, which ultimately is transformed into the proteins that make up your body. All of your DNA isn't turned on at once. It's a tightly regulated dance, and transcription factors, like NRF2, control which genes get turned on. In this case, when NRF2 senses oxidative stress caused by sulforaphane, it turns on a host of genes involved in combating this damage. Included in this group are enzymes that participate in the production and utilization of glutathione, like glutamate cysteine ligase and glutathione s-transferase.

Glutathione is a simple molecule, consisting of just three amino acids, but it's a real superhero that is tasked with donating electrons to the irascible free radicals formed when molecules like sulforaphane go running around our body. To further suggest what sort of characters sulforaphane and isothiocyanates are, let's think about the other types of things that can turn the NRF2 antioxidant response cascade on. Generally speaking, any type of molecule that causes oxidative stress in our body activates this pathway so we can ramp up our defenses. This includes tobacco smoke, heavy metals like lead, mercury, and arsenic, alcohol, oxidized vegetable oils, and hyperglycemia.[32,33,34-36] That's a pretty rough crowd, basically the "Bad News Gang" riding around on motorcycles and wearing leather jackets that say "Born To Be Bad." It's not exactly the type of folks you'd want your son or daughter to be hanging out with.

But this isn't the story we are told about broccoli and sulforaphane at all, is it? While it is true that sulforaphane does act as a pro-oxidant, by activating the NRF2 system it *induces the formation of our own endogenous antioxidants*, like glutathione. There are studies showing that administration of sulforaphane improves antioxidant status in the short term, but this is related to increased production of glutathione, not to any direct antioxidant capacity of sulforaphane. None of the other plant molecules like polyphenols act directly as antioxidants either—they also act as pro-oxidants and turn on the NRF2 system.

At first glance, this may seem like a good thing, but there's much more to this story that will unfold as we go deeper down this rabbit hole. For now, remember that these molecules are toxins that create oxidative stress, just like all of the other things that also induce the NRF2 cascade. No one would suggest that we might achieve better health by taking a small dose of lead every day or smoking a few cigarettes daily, but this is essentially what is happening when we ingest sulforaphane and other isothiocyanates. These are chemical weapons used by plants to discourage predation, not molecules that create health in humans.

Because we've been exposed to lots of toxic substances throughout our evolution, like heavy metals, plant defense molecules, and smoke from fire, we've benefited from the activity of the NRF2 system as it participates in the detoxification of our bodies after these exposures, but we shouldn't be purposefully exposing ourselves to pro-oxidants of any type if we can avoid it.

"But wait!" you say. "Isn't this the process of hormesis, by which a small amount of a toxin can be good for us?" To which I'd offer the following: do we consider cigarettes hormetic? Lead? Mercury? Alcohol?

Why do we believe that *because sulforaphane comes from a plant, it must somehow be a magical molecule with unique chemical properties that couldn't possibly be bad for us,* when in actuality, it acts precisely the same way that these other oxidizing toxins do?

I believe we've got the notion of hormesis all wrong, and there are two main issues I have with relying on this idea as a justification for consuming broccoli and its coterie or any other plant compounds described as "xenohormetic"— hormetic molecules of foreign origin.

First problem with xenohormesis: If we accept that sulforaphane and related isothiocyanates are hormetics, then we must also accept that tobacco smoke and the rest of the "Bad News Gang" are hormetics. If you still want to believe that broccoli is really healthy for you, then you can make it even healthier by drenching it in oxidized canola oil while smoking a cigarette and inhaling diesel exhaust. That sounds absurd, doesn't it? But all of these compounds turn the NRF2 pathway on, just like sulforaphane. They are *all* part of the same gang, but I'll leave it up to you to decide whether they are all heroes or villains.

Second problem with xenohormesis: The concept of xenohormesis assumes that we need the compounds found within vegetables to achieve optimal antioxidant status *and* that eating crucifers somehow elevates our glutathione above baseline levels long-term, thus, making us super-human. Sadly, these assumptions are not the case. There have been multiple *interventional* studies comparing diets rich in fruits and vegetables, including crucifers, to diets with low or zero amounts of these plant foods—and the results have shown *zero* benefit to eating such foods.[37,38,39]

The length of these studies ranged from twenty-four to twenty-eight days and each had two groups of people. One group ate around one-and-a-half pounds (ten servings!) of fruits and vegetables daily, and the other group ate either a much lower amount or NO fruits and vegetables. Other than this variable, participants followed their normal diet, which generally consisted of meat, bread, and some dairy products. At the end of these studies, investigators ran both groups through a battery of tests to examine inflammation, oxidative stress, and DNA damage— and across the board, they found no differences between the two groups!

Overall, the results measured absolutely *zero* benefits from the massive amount of fruits and vegetables consumed. Though short term studies with sulforaphane show a temporary bump in glutathione production, this doesn't appear to last longer than a few days, and as shown in these studies, there is no appreciable hormetic benefit from plant compounds four weeks after consumption.

For the icing on this cake, there is even a ten-week study of this sort that showed *improvements* in markers of oxidative stress and inflammation in the group *without* fruits and vegetables, concluding that:

> *"The overall effect of the 10-week period **without dietary fruits and vegetables** was a **decrease** in the oxidative damage to DNA, blood, proteins, and plasma lipids, concomitantly with marked changes in anti-oxidative defense."*[40]

While we are bombarded with mainstream messaging in the health space that tells us fruits and vegetables are good for us and that we benefit from "antioxidants" and "phytochemicals," scientific literature repeatedly states otherwise. We don't need fruits and vegetables to achieve robust antioxidant defenses, and there isn't any evidence that consuming these plant foods makes us healthier. As we discussed earlier in this chapter, however, there is significant evidence that these plant compounds are harmful, damaging DNA, and interfering with hormonal signaling throughout the body. Still think kale is a super food?

LIVING A RADICAL LIFE IS GOOD ENOUGH

My critique of xenohormesis does not mean that I don't believe hormesis exists in humans, only that consuming plant-defense chemicals is not the best way to leverage this process. Of hormesis, it is often said that the dose makes the poison. I believe this is true with environmental hormetics but not molecular hormetics like isothiocyanates, polyphenols, smoking, etc. Because of the often ignored side effects of these molecules on the body as a whole, they are toxic from the get go, even in small doses. Environmental hormetics and molecular hormetics do not operate the same way and should not be confused.

There are multiple examples of environmental hormetics—heat, cold, sunlight, exercise—and if we experience these in the setting of a nutrient-rich diet, they are all we need to obtain robust levels of antioxidant defense. Too much exposure to any of these will certainly be damaging to our body, but small amounts act as stressors that temporarily cause oxidative stress with glutathione depletion, followed shortly thereafter by a rebound to levels higher than baseline.[41,42]

A study in Berlin of cold water winter swimmers illustrates this well. Researchers measured glutathione levels in swimmers before and after they spent an hour in frigid waters, and they observed a post-swim drop in glutathione but a rebound to above baseline levels by the next day.[43] Heat, cold, and sunlight are known to create a small increase in reactive oxygen species, triggering the NRF2 pathway and increasing our endogenous antioxidant defenses. We don't need plant molecules to obtain a robust supply of glutathione or other endogenous antioxidants. We can accomplish the same result by eating animal foods and living a "radical life": exercising, spending time in the sauna, being in the sun, and jumping in cold water.

I'll mention one more study just to really drive this point home. In this randomized controlled trial, participants who reported low fruit and vegetable intake (<3 servings daily) continued their normal diet or increased these foods to 480 grams per day and drank an additional 300ml of fruit juice daily for 12 weeks.[44] At the end of the study, despite increased blood levels of vitamin C, the researchers found the following:

> *"There were no significant changes in antioxidant capacity, DNA damage and markers of vascular health...[Thus] a 12-week intervention was not associated with effects on antioxidant status or lymphocyte DNA damage."*

That pitches some cold water onto the xenohormesis campfire, doesn't it?

Much of the confusion here arises because the concept of environmental hormesis is incorrectly extended to molecules as xenohormesis. These are two fundamentally different entities. Though both create small amounts of oxidative stress, plant molecules also have collaterally damaging effects in the body that environmental hormetics do not. In the case of isothiocyanates, these molecules compete with iodine at the level of the thyroid and damage DNA in a similar fashion as compounds in tobacco smoke, heavy metals, and other known toxins. *Why would we ingest Brassica plants or other vegetables with no clear benefit (as demonstrated in the aforementioned vegetable intervention trials)—and when they may be harming us—when we can achieve robust antioxidant levels without them?*

We will see a similar pattern as we continue to examine claims of health benefits from polyphenols in the next chapter. Researchers appear much too eager to myopically focus on one aspect of a plant molecule's potential benefit, seldom pausing to consider the totality of that molecule's effect on the human body. Because these molecules are not from our operating system, there always seems to be a catch. Investigators may be able to show an apparent beneficial effect on one cellular process, but when more in depth studies are done, collaterally damaging effects appear elsewhere. The programs just aren't that compatible.

At a basic level, these plant compounds are only molecules, and just like synthetic pharmaceuticals, they should be viewed as such. Clinicians and patients alike both know that every pharmaceutical has side effects. Why then do we so easily forget this about plant molecules? Every molecule that is foreign to our operating system is going to have side effects, but with plant compounds, this concept isn't often taken into consideration. We've been told that plant molecules are intrinsically benevolent, can't harm us, and exist to improve our health—and we've blindly accepted these notions. In reality, nothing could be further from the truth. As we discussed in the previous chapter, plants have their own agenda, and it's definitely not getting eaten. The molecules they make do not have unique benefits in humans. They don't make us super-human. They just end up decreasing our health slowly or swiftly, but inevitably, nonetheless.

TYPES OF STUDIES

As we continue on our adventure and begin to dig into increasingly technical scientific literature, I'd like to take a moment to explain a bit about the different types of studies we may encounter. The most valuable type of study that we'll examine will be those that are interventional, which are studies that have multiple groups of humans or animals exposed to specific interventions like dietary change or the introduction of specific compounds. These groups are then observed for a set amount of time and monitored for changes in parameters like inflammation or DNA damage.

Interventional studies usually have a control group, also known as the placebo group, and both researchers and subjects may be "blinded" to which group is receiving the placebo or the active compound. In human trials, subjects are also randomly assigned to either the control or interventional groups. This process is known as "randomization," and is responsible for the nomenclature used in human trials like "randomized, double blind, placebo-controlled." Clearly, human studies are more valuable than animal studies, but in circumstances where animal studies are all we have to go on, we do the best we can.

The other major category of scientific literature we'll discuss is colloquially known as epidemiology. Epidemiology studios are *completely* different from interventional studies. In this type of research, there are no control or placebo groups and there's no actual intervention. These are population based studies in which researchers administer questionnaires to participants regarding various lifestyle factors like diet and exercise and then look either prospectively (forward) or retrospectively (backward) in an attempt to *correlate* dietary or behavioral patterns with health outcomes.

The limitations of this type of study quickly become apparent. As the website SpuriousCorrelations.com hilariously points out, correlation does not equal causation. Take a look at the graphic below for an illustration of this point.

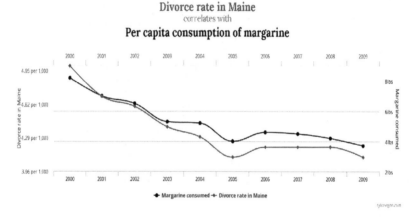

As you can see, the divorce rate in Maine from 2000–2009 was highly correlated (99.26%) with the per capita consumption of margarine. As rates of margarine consumption fell in those years, so too did the divorce rate in this northern state. Does this mean that eating margarine caused people in Maine to get divorced? Of course not, that would be an absurd assumption! Just because these two phenomena are highly correlated does *not* mean that we can draw causal conclusions.

See how misleading epidemiology can be? In later chapters of this book, we'll debunk the myths suggesting that meat is bad for humans and will refer back to this idea many times. As we'll soon see, just because those eating more meat appear to have worse health, it does not mean that it was the meat that caused the problem. *It's much more likely to have been the things most of the population eats with meat: refined grains, bread, sugars, and other junk foods.* Epidemiology simply can't distinguish between all of those possibilities—it can only show correlations, but cannot describe causal connections. That's what interventional studies are for, and when we look at this type of research with meat, *we find that it is clearly not bad for humans in ways that those misled by epidemiology might believe.*

AVOIDING THE BOOBY TRAPS

Throughout human history, when animals have been scarce or our hunts unsuccessful, we've needed to consume plants like those from the *Brassica* family in order to survive. It's quite interesting to note, however, that when indigenous cultures consume mostly plants, they employ special methods of preparation to detoxify them. Though cooking doesn't degrade glucosinolates, fermentation does. This is likely the origin of foods like Kim-chi and sauerkraut. When faced with the need to consume cruciferous vegetables, like cabbage, our ancestors discovered that they could detoxify many of the harmful compounds through fermentation.[45] Maybe they didn't know about toxic molecules in these foods, but surely they had a sense of feeling better overall when eating them fermented. As we'll see in future chapters, fermentation of foods like grains and beans also helps break down some (but not all) of the toxins, making them more suitable for consumption.

Fermentation also degrades most of the polyphenols present in plant foods.[46] Like sulforaphane and isothiocyanates, we've been told that these compounds are good for us, but as we'll see on our continued journey deeper into the wild lands of plant toxins in the next chapter, this narrative is also incorrect and these compounds can cause us significant harm. It should also be noted that cooking *Brassica* vegetables degrades myrosinase, but sulforaphane can still be formed by myrosinase from gut bacteria, so even with cooked broccoli, you'll be getting a dose of this isothiocyanate.

Our ancestors were a lot smarter than we often give them credit for, and they were clearly very resourceful in times of animal food scarcity. There's a huge amount of wisdom in the way that they sought out and consumed foods, and I believe that returning to ways of eating that mimic theirs will quickly bring us closer to optimal health. Let's move on to talk about polyphenols and how the mainstream story of these compounds is also very wrong!

CHAPTER FIVE

OF UNICORNS AND FAIRY TALES

Perhaps more than any other plant molecule, polyphenols have become associated with the term "superfoods." They are often dubbed "antioxidants," and we are told to consume as much of them as possible. It seems that every day, another company comes out with a supposedly magical supplement, juice, or powder with bold claims of decreased inflammation and longevity as it touts its robust polyphenol content. Let's talk about what polyphenols actually are and why we've been told they are good for us. Then we'll discuss why I'm going to take the radically contrary viewpoint that their purported benefits are nothing more than the stuff of imagination, just like unicorn fairy tales. To put the icing on the cake (or steak?), I'll then go further and show you how these molecules may actually be bad for us. If your head wasn't spinning after the last chapter, it surely will be after this one, so buckle up!

How about a quick chemistry lesson to start? I promise to make it as painless as possible! The field of chemistry is generally divided into two flavors: organic, which involves carbon-based molecules, and inorganic, which deals with all of the other elements. Most of the molecules we see in human biochemistry are of the organic sort. The term "polyphenol" refers to the molecular structure of a class of organic compounds. "Poly" means many, and "phenol" refers to the aromatic (multiple double-bonds between carbons) ring structure with an OH group attached. Examples of a few molecules we'll talk about in this chapter are noted below to help illustrate this. If you look closely, you'll be able to see the many aromatic phenol rings that comprise these compounds.

curcumin

genistein

resveratrol   catechin

In the plant kingdom, polyphenols serve unique roles as phytoalexins and as plant pigments. You'll recall from the last chapter that phytoalexins are weapons that plants marshal against attacking organisms like fungi, insects, or animals. Resveratrol, for instance, is produced as a defense molecule in the skin of grapes and other plants when they are attacked by pesky fungi. Intriguingly, but not surprisingly, humans and animals do not make molecules that are polyphenolic in structure within their biochemistry. Remember the concept of disparate operating systems? This is another illustration of the differences in the way that plants and humans work at a biochemical level. Polyphenols are like Porsche parts, which don't work in our human Tesla bodies, and the Tesla factory surely doesn't make Porsche parts.

As an aside, the whole premise that molecules that independently evolved in plants would somehow be beneficial in humans sounds a bit far-fetched to me. It would be highly unlikely for one molecule, let alone thousands of molecules, produced during plant evolution to truly be beneficial in humans after our evolutionary path diverged from theirs 1.5 billion years ago when we were little more than a single-celled blob. Imagine the odds against this!

If polyphenols are made by plants, for plants, why are we inundated with the notion of them as such magical compounds? The vast majority of the data suggesting benefits from polyphenols is derived from epidemiological research. But epidemiology doesn't actually involve any sort of intervention. The studies are no more than population diet surveys followed by observations of health outcomes. Although there are many epidemiology studies that show some degree of *correlation* between consumption of fruits and vegetables containing polyphenols and improved health outcomes,[1] many interventional studies don't reveal any iota of benefit.[2,3,4] We must not make the mistake of confusing correlation with causation. Epidemiology studies don't tell us anything about causation but instead leave us to hypothesize regarding possible causal connections. In a perfect world, epidemiology studies would be used to generate hypotheses about how diet and health outcomes might be related, which would then be tested with interventional studies.

Unfortunately, interventional studies in the world of nutrition are seldom done. They are quite expensive and work intensive, and who's going to profit from telling people to eat differently? Most of the interventional research that is done within medicine today is funded by the pharmaceutical companies who stand to profit handsomely if their molecule du jour generates compelling data. If an interventional study shows that meat is good for you, cattle farmers aren't exactly going to get rich. They might sell a few more ribeyes here and there, but their profits won't be anything like the billions garnered by pharma when it strikes molecular gold.

The good news is that there *have* been some interventional trials done with polyphenol-rich fruits and vegetables. I spoke about them in detail in the last chapter. As we saw, many of these trials have *failed* to show benefits—in terms of inflammation, DNA damage, or immunologic markers—from the inclusion of lots of fruits and vegetables in a diet, and in one case, this intervention was *harmful.*[5]

How can this be the case? How can many epidemiological studies show correlation between fruit and vegetable consumption and improved health outcomes, but the interventional trials clearly suggest the opposite? This scenario is actually quite common. When they are put to the test in interventional studies, hypotheses generated from epidemiological studies are wrong more often than they are right. In the case of fruits and vegetables and health outcomes, there's a big problem called "confounding" that invalidates much of this data. Confounders come in many forms, but in this case, the most likely confounders are healthy user bias and unhealthy user bias.

THE PROBLEM OF HEALTHY USER BIAS

Think about the narrative surrounding plant and animal foods in the Western World over the last seventy years during which these epidemiology studies have been conducted. During the 1930s and 1940s, meat, fat, and other animal foods were viewed as healthy dietary choices that would make you strong and vital. Then suddenly, around the 1950's, that narrative began to change dramatically. We were told that butter was bad for us, saturated fat from animals would give us heart attacks, and that we should be consuming more plant foods and vegetable oils. As a whole, this has been the overarching narrative since that time.

For decades, the American Heart Association and other organizations have been telling us to eat a low-fat diet and to favor carbohydrate-rich plant foods over animal foods. Meanwhile, rates of obesity, diabetes, and heart disease have soared. Oops! This story is described in great detail by Nina Teicholz in her amazing book, *The Big Fat Surprise*. Nina pulls back the curtain on the shoddy science, corporate gain, and political interest that were all in play during this time and were responsible for driving these anti-fat policies. Thankfully, much of this delusion is beginning to be washed away within the broader populace, but these ideas have pinned us down ideologically and physically for the last seven decades.

Over the last seventy years, what type of people were eating lots of vegetables? It was those who were listening to mainstream nutritional advice and trying to lead healthy lives! These people were also much more likely to have been practicing other types of healthy behaviors like meditation, stress-reduction, paying attention to sleep, exercising, and avoiding junk food. Because fruits and vegetables aren't cheap, they were also much more likely to be consumed by those of higher socioeconomic status with access to good medical care.

What if it were these healthy behaviors that resulted in better health outcomes *rather* than the fruits and vegetables suggested by these epidemiology studies? What if we could find a place in the world where the narrative for the last seventy years hasn't been that fruits and vegetables are salvation and that animal foods are damnation? What would we find if we did epidemiology studies on such a mythical population? Take heart, dear reader, because such a place *does* exist and epidemiology studies *have* been done looking at correlations between diet and health outcomes. The sad fact is that these studies are often ignored because they don't fit the story advanced by mainstream media in the Western world.

In Asia, the narrative around plant and animal foods over the last seven decades has been very different from the Western perspective. In Eastern cultures, meat and animal foods have been consistently valued as vital components of the diet and are ideologically associated with affluence and vigor. Not surprisingly, epidemiology studies done on Asian populations paint a very different picture from those done on Western populations. In one study, 112,310 men and 184,411 women from Bangladesh, China, Japan, and Korea were followed for an average of eleven years while researchers examined all causes of mortality, including cardiovascular disease (CVD) and cancer. The authors summed up the findings of this very large study as follows:

> *"Our pooled analysis did not provide evidence of a higher risk of mortality for total meat intake and provided evidence of an inverse association with red meat, poultry, and fish/seafood.* **Red meat intake was inversely associated with CVD mortality in men and with cancer mortality in women in Asian countries.**"[6]

In the Asian countries studied, intake of red meat was associated with *less* cardiovascular disease related death in men and a *lower* risk of cancer mortality in women. That throws a big fat monkey wrench into the notion that red meat is causing heart disease or cancer, and that only plants can save us from these ills, doesn't it?

Another study done on 3,731 men and women in Japan from 1984 to 2001 looked at rates of stroke and surveyed participants' diets over this time. It found that "a high consumption of animal fat and cholesterol was associated with a reduced risk of cerebral infarction death."[7]

Hmmmm....

Again we see that in an Asian population, consumption of animal foods was associated with better health outcomes, in this case with respect to stroke. Both of these studies are epidemiological, which always comes with limitations, but they and many other investigations paint a very different picture from those done in the West. This contrast calls into question the validity of the latter's findings and strongly suggests healthy user bias as a confounder.

The problem with healthy user bias is that despite the best efforts of super smart, number-crunching statisticians doing epidemiological research, these healthy behaviors cannot possibly all be accounted for, even in the most sophisticated statistical models.[8] Perhaps the best illustration of this phenomenon and how it can make interpreting epidemiological studies challenging is derived from a study of 21,000 citizens of the UK who were characterized as "health-conscious." Of this group, 8,000 were vegetarian, and the remaining 13,000 were eating both animal and plant foods. While British vegetarians in this study were found to have a low mortality rate relative to the general population, their death rates were similar to those of the non-vegetarians who were also participating in other healthy behaviors. This study found that:

> *"British vegetarians have a low mortality rate compared with the general population. Their death rates are similar to those of comparable non-vegetarians,* **suggesting that much of this benefit may be attributed to non-dietary lifestyle factors such as a low prevalence of smoking and a generally high socio-economic status, or to other aspects of the diet rather than the avoidance of meat and fish."***[9]*

Thus, the authors of this study came to the conclusion that it was probably the *healthy behaviors* in both groups of people that led to improved mortality rates, rather than the avoidance of meat and fish by the vegetarian group. If the investigators had only compared this vegetarian group to the general British population, it might have looked like it was their dietary choices that improved longevity, and this is exactly how healthy user bias can be misleading. It's quite common now for this type of study to be shared in the media without a clear explanation of the experimental methods used and without any explanation of potentially confounding factors or limitations in its research. This is not only a disservice to the general public but is also incredibly misleading, causing much unneeded confusion and widespread frustration when it comes to health advice.

THE JAMES DEAN TYPE

The other side of the proverbial coin is the unhealthy user bias. After our discussion of healthy user bias, I bet you can guess what this one means. It's the confounding fact that because meat has been associated with the potential for ill-health in Western culture for the last seventy years, those people who are eating more meat are the rebels. These are the James Dean type who don't care what they are told. They are going to eat meat even if they are told it's bad for them, and they are also probably going to smoke, ride motorcycles, not exercise, and eat a bunch of junk food with their meat. These are the folks doing very few of the healthy behaviors that we've previously seen as important contributors to health and longevity.

The premise of this book is that diet is the *most important* factor in determining whether we are healthy or sick, but independent of the food we eat, *other healthy behaviors* also play a significant role. Epidemiology studies done in the East and in the UK suggest that these behaviors are the beneficial factor for vegetarians rather than their diet. Furthermore, many epidemiology studies that suggest correlation between meat consumption and poor health probably reflect the absence of healthy behaviors and the presence of unhealthy behaviors rather than the negative effects of meat consumption. In other words, we must not blame the meat for what the soda, bread, junk food, smoking, and a sedentary lifestyle have done! This is the unhealthy user bias at play.

Now that we understand some of the nuances of epidemiology and its limitations with regard to the possible benefits of plant compounds like polyphenols, let's explore the research surrounding a few of the most widely touted molecules. We'll discuss resveratrol and the claim that it will help us live longer, as well as curcumin and the promise that this molecule will banish inflammation from our bodies. We'll also discuss a few other molecules, like the flavonoids found in soy, quercetin, tannins, and the polyphenols found in coffee, and illustrate why they aren't the fairy dust we've been told they are. There are too many polyphenolic plant molecules to discuss them all, but an examination of these will provide key themes that will prove illuminating.

TURMERIC HAS A DARK SIDE

You know those alien-looking roots in the grocery store that are bright orange inside? Yes, I'm referring to turmeric, a cousin of ginger containing the polyphenolic compound curcumin, which has been studied extensively for its biological activities. It is claimed to be valuable as an anti-inflammatory agent and in treating everything from Alzheimer's disease to erectile dysfunction—and basically everything else under the sun. But is there any validity to these claims? What does the research really show? In reviews of the therapeutic potential and the risks of curcumin, researchers have noted that most of the perceived benefits of this molecule are from test-tube studies that use doses much higher than what is found in the human body with normal turmeric ingestion.[10,11] These investigators also point to the large amount of evidence suggesting that curcumin also has harmful effects:

> *"A relatively high number of reports suggests that curcumin may cause toxicity under specific conditions…turmeric caused a dose and time-dependent induction of chromosome aberrations in several mammalian cell lines… Accumulating data have demonstrated since then that curcumin can induce DNA damage and chromosomal alterations both in vitro and in vivo at concentrations similar to those reported to exert beneficial effect. For instance, curcumin [was] shown to induce DNA damage to both the mitochondrial and nuclear genomes in cells. **These reports raise concern about curcumin safety, as the induction of DNA alterations is a common event in carcinogenesis.** "*[10,11]

As we've discussed previously, damaging DNA is a very bad thing. Curcumin appears to do this, as well as harming other cellular structures, by creating reactive oxygen species (free radicals) that result in oxidative stress. See a pattern here? In a horrid case of mistaken identity, the molecules that are marketed as being antioxidants are, yet again, actually pro-oxidants. With curcumin, part of the oxidative stress may occur because of its actions to irreversibly modify enzymes, like thioredoxin reductase, involved in our antioxidant defense system.[12] Curcumin has also been shown to induce DNA damage through inhibition of an enzyme called topoisomerase II, which helps unwind and repair DNA. Relevant to cancer, it's also been shown to **inactivate p53**, a very powerful tumor suppressor gene.[13,14]

Whoa! How could something so potentially dangerous be a part of the diets of some cultures for hundreds of years? Well, our body is actually pretty smart when it comes to plant compounds like curcumin, and under normal circumstances, it hardly absorbs them at all. Curcumin's bioavailability is vanishingly small, and what *is* absorbed is quickly detoxified in the liver and excreted. The amount of this molecule our body absorbs from eating turmeric is likely going to be pretty small, and our body gets rid of it quickly to avoid toxicity.

With all of the promises that curcumin would turn out to be a panacea, researchers and supplement manufacturers have gone to great lengths to try and circumvent our body's natural defense mechanisms. Most curcumin preparations now use piperine, a compound derived from black pepper, to highly increase absorption. Piperine works by inhibiting an enzyme called UDP glucuronosyltransferase, which is involved in the phase II detoxification of curcumin, thus increasing levels of this molecule.[15] With what we've now learned about curcumin, do we really want 2000 times more of it in our bodies to cause extensive oxidative stress, damage DNA, and turn off our tumor suppressor genes?

DETOXIFICATION PATHWAYS IN THE LIVER

Before we move on, let's discuss some of the detoxification systems for foreign molecules in our liver, which can be divided into two main groups of chemical reactions known as the phase I and phase II pathways. The phase I pathways are a large group of enzymes, known as the cytochrome p450 family, which generally convert lipid-soluble molecules into water-soluble forms through oxidation, reduction, hydrolysis, and cyclization (formation of ring structures). Once modified, foreign molecules and breakdown products from our body then undergo phase II detoxification in which they are conjugated with glucuronic acid, glutathione, sulfate, or glycine. Through this two-step process, our body transforms waste and toxins into forms that are ready to be excreted in the feces or urine—processes sometimes referred to as phase III detox.

As an aside, the astute reader may notice here that, contrary to popular belief, the liver does not store toxins but instead functions as the epicenter of toxin modification and excretion. Liver is an incredibly nutritious food that belongs in any diet and nothing like the "filter" it's so often made out to be. It is certainly not full of a lifetime of toxins, but you can thank this amazing organ for helping you get rid of them on a daily basis.

The liver is more accurately thought of as our "master detox control center" with dials and levers of the phase I and phase II detoxification pathways. A delicate balance is needed between all three phases of detoxification. If one isn't working well, we won't be able to excrete the harmful substances our body is trying to get rid of. Recall that the plant compound piperine inhibits the phase II detoxification process of glucuronidation. When you eat black pepper or take a curcumin supplement with piperine in it, the UDP glucuronosyltransferase enzyme is inhibited and can't detoxify curcumin by conjugating it to glucuronic acid. It also can't detoxify anything else that our liver wants to add a glucuronic acid molecule to. To add insult to injury, curcumin itself is also known to inhibit the CYP 450 enzymes that are part of phase I.[15] It's a double-whammy monkey wrench thrown into the delicate workings of our detoxification system.

But curcumin and piperine aren't the only plant molecules that mess with our liver's ability to detoxify. There are tens of thousands of plant and pharmaceutical compounds that do this. When these xenobiotic (foreign) molecules are suddenly given the key to the control room, they run amok, turning dials and pulling levers haphazardly, potentially causing some major metabolic chaos. No bueno!

TREATING THE ROOT CAUSE RATHER THAN SYMPTOMS

You've probably gathered by now that I don't think we should allow plant molecules like curcumin or piperine into the control room, but aren't there at least some studies which show benefits for curcumin? To be sure, there is some evidence of possible anti-inflammatory properties, but I have two big issues with the use of curcumin for this purpose. The first is that both plant compounds and *pharmaceuticals are just molecules*, and all foreign molecules have the potential for negative side effects in the human body. This concept is common knowledge when it comes to medications, but we seem to forget this when it comes to plant molecules. Even if curcumin does have some anti-inflammatory benefit, it also appears to have some nasty side effects. We wouldn't take ibuprofen (Motrin) or naproxen (Aleve) for inflammation under the delusion that these molecules have no side effects and we shouldn't make the same mistake with curcumin or other plant molecules. As you'll see throughout this section of the book, plant molecules can definitely harm us!

The second and even bigger issue I have is with how quickly we turn to curcumin or other "anti-inflammatory" plant compounds as the primary way to treat inflammation. Though inflammation isn't usually a good thing to have happening in our bodies, it's a valuable signal that things are out of balance. Rather than reflexively seeking to throw heaps of anti-inflammatory molecules at it, whether they be plant derived or synthetic, *we should first seek to understand where it's coming from*. Too often, I see clinicians of both mainstream and alternative sorts treating inflammation with anti-inflammatory molecules without first looking for its roots.

During a recent talk, I asked a room full of physicians and medical students for a definition of inflammation. Not one could come up with a good answer. In medical school, we're taught the word "inflammation" without ever being challenged to think deeply about what this actually means. It's pretty clear that inflammation is at the root of most chronic illnesses, but most of us don't really understand what this actually is.

At a biological level, inflammation is activation of the immune system, which is incredibly complex and made up of many types of cells. When activated, these various cells signal to each other that something is awry with molecules called cytokines that travel throughout the body and cross the blood/brain barrier. Simply put, inflammation occurs when our immune system is activated and pissed off. Rather than chilling on a beach with a Topo-Chico in hand watching the waves, our immune system is in a stinky gym, with heavy metal music blaring, hitting a punching bag as hard as it can.

Just like oxidative stress, inflammation isn't always bad. It's been an essential part of our human physiology for our entire existence. When you cut yourself, get sick, or break a bone, the immune system must be involved to repair these injuries and fight off invaders. That's what it's built for. But these aren't usually the things that kill us or decrease our quality of life any more. In recent history, humans have become increasingly afflicted by chronic diseases driven by inflammation. I strongly believe that most, if not all, chronic disease we suffer from today is inflammatory and autoimmune in nature. Autoimmunity occurs when the immune system begins to see our own body as foreign and attacks it as it would an invader. In both of these conditions, the immune system is the central player. In fact, I would suggest that in the setting of chronic disease, inflammation and autoimmunity are essentially describing the same process of inappropriate immune system activation.

Chronic diseases that plague Western civilization are inflammatory in nature, and in order to correct these, *we must understand what is triggering the immune system rather than using supplements and medications to mask its activation.* Using curcumin to "decrease inflammation" will only mask our body's natural response to an imbalance and is a misguided intervention until we know the original roots of the problem. Furthermore, reactive oxygen species serve invaluable signaling roles in the human body, and efforts to extinguish every last free radical invariably result in harm rather than good. The state of optimal health includes a balance between the processes of oxidation and reduction, not a complete abolition of these reactions in our body. Not surprisingly, many studies using antioxidant interventions reveal an increase in mortality outcomes.[16,17]

THE ROOTS OF INFLAMMATION

At this point, I bet you've already begun to ask the next logical question. You've followed my explanations of inflammation and autoimmunity and are willing to accept that these may indeed be at the root of chronic illness, *but what is at the root of inflammation and autoimmunity?* Kudos to you, dear reader. You've just discovered the **most important question** that this book seeks to answer. In fact, I believe this is the most important question that Western medicine should be seeking to answer as well, and what it was originally designed to do. Sadly, it appears that our medical system has been seduced by the promises of pharmaceuticals and technology, and it is too busy being distracted by the shiny new pill, supplement, or scanner to remember its original mission.

There are many things that can cause inflammation, but the food we put into our bodies is the greatest contributor of them all. Things like stress, inadequate sleep, and environmental toxins can contribute, but the impact of what we eat far outweighs these. Our physiology can be significantly impacted by quantities as low as a milligram (one-thousandth of a gram) or even a microgram (one-millionth of a gram) of a pharmaceutical molecule. How profoundly then could our physiology be affected by kilogram-quantities of food, which are over a million times more than these? This is why our search for the human user manual is so important.

Understanding what humans should be eating to thrive and avoid inflammation is *the goal* of my search, and the treasure we seek on our shared adventures within this book.

When food causes inflammation, the main pathway by which it does so is by *damaging the gut* with the subsequent activation of our immune system army that resides on the other side of the delicate intestinal epithelial cell layer. Antigens from food aren't supposed to get across the gut lining—but when they do, they look like invaders and cause the immune system to go into high alert. What results is the loss of gastrointestinal barrier function as well as subsequent immune activation, which colloquially is known as "leaky gut" and appears to be at the root of the majority of the chronic illnesses that we experience today.

So, which foods damage the gastrointestinal epithelium and cause "leaky gut" with its potential for downstream kindling of the immune system? Which foods are full of toxins, chemical weapons, and anti-nutrients designed to do exactly this? You guessed it: plant foods! Do animal foods have similar sorts of toxins and weapons in them? Nope. Animals don't need these because they can flee or fight. Sure, there are a few very rare exceptions like poisonous frogs and the puffer fish, but no one is eating those as a major portion of their diet. In the animal foods that compose our diets, there are no chemical toxins intrinsically present—end of story.

Surprised? I'll bet that even at this early point in the book, this conclusion might not come as a huge shocker. We'll talk much more about this as we continue on our journey, but for now, let's return to our scheduled program and examine a few other types of polyphenolic molecules as we continue to discover that they might not live up to all the hype.

AVOID THE FLAVONOIDS

Within the family of plant molecules with a polyphenolic structure, there's a group known as the flavonoids that garners the adulation of the masses. The flavonoid family is large and includes molecules like anthocyanins (found in the skin of berries as pigments), isoflavones (found in soy), catechins (compounds in tea), and flavan-3-ols (molecules present in cocoa). The mainstream narrative is that these compounds are "antioxidants" and are beneficial for health. As we've learned, however, these claims can be quite misleading. Invariably, plant molecules do not act directly as antioxidants in the human body, nor would this sort of disruption of our redox balance be advantageous. The story of flavonoids is similar to that of sulforaphane. When these molecules demonstrate improvements in oxidative stress parameters, they do so through the NRF2 system by first acting as pro-oxidants. They have also been shown to have other collaterally damaging effects throughout our body that are too often ignored. They should come with a package insert to warn us of these, but sadly, they don't.

One of the biggest problems with the flavonoids is their ability to act as endocrine disruptors.

Because their structure mimics that of estrogen, this entire family of molecules has been found to activate the 17B estradiol receptor.[18,19] In the pictures below, you can see the similarities between an estrogen molecule and the flavonoid molecules *quercetin* (from onions) and *genistein* (from soy) and understand how our body might get confused.

estradiol

genistein

quercetin

In a study of estrogen receptor-binding by flavonoid molecules, the authors state:

> *"Numerous reports have implicated flavonoid phytochemicals as possessing hormone-disrupting activity, in particular acting as environmental estrogens. The endocrine-disrupting effects of flavonoids are seen in examples of sheep grazing on flavonoid-rich clover, and cheetahs fed soy-rich diets have presented with **infertility, reproductive abnormalities, and tumors.**"[19]*

Yikes!

The isoflavones in soy are also well-known endocrine disruptors in both humans and animals.[20,21,22,23] In men, consumption of soy is associated with increased rates of infertility and poor sperm quality.[24] The authors of a review paper examining the potential risks of polyphenols note:

> *"**High intakes [of isoflavones] have been associated with reduced fertility in animals and with anti-luteinizing hormone effects among premenopausal women.** Furthermore, concerns have been expressed regarding sexual maturation of infants receiving very high levels of isoflavones in soy-based infant formula. This is of particular importance for baby boys, who normally exhibit luteinizing hormone secretion between birth and 6 mo of age."[25]*

For both males and females, disruption of hormonal signaling by plant compounds is clearly a very bad thing! In both sexes, proper balance between estrogen and testosterone is crucial for libido and the health of hormonally responsive tissues in the breasts, prostate, ovaries, and testicles. Even small doses of endocrine disrupting compounds from plants or the environment can cause things to go awry. As we'll see later in this chapter, resveratrol has also been found to have hormone-disrupting effects by activating the estrogen receptor. Do we really want to be ingesting plant compounds that can mess with our precious nether regions?

Soy is a really bad actor here, and isoflavones like genistein contained in it also affect hormonal processes negatively at the level of the thyroid:

> *"Furthermore, a reduction of thyroid peroxidase activity was observed in rats fed a diet supplemented with genistein. These effects of genistein on thyroid function are more pronounced in cases of iodine deficiency. **This is of particular concern for babies exposed to particularly high doses of isoflavones through soy feeding.**"[25]*

Thyroid peroxidase is one of the enzymes needed to make active thyroid hormones. Reducing or inhibiting its activity leads to a drop in these hormones and other negative effects throughout the body. Catechins in tea have also been connected with thyroid abnormalities as well as decreasing levels of thyroid peroxidase and other enzymes needed for thyroid hormone synthesis in animal models.[26] Inadequate levels of thyroid hormones cause fatigue, depression, weight gain, cold intolerance, brain fog, and many other symptoms that make it impossible to lead a radical life.

Soy and the flavonoid compounds within it also appear to worsen our inflammatory response to pathogens. In a recent study, 250 individuals were given a bacterial cell-wall component known to trigger the immune system. The resulting inflammatory markers, including IL-1, IL-6, and TNF-alpha were all higher in those eating the most soy-containing foods.[27] More research is needed here, but studies like this suggest that flavonoids and other compounds in soy are not playing nice with our immune system.

The flavonoid madness doesn't stop there, however. Quercetin, a molecule found in onions, berries, grapes, and peppers, is also known to trigger estrogenic signaling and act as an endocrine disrupter. It accomplishes this both by binding to the estrogen receptor and interfering with the breakdown of estrogen through inhibition of the enzyme catecholamine-O-methyltransferase, also known as COMT.[28] The authors of a review paper examining the estrogenic effects of quercetin with regard to possible promotion of cancer point out:

"Quercetin inhibits O-methylation of catecholestrogens and increases kidney concentrations of 2- and 4-hydroxyestradiol by 60-80%. This may result in enhanced redox cycling of catecholestrogens and estradiol-induced tumorigenesis."[29]

Guess what else are endocrine disruptors? Those shady characters from the last chapter, the "Born To Be Bad" isothiocyanate gang, also mess with our hormones. Extracts from raw cabbage, fermented cabbage, and Brussels sprouts stimulate estrogenic signaling in cell-culture breast cancer models.[30] When a compound stimulates estrogen signaling in cell-culture models, it's going to behave similarly in our bodies and will usually be damaging for both men and women. Hide your private parts from phytoestrogens of all shapes and sizes.

I'd also like to emphasize that the purported benefits of flavonoids are far from proven. The most studied flavonoid compounds are the flavanols from cocoa. These have shown benefits in some studies on arterial health but also failed to show benefit in this regard in many others.

> *"Although in one study cocoa flavanols (990/520 mg/d) reduced insulin resistance, blood pressure, and lipid peroxidation and improved performance on 2 of 3 cognitive tasks, **several studies failed to elicit any improvements in cognitive function.** For instance, there were no cognitive improvements reported after administration of chocolate products containing 750 mg/d flavanols for 6 wk in participants (43) and no improvement on a working memory task after 30-d administration of 250 or 500 mg cocoa flavanols to middle aged volunteers... Finally, a recently reported study also assessed the effects of both single doses and 30-d administration of 250/500 mg/d cocoa flavanols in healthy middle-aged participants and **failed to demonstrate any substantial cognitive effects.**"*[81]

If you're still on the fence about flavonoids due to mainstream claims of health benefits, remember that we previously discussed a striking study in which the removal of all flavonoids from the diet resulted in improvements in markers of oxidative stress and inflammation.[5]

So if curcumin can be damaging to our DNA, and flavonoids are messing with our hormones, are there any other ways that the supposedly magical unicorn polyphenols can harm us? You betcha! We are in some rough country right now, but let's continue our important examination of the dangers of this class of compounds.

MESSING WITH OUR DIGESTION

Tannins are another class of polyphenolic molecules that are widely distributed in plant foods. They are defense molecules produced to inhibit digestive enzymes of animals trying to eat them, making them harder to digest. I previously mentioned that many herbivorous ruminant animals, like moose and sheep, have developed proteins in their saliva that bind to tannins and inactivate them. Animals that have consistently evolved eating plants as their main source of food appear to have developed multiple mechanisms like this to help them deal with plant toxins, *but humans are lacking in this department.* Without such protection, these molecules inhibit our digestive enzymes when ingested and impair the digestive process.[32,33] The authors of a review on the topic of polyphenol and tannin studies state:

*"The ability of polyphenolic compounds to form insoluble complexes with other macro-molecules such as proteins has long been associated with the **observed reduction in nutritive value resulting from their inclusion in animal diets.** Naturally occurring polyphenols, and in particular condensed tannins isolated from various plant sources, have been shown to inhibit in vitro a number of digestive enzymes including trypsin, a-amylase and lipase. In addition, the results of various feeding trials suggest that **similar reductions in intestinal digestive enzyme activity may result from the feeding of high polyphenolic diets.**"*

Flavonoids can also act as digestive inhibitors, impairing the absorption of vitamin C and resulting in a significant decrease in net protein utilization.[34,35] If we want to absorb all of the nutrients from our food, *we have to be able to properly digest it*, and polyphenols inhibit this process.

As I'll talk about in Chapter Eight, not only are the nutrients in plant foods less bioavailable, but the presence of these digestive enzyme inhibitors, like tannins and other polyphenols, further contributes to the lower nutritive value of plant foods.

CELL DIVISION AND CHROMOSOMES

I've used some technical terms in this chapter that I want to be sure to explain. At the most basic level, our genetic code is written into our DNA with an alphabet of nucleic acid bases. Your "book of life" is written in A, T, C, G bases: adenine, thymine, cytosine, and guanine. Since DNA is a double-stranded molecule, bases on one strand pair with their complimentary partner on the other strand through hydrogen bonds. Generally speaking, A pairs with T, and C with G to create what might be imagined as a ladder, in which the rungs are the bonded base pairs. DNA molecules are huge, and in order to pack them neatly into cells, they are wound around proteins called histones, which are then neatly packed into chromosomes.

In order for DNA to be turned on and transcribed, portions of our chromosomes must be "unwound" to expose the DNA. Our DNA sequence constitutes our genetics, and the way genes are turned on and off through unwinding of chromosomes is known as **epigenetics**, a process controlled by the addition or subtraction of methyl groups and other molecules to histone proteins. We can't change our genes, but we absolutely *can* change the way they are turned on and off. How? Through diet and lifestyle! These are the most powerful tools we have to create health in our lives.

In this chapter, when I've discussed damage to our DNA, I'm referring to breaking the DNA strands that make up our chromosomes. Cellular structures known as **micronuclei** arise from chromosome fragments as a result of chromosomal breaks. When cells go to divide, these damaged fragments fail to be incorporated into daughter cell nuclei, and form micronuclei. All agents that cause double-stranded chromosomal breaks induce micronuclei, and as we'll see, there are lots of plant molecules in this group!

SALICYLATES—EVEN ASPARAGUS AND COCONUT CAN HARM US

Though salicylates are not technically polyphenols, these molecules do contain one aromatic ring and are used as plants as defense hormones in response to attack.[36] They don't get as much spotlight as many of the other plant toxins, but they are common and can definitely trigger reactions in many people, especially those who have polymorphisms in the phase II detoxification enzyme used to break them down, known as phenol sulfur transferase (PST).[37] These molecules do not occur in animal foods, and blood levels are known to be higher in vegetarians.[38] Common symptoms related to salicylate sensitivity are headaches, asthma, rashes and ringing in the ears, and elimination of these toxins from the diet has been shown to benefit those with asthma and other allergic conditions who are sensitive.[39]

Foods high in salicylates include asparagus, almonds, avocados, cherries, nectarines, dates, blackberries, coconuts and coconut oil, honey, tomatoes, potatoes and eggplants, though this is not an exhaustive list. We shouldn't forget about this class of compounds if symptoms persist on a carnivore-ish diet (discussed in detail in Chapter Twelve) when foods containing them remain in our diet.

THE PROMISE OF SUPERMODEL VAMPIRE STATUS

After curcumin, resveratrol is probably the most talked about plant compound these days. We must remember, however, that this molecule, and most polyphenols, are plant defense chemicals produced in response to attack. Just like the isothiocyanates and cyanogenic glycosides discussed in the previous chapter, this should be our first clue that these compounds are probably not going to be good for us. The media would have us believe otherwise, however, touting resveratrol as a "fountain of youth" that will promote vitality and longevity. By taking resveratrol, they claim, you can become a *supermodel vampire*—forever young and vital. Sadly, these claims were made prematurely and based entirely on animal studies. To be fair, the results in worms, fruit flies, and mice were impressive. They showed improvements in models of diabetes and increased longevity. The mechanism of resveratrol, which appears to turn on a family of genes called sirtuins involved in longevity, is intriguing. Be that as it may, in human trials, resveratrol has been a massive failure and also shown many potentially damaging side effects.

When studied in a randomized, placebo-controlled fashion in patients with metabolic syndrome, resveratrol failed to show any benefit and actually worsened markers of glycemic control.[40] In a trial of non-alcoholic fatty liver disease (NAFLD), the results with resveratrol were similarly disappointing, showing no clinical or histopathological (microscopic) benefits.[41] Another four-month interventional study in middle-aged men with metabolic syndrome again showed no benefit and revealed a decrease in the testosterone precursors androstenedione, DHEA, and DHEA-S.[42] Doesn't sound so magical to me.

Like all of the plant molecules touted as "antioxidants," resveratrol has also demonstrated pro-oxidant activity, with its capacity to oxidize membrane lipids, and to damage DNA.[43,44] Remember our friend NRF2 from the previous conversation in Chapter Four about induction of this transcription factor by isothiocyanates as pro-oxidants? Resveratrol also activates this pathway. My point here is not to say that activation of NRF2 is always a bad thing, but to highlight the following fact: isothiocyanates, smoking, alcohol, exercise, heat/cold, and polyphenolic molecules are pro-oxidants rather than antioxidants. As we touched on previously, molecular pro-oxidants, at even small doses, possess damaging side effects like endocrine disruption, and inhibition of detoxification systems, whereas the environmental inputs do not. *This is the key difference between hormetic plant compounds and environmental hormetics.*

So what do we have here with regard to resveratrol? A highly praised molecule that has repeatedly failed to show benefit in human studies, has repeatedly demonstrated negative effects in terms of glucose control and male sex hormone production, and that acts as a pro-oxidant with potential to cause DNA damage. Does that sound like something you want to put in your body?

Another interesting wrinkle to the resveratrol story is that we don't need this molecule to activate the sirtuins, which potentially improve longevity. Guess what else activates these genes? Ketosis! Ketones, like beta-hydroxy butyrate, turn on the sirtuins and many other genes associated with longevity. Remember at the end of the previous chapter when I said that we don't need plant molecules to activate the cellular mechanisms that help us achieve optimal health? In that chapter, I gave the example of glutathione formation and optimal antioxidant status, and now

I'm describing the epigenetic control of longevity genes—and both of these can be achieved without plant molecules *just by living a radical life*.

We don't need the empty promises of plant molecules to be optimal. Jumping in cold water, exercising, and fasting or eating a ketogenic diet like the carnivore diet allow us to achieve optimal health *and* avoid the negative side effects that come with plant molecules not compatible with our human "operating system."

We've been told that plant molecules can help us live better lives because of the magical "phytonutrients" they contain. Not only is this statement factually incorrect, it's short-sighted and ignores the fact that these compounds also cause us harm when we consider their *overall effects systemically in our body*. We can have these better lives by eliminating plants, consuming nutrient-rich animal foods, and "living radically." So many of the claimed benefits of plant molecules are available to us alternatively by fasting, ketogenic diets, and playing in the natural world—just like our ancestors did!

I'm certainly not suggesting here that plant molecules don't have therapeutic value or that we shouldn't study them as possible agents for cancer or other diseases, but there's a difference in using plants and plant compounds as food versus medicine. The former application suggests that we somehow need these molecules to function optimally, a premise I disagree with strongly.

There is a subtle message advanced by supplement manufacturers selling these molecules that claims they can make us super-human but that clearly ignores the well-documented potential downsides to ingesting these molecules on a routine basis. Why would we take foreign molecules with known toxicities in order to achieve unproven benefits when we know that we can attain optimal health just by eating and living well? **Avoiding inflammation, turning on longevity genes, and achieving healthy hormonal balance are all things that are easily discovered with a nose-to-tail carnivore diet—and all of which can be attained without harmful plant compounds.**

In the case of illness, I remain open to the possibility that both naturally and synthetically derived pharmaceuticals could offer efficacious therapies, but as I noted earlier, we must remain vigilant in our search for the root cause of diseases and not be too quick to ameliorate or mask symptoms with molecular interventions.

In the next chapter, we'll continue to explore the sordid world of plant molecules and how they negatively affect our health as we journey into the dangerous land of oxalates. It's a scary place, so please keep your arms and legs inside the vehicle, and do not feed the wildlife. They bite!

CHAPTER SIX

ATTACK OF THE OXALATES

In the previous two chapters, we talked about plant defense chemicals that can have damaging effects in our bodies because they're not compatible with our human operating system. In this chapter, we're going to talk about a molecule that is produced in small quantities as a waste product of human metabolism but occurs in very large amounts in some plants, and can cause serious pain, kidney stones, and other issues when it accumulates in our body.

I speak of oxalates, the colloquial term for a combination of oxalic acid and a mineral such as calcium or magnesium. In general chemistry terms, when a molecule or an atom with a positive charge connects to another molecule or atom with a negative charge through an ionic bond, a "salt" is formed. Technically, calcium plus oxalic acid is a calcium oxalate salt, but for the purposes of this discussion, I'll use the term oxalate to refer to both oxalic acid and its salts.

So what is oxalic acid? Hearkening back to our previous discussions of chemistry, oxalic acid is a two-carbon molecule with two carboxylic acid groups, which are made of carbon double-bonded to an oxygen and an OH group (the graphic below will help you visualize this). You may remember the OH group from the phenol molecule. You didn't know you were going to learn some organic chemistry in this book, did you? Go ahead, spin that propeller on your nerd hat, you've earned it.

oxalic acid

In humans, oxalic acid is produced as a waste product and excreted in the urine. It occurs as the result of the breakdown of the amino acids glycine and hydroxyproline and of a molecule called glyoxalate in a process termed the glyoxalate pathway. In a small number of individuals with a rare genetic disorder known as primary hyperoxaluria, or PH, mutations in this pathway lead to much larger endogenous formation and excretion of oxalates (100mg to 600mg per day). People with primary hyperoxaluria suffer from the formation of frequent and severe calcium oxalate kidney stones, often leading to permanent kidney damage or renal failure as well as oxalate deposition in bones, joints, bone marrow, and other tissues outside of the kidneys. This is a condition known as systemic oxalosis.[1]

Plants make and use oxalic acid in very different ways than humans, yet another illustration of the concept of different operating systems. In plant biochemistry, oxalic acid is actively formed during the process of photosynthesis and has many roles, for example, chelating ("biting") minerals such as calcium, magnesium, and zinc to regulate their concentrations within cells. Plants also use oxalic acid as a defense weapon against predators.[2,3] Oxalic acid crystalizes into multiple shapes in both plants and humans. One of these is the **raphide** form depicted in the graphic below that shows the foods with the highest concentrations of oxalates. Raphides are basically microscopic needles, not exactly the type of thing insects, animals, or humans want to be biting into.

HIGH OXALATE PLANT FOODS

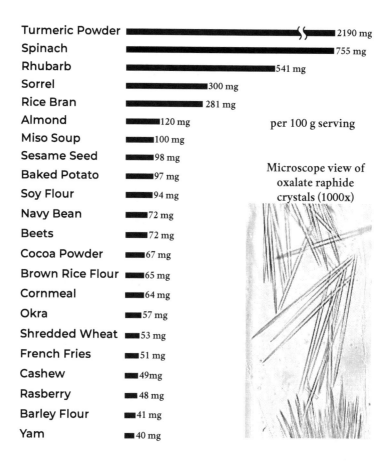

Turmeric Powder	2190 mg
Spinach	755 mg
Rhubarb	541 mg
Sorrel	300 mg
Rice Bran	281 mg
Almond	120 mg
Miso Soup	100 mg
Sesame Seed	98 mg
Baked Potato	97 mg
Soy Flour	94 mg
Navy Bean	72 mg
Beets	72 mg
Cocoa Powder	67 mg
Brown Rice Flour	65 mg
Cornmeal	64 mg
Okra	57 mg
Shredded Wheat	53 mg
French Fries	51 mg
Cashew	49mg
Rasberry	48 mg
Barley Flour	41 mg
Yam	40 mg

per 100 g serving

Microscope view of
oxalate raphide
crystals (1000x)

As you can see in the graphic above, some plants widely considered to be healthy contain huge amounts of oxalates relative to what we might naturally find in our bodies. Normally, humans produce 10–30 mg of oxalates per day through the glyoxalate pathway and amino acid breakdown. By simply downing one "healthy" green smoothie in the morning, we could be exposing ourselves to more than *two hundred times this amount!* Can we please stop the green smoothie madness? These things should really be called green sludge oxalate bombs.

OXALATE TOXICITY

What do most people put into their green smoothies? A concoction of spinach, almond milk, and blackberries, with a scoop of turmeric thrown in for good measure, could easily create a drink with over one thousand milligrams of highly absorbable oxalates. Is that a lot? You bet it is! There have been documented cases of *deaths* related to consumption of as little as five thousand milligrams of oxalates,[4,5,6,7] a dose that is attainable in one day from something like a "green smoothie cleanse."

"No," you say, "you're crazy! A green smoothie cleanse couldn't hurt someone!" Oh yes it could, and there are case reports documenting exactly this occurrence with such a misguided endeavor, resulting in permanent kidney damage:

> *"We report a case of acute oxalate nephropathy in a 65-year-old woman, temporally associated with the consumption of an oxalate-rich green smoothie juice "cleanse" prepared from juicing oxalate-rich green leafy vegetables and fruits...**Consumption of such juice cleanses increases oxalate absorption, causing hyperoxaluria and acute oxalate nephropathy in patients with predisposing risk factors.** Given the increasing popularity of juice cleanses, it is important that both **patients and physicians have greater awareness of the potential for acute oxalate nephropathy in susceptible individuals** with risk factors such as chronic kidney disease, gastric bypass, and antibiotic use."* [8]

The patient discussed in this case had the predisposing risk factors of gastric bypass surgery and recent antibiotic use, but prior to this "cleanse," her kidney function was normal. She consumed an average of 1300mg of oxalates daily, leading to acute renal failure and eventually leaving her with permanent kidney damage requiring ongoing dialysis.

In extreme cases, kidney damage due to oxalates has also been reported due to excess consumption of *peanuts*.[9] Oxalate toxicity is well known in the medical literature, and the nephrologists who authored the green smoothie case report go on to state:

> *"Diet-induced hyperoxaluria has been reported with star fruit, nuts (peanuts and almonds), rhubarb, iced tea, chaga mushroom, juicing from fruits and vegetables, and vitamin C."*

Furthermore, in children with genitourinary problems ranging from bloody urine to kidney stones, removal of almond milk has been shown to resolve these issues.[10] I'll talk more about dairy in Chapter Twelve, but alternative "nut milks" do not belong in any sort of healthy diet for children or adults.

Oxalate toxicity isn't a new thing, however. Reports of serious complications and even death related to excess consumption of oxalates have appeared in medical literature for over 100 years. In 1919, physician H.F Robb reported a case of death related to consumption of rhubarb leaves and roots.[4] Going back even further, oxalic acid has been known to be an extremely toxic agent since the early 1800s when experiments with it were done on dogs, who sadly suffered painful deaths as well.[11]

One of the foods I get asked about frequently as a possible inclusion in the carnivore diet is mushrooms. Technically, mushrooms are a different family from plants, but they do appear to have frequently evolved defense mechanisms that might give us pause in consuming them. I talk more about mushrooms in the frequently asked questions section, but here it's relevant to point out a case study showing renal failure requiring dialysis with frequent consumption of chaga mushroom powder:

> *"A 72-year-old Japanese female had been diagnosed with liver cancer one year prior to presenting at our department… Chaga mushroom powder (four–five teaspoons per day) had been ingested for the past six months for liver cancer. Renal function decreased and hemodialysis was initiated. Renal biopsy specimens showed diffuse tubular atrophy and interstitial fibrosis.* **Oxalate crystals were detected in the tubular lumina and urinary sediment and oxalate nephropathy was diagnosed.** *Chaga mushrooms contain extremely high oxalate concentrations."*[12]

Very specific methods are required to accurately measure the oxalate content of foods. In the case of chaga and other mushrooms, reliable numbers do not exist. Consequently, I have left them off the chart of foods with the highest amounts of oxalates depicted a few pages back. Case studies such as this remind us that medicinal mushrooms can be harmful in high doses as well. On a personal note, I'll point out that prior to discovering the carnivore diet and changing my own pattern of eating, consumption of mushroom powders including chaga, reishi, and lion's mane appeared to cause severe eczema flares.

Star fruit is another food that packs a whopping oxalate punch. It's not that common in the U.S., but in countries where it grows, there have been numerous reports of death and serious medical complications related to its consumption, especially among patients with impaired kidney function at baseline:

> *"Star fruit has been reported as containing neurotoxins that often cause severe neurological complications in patients with chronic renal disease. We report two patients with chronic renal failure at a pre-dialyzed stage who developed refractory status epilepticus after ingestion of star fruit. In addition, we review fifty-one cases in the literature. Among fifty-three patients, sixteen patients presented with epileptic seizures (30%). The mortality rate was as high as 75% in patients with seizures."*[13]

The neurotoxins mentioned in this article are most likely oxalates, which may also be able to affect our brain in negative ways.

NEEDLES EVERYWHERE!

So far, we've looked at some extreme examples of the toxicity of oxalates, and I bet you are asking if oxalates at lower doses are really a big deal or if our bodies can handle them. Remember that oxalates don't have any role in the human body, so any amount we take in via diet must be excreted in addition to what we produce. With this in mind, let's continue our oxalate safari and look at the harm lower doses of this carboxylic acid-containing critter might be causing.

Earlier, I mentioned primary hyperoxaluria and the fact that people with this genetic mutation make and secrete large amounts of oxalate in their urine, invariably leading to severe kidney stones and renal damage. In this condition, deposition of oxalate crystals outside of the kidneys is also observed, suggesting that when large amounts of oxalates are present in the body, they can become lodged in our tissues. Strikingly, systemic deposition of oxalates has been observed even in those without primary hyperoxaluria in cases of excess oxalate absorption or intake.

In healthy individuals, microscopic and macroscopic (large) oxalate crystals have been observed pathologically in the thymus, kidney, blood vessels, testicles, brain, eyes, thyroid, and breasts.[14] Oxalates do not serve a purpose in these tissues but appear to be deposited in them over our lifetime, which is likely connected with increased levels in the blood from consumption of high oxalate-containing foods. When examined at autopsy, a survey of 103 thyroid glands showed that *79 percent contained oxalate crystals.* A toxic compound is found in the vast majority of thyroid glands? People must be eating tons of this stuff throughout their lives. Oh wait, that's exactly what's happening! After all, we are told that many high oxalate foods are healthy, and we are encouraged to consume as many of them as possible. Maybe it's time to reconsider the mainstream health advice that spinach, almonds, beets, and chocolate are good for us?

This autopsy study and others have shown that oxalate levels in people with thyroid diseases, such as Hashimoto's thyroiditis or Grave's disease, were lower than those with normal thyroids. One compelling hypothesis for this trend is that these autoimmune illnesses may have been triggered in response to oxalate deposition in an effort to remove these crystals. There are probably many things that trigger autoimmune injury to the thyroid leading to hypothyroid and hyperthyroid conditions, but oxalates certainly might be a factor for some people. Not surprisingly, patients with primary hyperoxaluria also often develop hypothyroidism during the course of their illness, as described in numerous case studies:

> *"We describe four patients, aged three months to twenty-three years, with end-stage renal disease and severe, symptomatic hypothyroidism. All four had primary hyperoxaluria with diffuse tissue (kidneys, skeleton, eyes, heart) calcium-oxalate deposition, a condition known as oxalosis...* **Clinical hypothyroidism within the framework of primary hyperoxaluria oxalosis was probably caused by thyroid tissue damage from an abundance of calcium oxalate."**[15]

Is it possible that oxalates are depositing in many tissues in our bodies and causing damage or physical symptoms like pain? Though it's not recognized by the formal medical establishment as being connected with oxalates, many women with vulvovaginal pain syndrome, or vulvodynia, find significant relief when oxalates are removed from their diet. Women who suffer with this condition have pain with sex, urination, and prolonged sitting, resulting in significantly decreased overall quality of life. Data gathered by the Vulvar Pain Foundation suggests that a low oxalate diet is the most effective intervention for women who suffer from these issues.

Oxalates may also be involved in neurological diseases, including autism, though the pathogenesis of this condition is far from fully understood. A 2011 study found that children with autism displayed three-times greater levels of oxalate in their blood and two-and-a-half-times greater levels in their urine.[16] These researchers concluded:

> **"Hyperoxalemia and hyperoxaluria may be involved in the pathogenesis of Autism spectrum disorder in children.** *Whether this is a result of impaired renal excretion or an extensive intestinal absorption, or both, or whether oxalates may cross the blood brain barrier and disturb central nervous system function in the autistic children remains unclear."*

More research is clearly needed to elucidate the role of oxalate in autistic children, but it appears that there's something important going on here and that avoidance of oxalate-containing foods might be a reasonable strategy for the management of this disorder.

Deposition of oxalate crystals in breast tissue has also been documented in multiple studies and is associated with precancerous lesions known as lobular carcinoma in-situ, or LCIS.[17] Unhealthy breast tissue has consistently been found to contain higher levels of oxalate than healthy regions, and oxalates induce cancerous proliferation of breast cells in culture, turning on the cancer promoting gene *c-fos*. When injected into the mammary fat pads of mice, oxalates induced the formation of tumors:

> *"We found that the chronic exposure of breast epithelial cells to oxalate promotes the transformation of breast cells from normal to tumor cells, inducing the expression of a proto-oncogen as c-fos and proliferation in breast cancer cells. Furthermore, oxalate has a carcinogenic effect when injected into the mammary fatpad in mice, generating highly malignant and undifferentiated tumors with the characteristics of fibrosarcomas of the breast. As oxalates seem to promote these differences, it is expected that* **a significant reduction in the incidence of breast cancer tumors could be reached if it were possible to control oxalate production or its carcinogenic activity.** *"[18]*

What's the best way to control the amounts of oxalates in our bodies? Since we make only a very small amount per day, *the vast majority of our oxalate burden comes from the foods we eat.* There's no need for a multimillion dollar trial to tell us that the best way to decrease our levels of oxalates is to not consume them in our diets!

OXALATE KIDNEY STONES

Oxalates clearly get deposited into many tissues in our bodies in a pathological way, but the major burden of suffering related to them comes from calcium oxalate kidney stones. The mechanisms surrounding formation of these in the kidney aren't totally understood, but more oxalate in urine appears to be a major risk-factor. Oxalate also appears to cause damage to the tubules of the kidneys by creating free radicals that activate cascades of inflammatory genes, like the NLRP3 inflammasome, within the kidney and other tissues.[19,20]

If you or someone you know has had a kidney stone, you'll understand the enormous amount of suffering these little buggers cause.

Imagine trying to pee out a piece of glass the size of a gravel pebble. Ouch! And guess what? Over 75 percent of kidney stones are made from calcium oxalate. This means that around three-fourths of all kidney stones could possibly be prevented by avoiding oxalate-containing foods.

I mentioned my Dad in the introduction of this book. He's an amazing guy and one of my greatest heroes. Sadly, he's also struggled with kidney stones throughout his life and recently had a stent placed in his ureter, which is the tube that connects the kidney to the bladder. When I asked him if he had changed anything in his diet, he admitted that just before the stone formed, he'd begun eating large amounts of spinach again, forgetting how high this nasty leaf is in oxalates. I've since cautioned him against consuming too much of the foods highest in oxalates, since he appears to have a propensity for forming oxalate kidney stones.

When we eat food that is high in oxalates, how much can it raise the levels in our body? Urinary levels are the best proxy we have for levels of oxalate in the blood, and there have been some revealing studies examining how much oxalate is excreted after we consume certain high-oxalate foods. Recall that urinary excretion of oxalate in healthy individuals from endogenous production alone is around 30 milligrams per day. In other words, if we are fasting or not eating any foods with significant amounts of oxalates, we will produce and excrete about this amount on a daily basis in the urine.

On the other hand, someone with primary hyperoxaluria may excrete between 100–500 milligrams of oxalate in their urine per day—quite a bit more than a healthy individual. As observed in PH patients, we know that these levels of oxalate in the urine and corresponding levels in the blood significantly increase the risk of stone formation in the kidneys and oxalate deposition in tissues. High-oxalate foods cause an increase in urinary oxalate excretion observed two to four hours after they are eaten, and in studies with chocolate and turmeric, postprandial levels of urinary oxalate jumped substantially to levels that mirrored those found in PH patients:

> *"In six male subjects…the ingestion of chocolate caused a striking but transient increase in urinary oxalic acid excretion due to its absorption in the upper gastrointestinal tract. The peak excretion rates occurred 2–4 h after the intake of the chocolate. The peak values were 235% of the fasting excretion rate in the trial with 50 g chocolate and **289% in the trial with 100 g chocolate and reached the amounts found in cases with primary hyperoxaluria.** The transient hyperoxaluria observed*

*seems to be an important factor for the formation of calcium oxalate cal-
culi in patients at risk for stone disorders.'[21]*

Fifty to one hundred grams of chocolate is a moderate amount, but
it's completely doable. As this study illustrates, by consuming an ordinary amount of only one food that is high in oxalate, we can create levels
of oxalate in our bodies that are comparable to someone with primary
hyperoxaluria.

Other studies have shown that increasing the amount of oxalate in
the diet from 10 milligrams to 250 milligrams per day caused a doubling
in the urinary oxalate excretion.[22] There's going to be some variation
from person to person in terms of the degree of absorption and excretion of oxalates. Some people seem to be more prone to forming oxalate
kidney stones than others, but generally speaking, it's pretty easy to bump
the amount of oxalate in your body to potentially damaging levels by eating normal quantities of common foods.

Remember our old frenemy, turmeric? It is very high in oxalates and
has also been shown to significantly raise urinary excretion to potentially
harmful levels:

*"The consumption of supplemental doses of turmeric… can significantly
increase urinary oxalate levels, thereby increasing risk of kidney stone
formation in susceptible individuals.'[23]*

As you can see from the oxalates chart, turmeric, spinach, and almonds are major contributors of this molecule, but potatoes, beans,
beets, and chocolate also contain significant amounts. Those with a history of kidney stones are widely advised to avoid these food items. Many
studies have also shown that green tea and black tea contain significant
amounts of oxalates, and tea is further problematic due to its high-tannin
content, which acts as a digestive enzyme inhibitor and could potentially
cause damage to the lining of our gut.[24] Danger lies around every corner
in the plant kingdom!

OXALATE DETOXIFICATION

Well, that was a wild little safari through the land of oxalates. They do
indeed have sharp teeth, don't they! Let's recap all that we've learned in
this chapter.

Oxalates are produced in very small amounts as a part of normal
human metabolism and the breakdown of amino acids like hydroxyproline. They aren't used in our biochemistry and are excreted after they

are produced. Plants, on the other hand, make lots of oxalates. They are used by plants for various cellular processes, as well as in a defensive function to discourage predation. Oxalates can cause issues for animals and humans eating them and are known to be involved in the formation of calcium oxalate kidney stones. We have also seen that oxalates can be deposited in tissues such as the breast and thyroid, causing severe damage, and excessive amounts can potentially contribute to the development of inflammation or even cancers. Remind me again why you would ever want to eat spinach or make a green smoothie?

Despite all of this evidence, we still really don't know as much as we need to about oxalates and how to detoxify them. The best strategy is to completely avoid them or to educate ourselves and avoid the foods that contain the highest amounts. Once we stop ingesting oxalates, our bodies appear to be able to start removing them from tissues, though this an area that requires much more research. At times when individuals stop eating oxalates, they may experience a "dumping" phenomenon with various symptoms. It's been suggested that citrate minerals like calcium citrate in supplemental form may aid with the process of "oxalate dumping." Since oxalates don't have any role in our bodies, the sudden onset of unusual symptoms after stopping consumption of them could be a dumping process occurring, and in such a case, a visit to your primary physician may be advisable.

There is research suggesting that a species of bacteria called *oxalobacter formigenes* might help break down oxalate in our gut.[25] The problem is that not everyone is colonized with this bacteria, and the over-abundance of antibiotic exposure that we've all suffered throughout our lives might have eliminated this guy from our microbiome. Perhaps in the future we'll discover a way to successfully reintroduce *oxalobacter* back into the populations of our gut flora, but for now, I wouldn't bet on this microbe to protect us from oxalates.

It's pretty darn clear that oxalates don't do good things in our body and that consuming them is only going to be damaging. But also remember that oxalates are just one form of plant toxins among many. So far, we've talked about multiple plant toxins including isothiocyanates, polyphenols, salicylates, and now oxalates, but that's not the end of the plant mayhem story. In the next chapter, we'll talk about carbohydrate-binding proteins, known as **lectins**, which may also cause inflammation and trigger the immune system in negative ways. Plants are crafty little fellows who have truly evolved multiple systems of defense to discourage us from eating them. Onward!

CHAPTER SEVEN

OF KIDNEY BEANS AND PARKINSON'S DISEASE

On a chilly fall day in November of 2003, a letter addressed to the White House arrived at the off-site processing facility. On the outside, this letter looked like thousands of others sent to the president, though the handwriting was a bit messy. Upon opening it, however, workers at the mail facility quickly discovered the letter was anything but ordinary. It contained a vial full of white powder, and a typewritten note that read:

> Department of Transportation,
> If you change the hours of service on
> January 4, 2004, I will turn D.C. into a ghost town.
> The powder on the letter is RICIN.
> Have a nice day,
>
> > Fallen Angel

Subsequent tests confirmed the contents of the vial were, in fact, the potent lectin toxin known as ricin. Other letters with similar white powders followed in what came to be known as the 2003 Ricin Letters. Because I know you must be curious about the rest of the story, the "Fallen Angel" turned out to be the owner of a cross-country trucking company who feared that his profits would dwindle if the Department of Transportation changed the law to limit the number of hours drivers were allowed to work each day. Though the sender of these letters was never captured, he never succeeded in turning Washington, D.C. into a ghost town, nor was anyone harmed by his attempts at intimidation.

Ricin is a poison derived from castor beans and is the most deadly lectin known. A dose the size of a few grains of salt can kill an adult human. During WWI, the U.S. military considered coating bullets with ricin, and it has been used for many covert assassinations within the last seventy years. A famous example of this was the death of Bulgarian dissident Georgi Markov in 1978 after he was struck by a ricin pellet fired from a modified umbrella air gun by the Bulgarian secret police. Perhaps the most colorful incident involving ricin occurred in 2013 when another ricin letter was sent to President Obama. This one didn't contain well-purified ricin, and it never reached the president; but the story behind it is entertaining, to say the least. In the interest of brevity, I won't detail the whole backstory here, but it involved a plot to frame an Elvis impersonator by a Tae Kwon Do instructor in Tupelo, Mississippi. The incident also included a dog named "Moo Cow" and an illegal human-organ-selling operation. You can read the whole story in GQ magazine in an article titled, "The Elvis Impersonator, the Karate Instructor, a Fridge Full of Severed Heads, and the Plot 2 Kill the President."[1] Reality is truly stranger than fiction.

Whether it's inhaled from a letter in a powdered form or injected as a pellet by a devious secret police agent, ricin kills victims over the course of a few painful hours by inhibiting the function of ribosomes—cellular organelles where RNA fragments are made into proteins.[2] It basically gums-up our cellular factories, grinding them to a screeching halt and slowly ending the life of any organism unlucky enough to ingest it. Not surprisingly, castor beans do not make good food, and the consumption of five to twenty castor beans has proven fatal to humans.[3]

The concept of lectins can be a bit confusing, but simply put, they are a special type of protein that binds to glycoproteins on the surface of or within our cells. In the case of ricin, this lectin binds to a carbohydrate portion of the ribosome and prevents it from doing the crucial work of protein formation.

Lectins occur across all kingdoms of life, but lectins from plants often do not behave well in humans. This is yet another example of the disparate operating systems that exist between these two kingdoms of life. Generally speaking, lectins tend to be highest in the roots and seeds of plants, and foods with the highest content of these disruptive proteins are usually legumes, grains, seeds, nuts, and tubers.

The Toxic Lectin in Beans

The history and chemistry of ricin illustrates just how toxic lectins can be in animals and humans. Though usually not as potent, many other plant lectins can also be toxic and have caused poisonings. Acute nausea, vomiting, and diarrhea have occurred in humans who have consumed undercooked kidney beans, which contain a lectin known as phytohemagglutinin, or PHA. There are hundreds of recorded food poisoning outbreaks related to this seemingly innocuous bean and its powerful lectin. Between 1976 and 1989, there were fifty incidents of poisoning related to red kidney beans recorded in the United Kingdom:

> *"These and subsequent incidents in the UK have followed the consumption of raw or incompletely cooked red kidney beans. Symptoms develop after a 1-3 h incubation period and include nausea and vomiting, followed by diarrhea and sometimes abdominal pain... Outbreaks have also been reported in Canada and Australia."*[4]

Consumption of raw kidney beans and many other types of legumes will similarly lead to the rapid onset of severe gastrointestinal distress and will result in a horrible day for whatever hapless animal decides to nibble on them. In experiments with rats fed PHA, researchers observed damage to the intestines, pancreas, liver, and the thymus. A loss of muscle mass in direct proportion to the amount of lectins ingested was also observed.[5] Further experiments across multiple animal species that include mice, quail, and chickens have shown similar negative effects:

> *"**PHA, the lectin derived from red kidney beans (Phaseolus vulgaris) causes reduced growth rates in several animal species, when incorporated at 0.5-5% of dietary protein.** Lectin feeding results in diarrhea, impaired nutrient absorption, growth rate inhibition, and can even lead to the eventual death of PHA-fed animals."*[6]

Clearly, this stuff is highly toxic to both animals and unsuspecting humans that consume undercooked beans.

One of the ways in which PHA appears to be causing these severe effects is by negatively affecting the balance of microbes in the gut, and animals raised without gut flora (known as gnotobiotic animals) do not experience the same issues when exposed to this lectin:

> *"It is established that these adverse effects are the result of PHA-induced changes in the normal endogenous [bacterial] flora and are not due to lectin selection of specific pathogenic bacteria. The major change appears*

> *in the levels of facultative aerobes, which increase in PHA-fed animals without an increase in obligate anaerobes.*[6]

Among the bacteria living within us, broad divisions can be constructed based on whether these organisms use oxygen for respiration or not. Those that use oxygen are known as aerobic organisms, while those that do not are considered anaerobic. Facultative aerobes, like those observed to proliferate in these lectin studies, are organisms that don't have to use oxygen but can use it when it's around.

Bacteria are also divided into groups based on the structure of their cell wall. Gram-positive organisms possess a thick outer cell wall that is made of sugars and amino acids known as peptidoglycans. During the process of gram staining, these peptidoglycans hold onto the dye used, coloring these bacteria purple. Gram-negative bacteria, on the other hand, do not retain this dye, because the peptidoglycans within their cell wall are hidden between two cell membranes. This type of bacteria possesses a unique coating of glycolipids known as lipopolysaccharide, or endotoxin. This fragment of gram-negative bacterial cell walls can be quite inflammatory in our body if it enters through a damaged gut lining, and we'll hear more about it later in this book.

Having a diverse array of microbes within our gastrointestinal microbiome is crucial for optimal health, and low diversity has been associated with a variety of chronic diseases, including diabetes and inflammatory bowel illnesses. PHA and many other plant lectins *appear to be damaging to our gastrointestinal tract by decreasing the diversity of organisms* there through interacting with our gastrointestinal epithelial cells.[7,8]

In these experiments with PHA, the damaging effects to the animals appeared to be due to selective overgrowth of facultative aerobes like *E. coli*, resulting in a loss of diversity within the gastrointestinal tract.[9] The researchers astutely asked: How exactly did this lectin cause such a damaging shift in the microbiome to occur? This is where things really get interesting!

Researchers knew from previous experiments that this lectin could bind directly to gastrointestinal epithelial cells in a region known as the brush border, the outermost membrane of the cells where they come into contact with the contents of the gut. In their experiments, they discovered that PHA did not interact with organisms like *E. coli* directly, but rather appeared to induce changes in cells of the intestine, leading to lessening of the mucus layer that coats these cells. This depleted mucus layer then allowed pathogenic bacteria to proliferate and cause damage:

*"These findings would suggest that PHA does not function as a direct ligand for bacterial adhesion to the mucosal surface, **but may induce changes to the intestine that facilitate bacterial colonization.** Scanning electron microscopy of the mucosal surfaces of PHA-fed rat intestines suggested that bacteria found on the mucosal surface may gain access through windows in the mucous blanket."*[10]

When a molecule binds to a receptor on the surface of a cell, we call that molecule a "ligand" for the receptor. PHA doesn't bind to bacteria but instead appears to bind to the surface of the gut, inducing pathological changes that allow certain bacteria to breach the protective mucus layer. To fully understand the significance of these findings, let's take a brief detour and explore how our gut works and interact with the microbiome within them.

THE WORKINGS OF OUR GASTROINTESTINAL TRACT

Let's use a shrinking machine to become the size of a particle of swallowed food that passes through our stomach and winds up in the small bowel. Eventually, we pass through the ileocecal valve and into the first portion of the large bowel known as the cecum—a large, low-pressure portion of the colon that can expand to hold food waste as it arrives via the ileum.

Most of the organisms of the gastrointestinal microbiome hang out on the surface of the gut atop a protective layer of mucus, beneath which there's a single layer of cells known as the gastrointestinal epithelium. This layer separates the food molecules and organisms that are *outside* of us, but inside our gut, from the majority of our immune cells. Those cells reside in the lamina propria, a layer just beyond the lining of our gut contained deeper within the intestinal wall.

Isn't that a little mind bending to think about? Everything we eat, and the trillions of organisms that live inside of us throughout our life, are separated from armies of our immune cells and the inside of our body by *one* cell layer. This is a *very* important layer of cells!

This gastrointestinal epithelium has the critical job of absorbing the nutrients we need to grow and thrive while simultaneously keeping pathogens out. It is composed of a variety of unique cell types that all originate from progenitor stem cells found in the base of folds within the membrane of the small intestine as can be seen in the following image.[11]

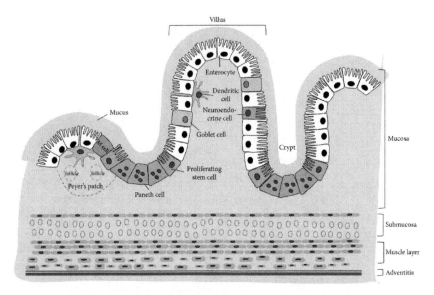

Shanshan Kong, Yanhui H. Zhang, and Weiqiang Zhang, "Regulation of Intestinal Epithelial Cells Properties and Functions by Amino Acids," *BioMed Research International*, vol. 2018, Article ID 2819154, 10 pages, 2018. https://doi. org/10.1155/2018/2819154.

The main cells within the epithelium are known as enterocytes and possess tiny finger like projections called microvilli, which exponentially increases the surface area of the small bowel. They are crucial for the proper absorption of nutrients from your food. In autoimmune conditions like celiac disease, regression of these microvilli is observed and the surface of the small intestine becomes pathologically smooth, causing malabsorption of nutrients and leading to profound nutritional deficiencies.

Other cell types of the gastrointestinal epithelium include mucus-secreting goblet cells, hormone-secreting enteroendocrine cells, and those with immunologic functions like paneth, tuft, and microfold cells. As they reside shoulder to shoulder to form the lining of the gut, these various cell types are connected to each other in multiple ways. The most important of these are called tight junctions, which bind adjacent cells together. They selectively allow certain molecules to pass between them and into the immune-cell-containing lamina propria. The cells that make up our gut lining must be very particular about the things they let in and keep out in order to maintain a healthy, peaceful environment at this intersection between the interior and exterior worlds.

How Lectins Damage the Gut

Now that we understand the lay of the land within the gut, let's return to our discussion of the lectin PHA from red kidney beans and the damage it causes. As mentioned, researchers observed changes in populations of aerobic bacteria, like *E. coli*, due to alterations in the mucus layer that allowed these organisms to thrive. They also noted that PHA is able to bind directly to the gastrointestinal epithelium in a manner that induces these changes. It appears that PHA is binding directly to the gut lining and damaging the cells there, including the goblet cells that help create and maintain a healthy mucus layer. As this mucus layer is eroded by the actions of PHA, bacteria come into direct contact with the gut epithelium, which causes our body to sound the alarm to mount an immune response.

One of the ways that our body does this is by releasing a protein known as zonulin, which triggers an opening of the tight junctions between the epithelial cells.[12] This allows immune cells from the lamina propria to move into the gut and fight off invaders so that the mucus layer can be reestablished and peace can be restored to the lands of our gastrointestinal tract. In animals and humans, *lectins like PHA appear to be causing harm by damaging the integrity of our gastrointestinal epithelia and creating leaky gut.* The researcher who discovered zonulin, Dr. Alessio Fasano notes that elevated levels of this molecule have been found to correlate strongly with autoimmune disease:

> *"Zonulin expression is **augmented in autoimmune conditions associated with tight junction dysfunction**, including celiac disease and Type 1 diabetes. Both animal studies and human trials using the zonulin synthetic peptide inhibitor established that zonulin is integrally involved in the pathogenesis of autoimmune diseases."*[13]

Celiac disease is an illness in which autoimmune injury to the small intestinal microvilli is triggered by the lectin called *gluten*. In type 1 diabetes, an autoimmune attack on the pancreas destroys the insulin secreting cells. The trigger for this is not known, but as Dr. Fasano suggests, leaky gut appears to play a powerful role in both of these conditions. He goes on to describe common triggers of zonulin release, and his comments recapitulate our previous discussions of lectins and how they lead to the exposure of bacteria to the gastrointestinal epithelium—thereby initiating an immune response.

*"Among the several potential intestinal luminal stimuli that can trigger zonulin release, we identified small intestinal **exposure to bacteria and gluten as the two more powerful triggers**. Enteric infections have been implicated in the pathogenesis of several pathological conditions, including allergic, autoimmune, and inflammatory diseases, **by causing impairment of the intestinal barrier**. We have generated evidence that small intestines exposed to enteric bacteria secrete zonulin."*

Let's summarize what we've discussed so far to emphasize a few points. A single layer of cells composing the gastrointestinal epithelium serves the invaluable role of keeping bad stuff out and bringing good stuff in. Specialized cells within it create the mucus layer that serves as a buffer between microorganisms inside our gut and the epithelial surface, beyond which a large amount of our immune system resides. When the mucus layer breaks down, bacteria can come into contact with cells of the gut epithelium, which triggers an inflammatory response that involves the release of zonulin and the opening of tight junctions. This allows the immune system to step in and fix things when they have gone awry. Lectins like PHA and gluten appear to trigger this inflammatory state of leaky gut by interfering with our body's ability to produce a healthy mucus layer as they bind to goblet cells and inhibit their functioning.

Not surprisingly, "Western diets" are associated with a dysfunctional mucus layer in humans, an association often blamed on the fact that they are relatively low in fiber.[13] But is it really the lack of fiber that is causing a lackluster mucus layer in those eating the standard American diet? Or might it be something else, like the hefty doses of lectins and processed sugars inherent in this way of eating? The findings we've just discussed with PHA, and from Dr. Fasano, argue that lectins are playing a significant role in gut barrier and mucus layer dysfunction, and we'll see later in Chapter Ten that fiber is definitely not the magical substance it's been made out to be, either!

GLUTEN AND OTHER LECTINS

PHA isn't the only lectin from plant foods that is known to cause damage. The aforementioned luten is another lectin found in wheat, rye, and barley that is responsible for a huge amount of suffering. It causes celiac disease and lesser know illnesses such as non-celiac gluten sensitivity. Wheat is full of lectins and also possesses wheat germ agglutinin (WGA). A substantial amount of research has been done on the negative effects that both of these lectins can have on animals and humans.

In a cell culture model mimicking the small intestinal epithelium, studies with WGA have shown that it induces both leaky gut and an inflammatory response when very low concentrations are administered:

*"In the micromolar (10-6) range of concentrations WGA could alter the integrity of the epithelium layer and increase its permeability…We show that at nanomolar [10-9] concentrations WGA is **unexpectedly bioactive on immune cells**….At nanomolar concentrations **WGA stimulates the synthesis of proinflammatory cytokines and thus the biological activity of WGA should be reconsidered by taking into account the effects of WGA on the immune system at the gastrointestinal interface.** These results shed new light onto the molecular mechanisms underlying the onset of gastrointestinal disorders observed in vivo upon dietary intake of wheat-based foods."*[15]

Gliadin, a fragment of the gluten molecule, also stimulates the release of zonulin in small intestinal epithelial cell culture models. It causes damage to the cytoskeleton, DNA/RNA and increased oxidative stress, often resulting in programmed cell death[16,17]

"Gliadin induces zonulin release in intestinal epithelial cells in vitro. Activation of the zonulin pathway by… cytoskeleton reorganisation and tight junction opening leads to a rapid increase in intestinal permeability." [18]

Whether by inducing the release of zonulin or by directly damaging cellular components and inducing oxidative stress, the gliadin molecule is clearly quite toxic to intestinal cells. This toxicity appears to occur in *all humans*, not just those with celiac disease, and Dr. Fasano and many other gluten researchers now believe that gluten invariably damages the intestinal epithelium and causes leaky gut. Within clinical practice, there is growing awareness of this, with diagnoses like non-celiac gluten sensitivity becoming more common.

I would go further to suggest that in addition to gluten and PHA, many other plant lectins also cause transient injury to the gut epithelium. I also believe that oxalates, polyphenols, and isothiocyanates may be creating intestinal damage, with varying degrees of immune activation, and that this could be yet another driving factor in most autoimmune and inflammatory illnesses.

So far we've talked about lectins from wheat and red kidney beans, but there are many other lectins in plant foods that can be damaging to humans. A lectin found in peanuts, known as peanut agglutinin (PNA), has been shown to alter the growth of rectal mucosa in a manner consistent with the possible induction of pre-cancerous lesions.[19] After ingestion of peanuts, PNA has also been found to be detectable in the blood, as have the lectins from kidney beans and tomatoes, where they are likely to be affecting cellular processes in negative ways.[20]

Tomatoes aren't seeds or tubers, but they belong to the nightshade family of vegetables, which possess many toxins known to be particularly harmful. Also included in this group are white potatos, eggplants, bell peppers, chili peppers, tobacco, and goji berries. Not only do members of this lineage contain the toxic glycoalkaloid solanine in their leaves and roots, they also contain many potentially harmful lectins. Removal of these vegetables from the diet often results in significant improvements in joint pain, arthritis, and other autoimmune symptoms. A lectin found in potatoes, *Solanum tuberosum* agglutinin (STA), activates basophil cells of the immune system, releasing histamine and leading to swelling, itching, hives, and an inflammatory response.[21] Consumption of this food may worsen symptoms in those with asthma, eczema, or hives—it makes me a bit itchy just to think about.

Further studies of multiple foods, including soybeans, lentils, wheat germ, and kidney beans, showed that many lectins from these could bind white blood cells, causing them to sound the cellular alarm by releasing inflammatory cytokines.[22] From previous discussions in this book, we know that cytokines are chemical signals our immune system uses to indicate to their comrades that something is wrong. Just like a fire alarm, they serve an invaluable role in our body when there's really a fire, but they're not such a good thing when there's no invader there, and it's just a false alarm. Remember those false fire alarms in your college dormitory that woke you and everyone else up in the middle of the night? Yeah, those were zero fun! Similarly, it's a real bummer when our immune system gets all hyped up responding to the false signals from lectins or from the other plant toxins and ends up *causing inflammation for no reason, potentially leading to a host of autoimmune diseases.*

COULD LECTINS PLAY A ROLE IN PARKINSON'S DISEASE?

So far, we've seen the havoc that lectins from plants like legumes, wheat, nightshades, and peanuts can wreak on our gut and our immune system, but lectins also appear to be able to negatively affect our brains and have been hypothesized to play a role in Parkinson's disease. This illness is a neurodegenerative condition in which dopamine-producing neurons from a region known as the basal ganglia are damaged, leading to problems with movement, speech, and cognitive processing. Many Parkinson's patients progress to dementia and experience depression as their illness worsens. The impact of this disease on quality of life is substantial. The cause of neuronal cell death and depletion of dopamine signaling in the midbrain is not fully understood, but characteristic aggregates known as Lewy bodies occur and are composed of the protein alpha-synuclein.

In 2015, an intriguing study was done in Denmark showing that people who had undergone surgical severing of the vagus nerve during the previous forty years developed Parkinson's disease at a much lower rate than the general population.[23] In order to understand what this may have to do with lectins, let's dig a bit deeper into what could be going on here.

The vagus nerve originates in the brain stem and sends signals to many portions of the body and much of the digestive tract, including the stomach, liver, pancreas, and intestines. It is a large nerve and serves as a bidirectional information superhighway between our gastrointestinal organs and our brain, with signals from the brain traveling through the vagus nerve to the digestive organs, and back again. You may have heard the term "gut-brain axis" in reference to the notion that our gut and brain communicate in many ways. In addition to the signals transmitted to the brain through cytokines in the bloodstream, the vagus nerve is also a big part of this cross talk.

Within surgical medicine, this nerve is sometimes cut to treat patients with severe peptic ulcer disease because signals from the vagus nerve to the stomach cause the release of acid during the digestive process. In the aforementioned study from Denmark, investigators compared people who had truncal vagotomy, a complete severing of the vagus nerve, with those who had superselective vagotomy in which only the vagus nerve's connection to the stomach was cut. Reduction in the incidence of Parkinson's disease was only observed with truncal rather than superselective vagotomy, suggesting that it was the connection between *both* the intestines and the stomach that accounted for this finding. Why would severing the neural connection between the gut and the brain affect a neurodegenerative condition like Parkinson's disease? Is it possible that a substance from the gastrointestinal tract could move to the brain through the vagus nerve?

This is truly a fascinating question, and I believe that a couple of studies in animal models of Parkinson's disease will help shed light on this mystery.

One of the coolest innovations in molecular biology over the last twenty years is the use of a bioluminescent protein from jellyfish, called green fluorescent protein (GFP). This molecule can be used to visualize the movement of proteins within living organisms. When a savvy group of investigators fed the invertebrate worm *C. elegans* green-fluorescent-protein labeled PHA and other lectins, they were able to visualize exactly where these lectins went in that organism after they were ingested. Their findings were striking. Not only did a number of lectins appear to be transported from the *guts to the brains of these worms through the vagus nerve*, the lectins then *clustered in the dopamine secreting neurons*. In the case of PHA, this lectin appeared to be toxic to neurons, reducing their number and function.[24] Referencing the aforementioned Danish study, the authors concluded:

> *"These observations suggest that **dietary plant lectins are transported to and affect dopaminergic neurons in C. elegans**, which support Braak and Hawkes' hypothesis, suggesting **one alternate potential dietary etiology of Parkinson's disease** (PD). A recent Danish study showed that vagotomy resulted in 40% lower incidence of PD over 20 years. Differences in inherited sugar structures of gut and neuronal cell surfaces may make some individuals more susceptible in this conceptual disease etiology model."*

As mentioned in the previous excerpt, Braak and Hawkes, had previously hypothesized that an ingested "unknown pathogen" enters the gastrointestinal tract and transports via the vagus nerve to the brainstem, inducing a spreading neural dysfunction.[25] The authors of this study suggest, based on the Danish vagotomy cohort and their own findings, that ingested lectins may be damaging the gut and traveling through the vagus nerve to the brain, where they appear to be toxic to dopaminergic neurons.

These researchers make another very interesting observation:

> *"Lectins from dietary plants have been shown to enhance drug absorption in the gastrointestinal tract of rats, **be transported trans-synaptically as shown by tracing of axonal and dendritic paths**...and other carbohydrate-binding protein toxins are known to **traverse the gut intact** in dogs."*

Enhanced drug delivery sounds like a good thing, until we realize that the way lectins do this is by increasing the permeability of the gut lining! As noted by these investigators, lectins have been found to damage the gut and traverse the small intestinal epithelium in animals like dogs, and the appearance of peanut, kidney bean, and tomato lectins in samples of human blood indicates that lectins are doing the same things in us.

C. elegans is not the only organism in which ingestion of lectins has been linked to damage in dopaminergic neurons in the brain. In a study with rats, researchers administered a lectin from peas and looked for Parkinsonian behavior or changes in gastric motility.[26] Their findings were striking and were published in the prestigious journal *Nature* in 2018:

> *"These data demonstrate that co-administration of sub-threshold doses of paraquat and lectin induces progressive, L-dopa-responsive parkinsonism that is preceded by gastric dysmotility. This novel preclinical model of environmentally triggered Parkinson's disease provides functional support for Braak's staging hypothesis of idiopathic Parkinon's disease."*

Paralleling the study from Denmark discussed earlier, these authors also included a group of rats that underwent vagotomy prior to exposure to pea lectins, and these rats did not demonstrate any of the neuronal damage or gastric dysmotility issues observed in the other experimental groups.

The possibility of plant lectins contributing to the pathogenesis of this disease is striking and is a potential paradigm shift in the world of neurodegenerative illness. It is important to highlight, however, that certain individuals are more likely to be susceptible to this type of neuronal injury. Not everyone who eats beans, tomatoes, or peanuts develops Parkinson's disease, but in those with genetics susceptible to this type of lectin-induced damage, consumption of plant foods could be a contributing factor to the development and progression of neurodegenerative illness.

More studies are needed here, but based on the these findings, it seems reasonable to hypothesize the following: lectins in the gut could cause damage there, travel to the brain through the vagus nerve in a retrograde fashion, and trigger injury of dopamine-secreting neurons in the regions of the basal ganglia that control movement and other complex tasks. Scary! Maybe this will make us think twice about adding beans to that chili.

THE PLINKO MODEL OF AUTOIMMUNE DISEASE

You may be familiar with Plinko from the game show, *The Price Is Right*. I used to love this show when I was a kid and always hoped someone would win the car. When playing Plinko, participants stand over a slanted board full of pins and release a disk, which slides down through the pins in a random fashion before ending up in one of the bottom wells that are each marked with different dollar amounts. I think of the combination of our genetic susceptibility to disease and our environment like the game of Plinko.

In this model, our genetics create a unique pattern of pins on the board through which the disk (inflammation) travels in a unique pattern leading to one of a variety of chronic diseases. As I mentioned previously, not everyone will be susceptible to Parkinson's disease when they eat lectins, but some might be. We all possess different genetics that make us uniquely susceptible to different diseases. We've all got holes in our armor—they're just in different places. I strongly believe that inflammation is at the root of most chronic disease but is manifested differently in each person based on their own unique genetic susceptibilities. Thus, eating lectins and other plant toxins might contribute to Parkinson's disease in some people, heart disease in others, and skin issues or joint pain for others still. All of these diseases have a common root trigger, which is inflammation, but it shows up differently in all of us based on our individual genetic Plinko board of susceptibilities.

Because we've been eating tons of plants and living in toxic environments for most of our lives, we've all been exposed to inflammatory stimuli, but the results show up in different ways. When I am exposed to such stimuli, I get asthma and eczema and become a bit irritable. These are my genetic weaknesses, not yours. When you are exposed to inflammatory insults, you might develop autoimmune thyroid disease, like Hasimoto's thyroiditis, or you might develop lupus, rheumatoid arthritis, or diabetes. Western medicine becomes flummoxed when it tries to think of these diseases as thousands of different entities, often leaving it powerless to bring real change in the lives of those who suffer with such maladies. **The critical error of judgment that Western medicine is making is in imagining that there are thousands of different chronic illnesses, when in fact there's really only one big one—inflammation.**

So how do we correct this one major cause of chronic illness? We search for its roots and remove them! One of the radical notions this book advances is that, because of all of their intrinsic toxins, plants might be triggering such inflammation in ways never before considered. Wild, right? Let's continue our journey through the lectin jungle; there's more to see!

COULD LECTINS BE CAUSING US TO GAIN WEIGHT?

One of the more positive effects experienced by those on a carnivore diet is weight loss. There are now thousands of stories of people easily losing weight when plants are eliminated from their diet and high-quality animal foods become the focus. Many of these people began with ketogenic diets, which still include some plants, but they found weight loss even easier and had fewer cravings when they fully eliminated all plants. One of the reasons for this may be that lectins have also been found to negatively affect fat storage and satiety mechanisms in humans.

Insulin is a hormone released from the pancreas primarily in response to the ingestion of carbohydrates or protein. Its actions in the human body are complex but, in general, insulin is an anti-catabolic hormone that signals our muscles and liver to take up and store glucose. It also signals our fat cells to store fat rather than burn it. If you know people who are using large amounts of insulin to treat type II diabetes, you may observe that this often causes significant weight gain for these reasons.

Studies with the lectin wheat germ agglutinin have shown that it can bind to the insulin receptor, stimulate growth of fat cells, and inhibit lipolysis.[27] Plant lectins appear to mimic the actions of insulin—signaling fat cells to grow, potentially leading to weight gain in those consuming them, and hampering efforts to attain a healthy body composition.

Those eating a carnivore diet also note significantly improved satiety and often find benefits beyond those experienced on ketogenic diets, which usually include many foods that are quite high in lectins, such as nuts, seeds, and nightshade vegetables. Lectins have also been found to negatively affect signaling of a satiety hormone known as leptin. In a simplified model, leptin is a hormone that is released when we eat to tell our brain that we've had enough and are full. The full cascade of hormones involved in the satiety response is much more complex than this, but at a basic level, leptin signals satiety.

When researchers remove the gene for leptin from mice, preventing their satiety signals, these poor critters overeat tremendous amounts of food and become quite obese. Similarly, when our body becomes resistant to the signals of leptin, we also tend to gain weight because we do not feel full and are constantly seeking food.

With all of this in mind, plant lectins look like the perfect storm for creating obesity. Not only do they appear to damage the gut, potentially leading to systemic inflammation, they also negatively affect the signaling of hormones, such as insulin and leptin, which are centrally involved in regulation of proper body composition and hunger.[28] It's no surprise, then, that removal of all plant lectins in a carnivore diet is so effective for gastrointestinal issues, autoimmune illness, and weight loss.

THE PARADOX OF PLANTS

To wrap up our discussion of lectins, let's take a look at the work of Dr. Steven Gundry, author of *The Plant Paradox*. Though he and I don't see eye to eye about animal foods, we agree on the importance of avoiding lectins. Dr. Gundry has published an impressive case series describing significant improvements in a large group of patients with autoimmune disease who were treated with a very low-lectin diet that involved the removal of all grains, beans, legumes, peanuts, cashews, nightshades, squashes, and dairy products.

> *"95/102 patients achieved complete resolution of autoimmune markers and inflammatory markers within 9 months. The other 7/102 patients all had reduced markers, but incomplete resolution. 80/102 patients were weaned from all immunosuppressive and/or biologic medications without rebound ....We conclude that a lectin limited diet, supplemented with pro- and prebiotics and polyphenols are capable of curing or putting into remission most autoimmune diseases."*[29]

Dr. Gundry and I will disagree on the utility of polyphenols within this protocol, but I agree with him that the elimination of foods with high-lectin content was likely at the root of the reversal of these patients' autoimmune issues.

The foods that appear to be highest in lectins that can trigger our immune system are seeds, grains, nuts, legumes, nightshade vegetables, the skin and seeds of squashes, and traditional dairy products.[30] Since dairy is an animal product, I haven't talked about it yet, but it also contains many proteins, including lectins, which can cause inflammation and immune issues in humans. I'll go into detail about dairy in Chapter Twelve when we discuss what to eat on a carnivore diet and the difference between A1 and A2 forms of the milk protein, casein. It's also important to remember that even aside from these foods, lectins are pervasive in all plant foods and many could be causing immunologic reactions. A review of lectins in commonly-consumed foods echoed this sentiment:

> *"In the present study the edible parts of 29 of 88 foods tested, including common salad ingredients, fresh fruits, roasted nuts, and processed cereals were found to possess significant lectin-like activity as assessed by hemagglutination and bacterial agglutination assays. Based on this survey and a review of the literature* **we conclude that dietary exposure to plant lectins is widespread.** *"* [31]

Just like all of the other molecules from plants we have talked about, lectins are plant weapons. They are designed to discourage predators, and the objective of plants is clear in this case. It is true that some lectins can be denatured with cooking, especially at high pressures and temperatures, but lectins are pervasive in the plant kingdom and occur in many foods that are commonly eaten raw or lightly cooked. It is also true that lectins occur in animal foods as well as in the human body. Reinforcing the concept of disparate operating systems, the majority of research on lectins suggests that plant lectins have the potential to damage our gut and trigger our immune system much more so than those from animal meat and organs.

The first step to decreasing our exposure to lectins is to eliminate those foods with the highest lectin content. If this does not significantly improve our symptoms, it's possible that lectins or other plant toxins in the remaining plant foods that we consume are still triggering the immune system, and a trial of complete elimination of these within a carnivore diet would likely be helpful. As we'll continue to see in the following chapters, this way of eating is a very powerful tool toward achieving profound health.

CONCLUDING SECTION II OF OUR JOURNEY

This portion of our journey to rediscover how humans are meant to eat has been a wild ride through the turbulent waters of the many types of plant toxins. As we prepare to conclude the second part of our adventures together and move on to an exploration of the merits of animal foods, let's recall the predicament of plants we imagined at the beginning of Chapter Three. When thinking about the dizzying array of plant chemicals that can harm us, remember that plants are rooted in the ground and have been for the entirety of their evolution. Animal and plant evolution split over 1.5 billion years ago, and our respective biochemistries have diverged massively over this time. For the 470 million years that plants have lived on land, they have been in a constant arms race with animals for their survival, and they developed many defense mechanisms out of necessity in order to survive. They've gotten pretty good at it and have created molecules like the isothiocyanates, polyphenols, oxalates, and lectins. All of these molecules have allowed them to maintain their place in the delicately balanced ecosystem of the Earth and prevented them from being over-consumed by animals or humans. As I stated earlier, it's clear that our ancestors ate some plants, but I believe that when they could get animals, these were always the preferred foods. Plants were likely eaten in much smaller quantities than we've previously been led to believe—and only as survival foods between successful hunts of more caloric and nutrient-rich animals.

In this section of the book, we've talked about why plants don't make great staple foods because of how they are riddled with toxins. Next, we'll dive deeply into how plant foods are also vastly inferior to animal foods from a nutritional perspective. It will quickly become clear that it's high-time for kale and goji berries to move aside and allow animal meat and organs to ascend the throne as the only true superfoods.

SECTION III

CHAPTER EIGHT

MYTH I
PLANT FOODS ARE SUPERFOODS

As you saunter down the aisles of any grocery store, it doesn't take long before you see signs claiming that foods like broccoli, spinach, kale, or goji berries are "superfoods." Fruits and vegetables are often marketed in this way, but what does this really mean? Where do these claims come from and what real evidence backs them up? What exactly makes these foods so "super?"

In the previous section of this book, we debunked many of the myths surrounding supposedly magical chemicals like "antioxidants" from the isothiocyanate or polyphenol families and showed that these plant toxins can damage DNA, inhibit digestion, disrupt hormonal balance, and trigger the immune system's inflammatory response. We also touched on compounds like lectins and oxalates. The former are common in nightshade plants like goji berries, and the latter are abundant in spinach and many other plant foods often labeled as "super." If we harbor any notions that it's the fiber in fruits and vegetables that makes them special, I'll do my best to thoroughly debunk that notion in the next chapter as well.

Discarding all notions of magical unicorn "phytonutrients" that make fruits and vegetables super, how might we theoretically define a "superfood?" Hearkening back to the concepts in the introduction of this book, I suggest that in order to earn this designation, a food must be rich in the micronutrients that humans need to thrive. In addition, these micronutrients must be in the most useable form for human biochemistry and they must be bioavailable. In this chapter, we will take a detailed look at the actual nutrient content and quality in animal foods versus plant foods. We're going to let these two duke it out in the boxing ring in order to see who the real champion is—and at the end of it all, we'll see who really deserves the superfood title belt.

MAGICAL NUTRIENTS IN ANIMAL FOODS

I've shared with you my conviction that unicorns don't actually exist and that there are no "magical" compounds in plants that are uniquely beneficial to humans. But what about magical compounds in animal foods? Could Sasquatch be real? A careful examination of animal foods reveals that they do contain many compounds that are known to be vital for optimal human health and performance that do *not* occur in plants. Many readers already know that cobalamin, or vitamin B_{12}, does not occur in any plant foods, but this is just the tip of the iceberg when it comes to unique nutrients in animal foods. Creatine, carnitine, choline, taurine, and carnosine are also found in appreciable quantities only in animal foods and are absolutely necessary for optimal health.

CREATINE: MAKING US SMART AND STRONG

What if I told you of a substance that could increase intelligence, working memory, reaction time, and strength when given to humans? Sounds pretty magical right? You might even think I was spinning a yarn. But this is no fairy tale, my friends, this is creatine. Creatine is just about as magical as it gets, and it's only present in meat. It's a molecule that helps us store energy in the form of phosphate bonds, which can be used when we need more ATP quickly. ATP is used by our muscles to contract and in all of the cells of our body during the protection and repair of our delicate genetic material. We can produce a small amount of creatine endogenously, on the order of one gram per day, but it's not enough for optimal performance of our brains, muscles, or DNA protection and repair.

A striking study of forty-five adult vegetarians found significantly improved mental performance when they were given five grams of creatine per day (the amount found in 1 pound of red meat) for six weeks in a double blind, placebo controlled intervention:

> *"Creatine supplementation had a significant positive effect on both working memory (backward digit span) and intelligence, both tasks that require speed of processing. These findings underline a dynamic and significant role of brain energy capacity in influencing brain performance."*[1]

Another study of 128 adult females who were supplemented with twenty grams of creatine for five days found similar improvements in cognitive function in the subjects who were vegetarians.[2] This suggests that those eating meat already had adequate creatine stores and that a vegetarian diet can result in mental performance deficits due to the lack of this nutrient.

Inadequate stores of creatine in the muscle also lead to decreased strength and explosive power. When supplementation with creatine was compared in eighteen vegetarians, and twenty-four non-vegetarians over a six-week period of time, investigators found that lean muscle-mass gain and overall relative strength gains were higher in the vegetarian group compared to the non-vegetarian group.[3] That is, vegetarians benefited more from creatine supplementation with regard to these measures. It was also noted that at baseline before supplementation, vegetarians had lower intramuscular creatine levels:

> *"Vegetarians who took creatine had a greater increase in total creatine, plasma creatine, lean tissue, and total work performance than nonvegetarians who took creatine. The change in muscle total creatine was significantly correlated with initial muscle total creatine, and the change in lean tissue mass and exercise performance. These findings confirm an ergogenic effect of creatine during resistance training* **and suggest that subjects with initially low levels of intramuscular creatine (vegetarians) are more responsive to supplementation.**"

See? I told you Bigfoot was real, but creatine is just the beginning of this rabbit hole of magical animal based nutrients.

CHOLINE

Choline is another amazing nutrient that isn't found in plant foods in significant amounts. The recommended intake for choline in humans is about 500 milligrams per day, but those with polymorphisms in genes involved in methylation probably benefit from even more than this amount. Without getting too complex, choline is used as a methyl donor during the methylation of homocysteine to methionine, and is also a downstream product of methylation by the methyl donor, SAMe. If all of that sounds like gibberish to you, don't worry about the details. What's important to know is that choline is crucial for kicking butt. A small amount of it can be made in our bodies, but just like creatine, this amount isn't adequate for optimal health.

Choline is used in the formation of the neurotransmitter acetylcholine. It is also needed for the production of membrane phospholipids like phosphatidylcholine and sphingomyelin that enclose every cell in our body. Although we may have heard that choline in food can raise levels of TMAO, a substance that has been associated with adverse cardiovascular outcomes, rest assured these notions are pure rubbish. We will thoroughly debunk these and other misconceptions regarding red meat and heart disease risk in Chapter Eleven.

Deficiencies of choline are associated with non-alcoholic fatty liver disease, neurodegenerative disease, and heart disease.[4] The need for this nutrient is also particularly high in pregnant and nursing mothers, and deficiencies have been associated with neural tube defects, poor fetal brain development, premature birth, and preeclampsia. A recently published article by English physician Emily Derbyshire titled "Could we be Overlooking a Potential Choline Crisis in the United Kingdom?" notes that choline is not included in nutritional databases there.[5] It has been largely ignored for the past few decades, and deficiency may be responsible for significant, unnoticed health consequences in the general population of Britain. Similarly, in the United States, choline has been largely forgotten, and many estimate that a large majority of Americans do not get enough choline daily.

Where can we get choline in our diets and avoid all of these dismal fates? The best sources are clearly animal foods—five egg yolks provide a robust 600 milligrams, and liver and kidney aren't far behind with about 350 milligrams per 100-gram portion. Muscle meat also has a moderate amount of choline, and when combined with organ meats or eggs on a carnivore diet, we will more than meet our choline requirements. Within the plant kingdom, broccoli is the richest source of choline, but guess how much of this you'd have to eat in order to achieve the 500 milligram mark? More than a pound! That's a lot of broccoli, replete with a whole bunch of toxic isothiocyanates and gas-producing fiber. You will not be popular in an olfactory manner if you eat a pound of broccoli per day, and you might just become iodine deficient as we learned about in Chapter Four.

CARNITINE AND MENTAL HEALTH

It just so happens that most of the powerful nutrients unique to animal foods all begin with the letter "C." I guess that makes them easier to remember, so let's go with it! The next "C's" in this illustrious group are carnitine and carnosine. The latin root of their names quickly alludes to the fact that these nutrients are almost entirely found in animal meat and organs. Plants don't use these molecules in their biochemistry because they have a different operating system from humans, as we've discussed multiple times thus far.

Like choline and creatine, our bodies produce some carnitine, but it isn't enough for optimal health. This nutrient helps shuttle fatty acids across the mitochondrial membrane to the interior of this organelle, where they can be used as fuel in the biochemical process of beta-oxidation. Carnitine helps us use our fat-stores for energy. This is a very good thing, because we have lots of fat to burn, but only a limited supply of available carbohydrates stored in the form of glycogen in our muscles and liver. Using fat for fuel also results in the formation of ketones, which benefit our body in many ways, including turning on genes associated with longevity (sirtuins and FOXO3) and improving mitochondrial function.[6,7]

In studies examining muscle carnitine content, significantly reduced levels have been found in vegetarians relative to meat eaters, as well as a reduced ability to transport carnitine into muscles when it is administered intravenously or through diet.[8] When carnitine levels drop, we aren't able to use fats for energy, and a fundamental part of our metabolism is disrupted with many negative consequences.

Fat-based metabolism is particularly important in the brain, and levels of carnitine are lower in the brains of humans during periods of depression. In animal models, the brains of mice and rats exhibit similar lower levels with depression.[9] Studies in geriatric rats have also shown that administration of carnitine improves their mitochondrial function and metabolism, resulting in more youthful behavior.[10] In humans, a study that compared seventy patients with major depression to forty-five healthy controls found significantly lower levels of carnitine in the brains of those who were depressed:

> *"We found that carnitine levels...were decreased in patients with major depression compared with age- and sex-matched healthy controls in two independent study centers. Secondary exploratory analyses showed that*

the degree of carnitine deficiency reflected both the severity and age of onset of Major Depressive Disorder."[9]

As noted by the authors here, not only were the levels lower in depressed patients, the degree of this deficiency correlated directly with the severity of illness. That is, the levels of carnitine were lowest in those with the worst cases of depression. Mechanistically, lower levels of carnitine are hypothesized to change the way genes in the brain are turned on and off, negatively affecting neurotransmitter levels and causing inflammation.

Strengthening the case that carnitine deficiency may be involved in some cases of depression, numerous trials have demonstrated improvements in this illness when carnitine is supplemented. In 2013, the authors of a review paper summarizing these findings stated:

*"Four randomized clinical studies demonstrated the **superior efficacy of carnitine over placebo in patients with depression**. Two trials showed its superior efficacy over placebo in dysthymic disorder, and 2 other trials showed that it is **equally effective as [antidepressant medications]** in treatment of dysthymic disorder. Carnitine was also effective in improving depressive symptoms in patients with fibromyalgia and minimal hepatic encephalopathy...In conclusion, carnitine may be a potentially effective and tolerable next treatment option with novel action mechanisms for patients with depression."*[11]

Another review paper from 2017, considering twelve randomized controlled trials involving 791 participants, echoed these findings:

"Carnitine supplementation significantly decreases depressive symptoms compared to placebo/no intervention, whilst offering a comparable effect to established anti-depressant agents with fewer side effects."[12]

Thus, the evidence that carnitine deficiency can play a role in depression is strong, and research supports the notion that increasing levels of this nutrient can ameliorate this illness in cases of deficiency with fewer side effects than anti-depressant medications. How did people in these studies get deficient in such an important nutrient? A dietary deficiency appears to be the most probable explanation. Sadly, the authors did not survey study participants to quantify their dietary preferences, but as we've seen, those avoiding animal products possess lower levels of carnitine. I'd be willing to bet a mountain of ribeyes that low-carnitine levels were caused by inadequate consumption of animal meat and organs. Steak and liver might just be the best antidepressants!

CARNOSINE

Carnosine is a molecule that acts as an endogenous antioxidant, much like our old friend glutathione. We can make a small amount, but the story remains the same: multiple studies have found that if we don't get enough through diet, our levels will be suboptimal, and because it's only found in animal foods, vegetarians have repeatedly been shown to possess lower levels.[13,14]

Carnosine appears to be far more that just another antioxidant, however. This little gem of a molecule has also been shown to reduce the formation of **advanced glycation end products** (AGEs) that can be formed in our body when sugar molecules are added to proteins or lipids. Elevated levels of AGEs have been associated with diabetes, heart disease, and dementia—a motley crew to be sure! Endogenous formation of AGEs is a complex process that isn't fully understood, but robust intake of molecules like carnosine can help to manage cellular levels, and play a valuable role in disease prevention. Consistent with these ideas, vegetarians demonstrate higher levels of AGEs, which may be due to a combination of increased consumption of sugars, like fructose, and lower levels of protective molecules like carnosine.[15]

Taurine is yet another valuable nutrient only found in animal foods that also functions to reduce AGEs.[16] Its functions in the human body aren't fully understood, but it is known to act as an endogenous antioxidant in the functioning of muscles and as an anxiety-reducing neurotransmitter.[17] The rest of the story? You guessed it! We can make a small amount, but not enough to be optimal; and, once again, it's very low in those who don't eat meat.[18]

The pattern here is clear. Animal foods uniquely provide numerous nutrients that we need to kick a lot of butt. Those who eschew these foods invariably suffer from a lower quality of life and unnecessary negative health consequences.

DECLINE IN MENTAL HEALTH WITH PLANT-BASED DIETS

Since we already know that vegetarians and vegans are likely to be deficient in many nutrients crucial for vibrant health, like creatine, choline, and carnitine, it will come as no surprise that the incidence of mental health disorders is much higher in vegetarian populations. Though the correlations in the following studies are suggestive, it's important to note this research is epidemiology, so we can't make causal conclusions. Based on what we know about deficiencies in vegetarians and vegans of several nutrients involved in brain health, however, we can definitely form some strong hypotheses.

In an analysis of over 9,000 Australian women, vegetarians had significantly more mental health issues, possessed higher levels of iron deficiency, and were more likely to be taking prescription and non-prescription medications than those who were not vegetarians.[19] Another Australian study found that vegetarians of both sexes were twice as likely to suffer from depression, anxiety, and other adverse health outcomes than was a non-vegetarian group matched in age and gender ratios. These investigators stated:

> *"Our results showed that a vegetarian diet is associated with poorer health (higher incidences of cancer, allergies, and mental health disorders), a higher need for health care, and poorer quality of life."*[20]

Well, that puts things in perspective, doesn't it?

The same trends have been observed in European populations. In a very large cross-sectional study in France, depressive symptoms were significantly more common in vegetarians and those who excluded red meat from their diet. These researchers showed that as more animal foods were excluded, participants were more likely to experience depression.[21] A similar trend was observed in Germany, where vegetarians demonstrated higher rates of mental disorders than those eating meat.[22] Finally, studies in Finland and Sweden have shown that vegetarians are three to four times more likely to experience seasonal affective disorder.[23] Remember when I said red meat might just be the best anti-depressant? I wasn't joking!

The studies noted above encompass more than 130,000 participants and consistently show a correlation between plant-based diets and mental health issues like depression and anxiety. This mountain of evidence suggests that nutritional deficiencies associated with vegetarian diets could be causing issues in the brain. If we truly want to achieve optimal health of our body and mind, high-quality animal foods simply must be a significant portion of our diet.

THE ROOTS OF DEPRESSION AND ANXIETY

As we explore the connections between nutrient deficiency and mental illness, now is probably a good time to pause for a moment and examine the roots of psychiatric disease more deeply. Depression causes a huge loss of quality of life throughout the world, and it's the single greatest cause of morbidity in the world today, recently surpassing heart disease and cancer for this dubious honor. In medical school, I found mental illness particularly fascinating and decided to do my residency in psychiatry when I graduated. Throughout my training, I was constantly bothered by the fact that the medicines we used didn't seem to be treating the root cause of the illnesses. The antiquated paradigm of psychiatric disease is that imbalances in neurotransmitters lead to illness and that we can "rebalance" these with pharmaceutical medications. The problem is that this paradigm is mostly incorrect. These types of approaches don't usually work, and they certainly don't treat the underlying causes of psychiatric illness, which are much more complex than a neurotransmitter deficiency.

Mental health is a complex field, and there are many disease entities, but when I explored the literature on my own and tried to understand the true roots of these illnesses, I discovered something amazing. There was a large body of research showing that in addition to being triggered by nutrient deficiencies, psychiatric disease is *also largely inflammatory in nature*. I wasn't being told about these possibilities, likely because we didn't have any drugs to treat inflammation in the brain, and there's little focus on nutrition in medical training. In the brain of people with depression, anxiety, and many other mental health issues, however, the immune system is activated with evidence for elevated levels of inflammatory cytokines, like IL-6 and TNF-alpha.[24,25,26] Psychiatric illnesses are no different from chronic illnesses found elsewhere in the body. Both can be related to inflammation and activation of the immune system. As rheumatoid arthritis and Crohn's disease represent inflammation in the joints and gut, respectively, most psychiatric illness is inflammation in the brain and must be treated in this way if we truly hope to fundamentally reverse it.

Sadly, in Western medicine, if we don't have a drug for something, we largely ignore it. Consequently, we often discard key clues to the roots of an illness. This is exactly what has happened in psychiatry over the last fifty years. Since the advent of anti-depressant medications, we've become enamored with a neurotransmitter model that doesn't work, because that's all we know how to do. As we've already discovered, however, we have a very powerful weapon to combat inflammation, but it's just something Western medicine continues to overlook: food!

Another fundamental flaw of the Western medical paradigm is its myopia. In medical school, and throughout our speciality training as physicians, we are taught to think of the body in terms of discrete organ systems. Gastroenterologists deal with the gut, cardiologists with the heart, and neurologists and psychiatrists with the brain. But our body doesn't work this way, it's entirely interconnected, and often the roots of a problem lie outside of the organ system in which symptoms of a disease may be manifested. In order to truly correct the roots of inflammation in the brain, joints, thyroid, or heart, we need to think about where this is coming from—and for most illnesses, ground zero appears to be the gastrointestinal tract.

We shouldn't be surprised by this. In the previous section of this book, we saw how damaging plant toxins can be to the gut and how they appear to trigger the cells of the immune system within the lamina propria. Once these immune cells are activated, systemic inflammation often follows, and cytokines circulate throughout the body, including into the brain. If we seek optimal health, we must be sure our gut is healthy and avoid consuming foods that may contribute to damage there.

VITAMINS AND MINERALS IN ANIMAL FOODS VS. PLANT FOODS

So far, we've talked about creatine, choline, carnitine, carnosine, and taurine, all of which demonstrate profound benefits in the human body when present in adequate amounts, and none of which are present in any appreciable quantity in plant foods. In contrast to these *magical animal nutrients*, minerals like zinc, iron, magnesium, and selenium are found in plant foods, but because of a molecule called *phytic acid*, and that shady character *oxalate*, our ability to absorb them is significantly reduced relative to animal foods.[27] Studies examining the absorption of minerals when foods with and without phytic acid are consumed indicate clearly that there is significantly decreased bioavailability from plant foods.

For example, oysters are the richest known food source of zinc, and when eaten alone, produce large increases in plasma zinc within two to three hours of ingestion. In contrast, when researchers added beans or tortillas, absorption of zinc was significantly impaired.[28] Both beans and tortillas are foods known to possess high concentrations of phytic acid. When black beans were combined with oysters, plasma levels of zinc decreased to one-third of the normal amount, and when tortillas were consumed, they *completely inhibited* zinc absorption. A similar pattern is observed for magnesium and calcium, with significantly decreased absorption of these important minerals when eaten with high-oxalate-containing vegetables like spinach.[29,30]

Both oxalate and phytic acid are used in plants to chelate, or "bite," minerals. These molecules wrap themselves around positively charged atoms like magnesium, phosphorus, zinc, selenium, or calcium to allow for storage within plant cells. The problem is that when we consume phytic acid or oxalate from plants, these molecules can also bind to these minerals in our digestive tracts, preventing their absorption.

Predictably, studies of plant-based dieters consistently show lower levels of minerals like iron, zinc, and calcium.[31,32,33-35] The authors of a study that examined the mineral levels of vegetarians state:

> "*Vegetarians had statistically significant lower levels of plasma zinc and copper than nonvegetarians, which may be the result of lower bioavailability of zinc and copper from this type of diet…Selenium status was significantly lower in vegetarians when compared to nonvegetarians…A vegetarian diet does not provide a sufficient supply of essential antioxidant trace elements, like zinc, copper, and especially selenium.*"

Looks like bad news for those hoping to obtain these minerals from plants.

Concerns about the nutritional inadequacy of plant-based diets are echoed in a recent review published by the Mayo Clinic:

> "*We found that some of these nutrients, which can have implications in neurologic disorders, anemia, bone strength and other health concerns, can be deficient in poorly planned vegan diets… Vegans may be at increased risk for deficiencies in vitamin B$_{12}$, iron, calcium, vitamin D, omega-3 fatty acids, and protein.*"[36]

Vegans have also been found to have very high rates of iodine deficiency,[37,38] a problem that could inhibit proper formation of thyroid hormones. Some studies have indicated rates of deficiency as high as 80 percent. Such a problem is especially possible in those consuming large amounts of isothiocyanate-containing *Brassica* vegetables.

Iron is yet another mineral that is known to be much more difficult to obtain from plants, and many studies show higher rates of deficiency in vegetarians and vegans.[39,40] In animal foods, iron is present in the "heme" form in which it is part of a larger molecule known as a porphyrin ring. Red blood cells carry oxygen bound to hemoglobin, a large protein composed of four subunits, each of which possesses a heme group containing iron and porphyrin ring. Because iron within this porphyrin ring has so many valuable roles in the human body, we absorb this form very avidly. In plant foods, however, the iron atom is naked, and isn't nearly as well taken up within the gut.[41] Therefore, relying on only plant foods definitely puts us at a much greater risk of iron deficiency anemia, a condition easily corrected with the heme iron present in animal meat and organs.[42] In the graphic below, you can see how drastically different the absorption of iron from animal and plant foods really is!

BIOAVAILABILITY OF IRON

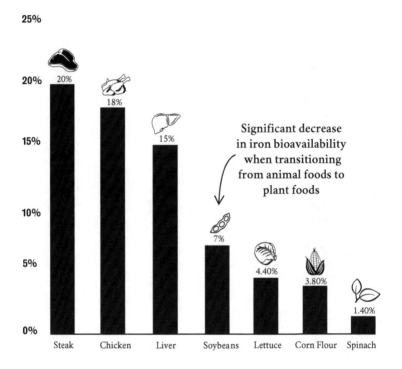

Insel, Ross, et al., *Nutrition*. Jones & Bartlett Publishers, 2010. Print

While we are talking about iron deficiency anemia, I will also add that in rare cases, such a condition may persist even in the setting of adequate iron consumption if there's a deficiency of riboflavin. As we'll see in the next section, this crucial B vitamin is only present in reasonable quantities in animal foods!

Clearly, choosing to rely on plant foods for these important minerals will invariably lead to a deficiency with many negative impacts on our health. Again, the solution is clear. Animal foods are far superior in providing us with the minerals we need to function optimally, and the phytic acid, oxalate, and fiber in plant foods only inhibit the absorption of these nutrients.

B Vitamins and Methylation

The first B vitamin that comes to mind when thinking about nutrients lacking in plants is B_{12}. This vitamin is needed for our cellular metabolism and proper cell division as it participates in the process of methylation (the movement of methyl groups between molecules within cells).

There are hundreds of methylation reactions in human biochemistry, and they all depend on a steady supply of these methyl groups from our diet to run smoothly. One of the main sources of these is folate, which exists in both plant and animal foods, but is more bioavailable in the latter. Adequate folate is essential for the formation of DNA and the synthesis of L-methylfolate, a molecule used to donate a methyl group to homocysteine during it's conversion to methionine. As it helps convert homocysteine to methionine in a reaction that also requires B_{12}, L-methylfolate is recycled to tetrahydrofolate, which is involved in the synthesis of DNA. When B_{12} levels are insufficient, however, L-methylfolate gets "trapped," and tetrahydrofolate cannot be formed, leading to inadequate levels of the building blocks for DNA and impairing normal cellular growth and division. Cells without enough B_{12} or folate can't divide properly, resulting in megaloblastic anemia, a condition in which red blood cells are much larger than normal. Deficiencies of B_{12} can also lead to neurological disease, which presents as balance issues and can progress to frank dementia.

It is important to note that homocysteine levels are known to be elevated more frequently when relying on plant-based nutrition, suggesting impaired methylation.[43] Elevated levels of this compound can indicate a deficiency in many B vitamins, including B_{12}, B_6, and folate, and have been correlated with reduced brain size in both healthy individuals and those with Alzheimer's dementia.[44] In a recent review paper on this topic, the authors stated:

> "*Vitamin B_{12} levels in the subclinical low-normal range (<250 ǫmol/L) are associated with Alzheimer's disease, vascular dementia, and Parkinson's disease.* **Vegetarianism and metformin use contribute to depressed vitamin B_{12} levels and may independently increase the risk for cognitive impairment.**"[45]

Remember in the first chapter of this book when we talked about the declining size of the human brain in the last 40,000 years? Declining levels of B_{12} and other B vitamins related to decreased consumption of animal foods may be playing a role in this unfortunate shrinkage. In an interesting study done at Oxford University, the brain size and B_{12} status of 107 elderly patients was monitored by MRI over a five-year period with striking conclusions:

"The decrease in brain volume was greater among those with lower vitamin B_{12} levels and higher plasma homocysteine and methylmalonic acid levels at baseline…Low vitamin B_{12} status should be further investigated as a modifiable cause of brain atrophy and of likely subsequent cognitive impairment in the elderly."[46]

As a whole, B vitamins appear to be less bioavailable from plants relative to animal foods. In the case of pyridoxine, or vitamin B_6, this is due to it being bound in a glycoprotein known as pyridoxine glucoside.

"The bioavailability of vitamin B_6 from animal products is quite high, reaching 100% for many foods. In general the bioavailability from plant foods is lower. The presence of fiber reduces the bioavailability by 5-10% whereas the presence of pyridoxine glucoside reduces the bioavailability by 75-80%. This glucoside is found in a variety of plant foods, with the highest content occurring in the crucifers."[47]

Well, well, well, those crazy crucifers make an appearance again, as does the notion that fiber also reduces nutrient bioavailability. I'm telling you, plants don't love us back.

Some B vitamins, like riboflavin or vitamin B2, are very hard to obtain in optimal amounts from plants alone. Riboflavin also plays a key role in the methylation process, allowing the aforementioned enzyme MTHFR to function properly to form L-methylfolate. Single nucleotide polymorphisms (SNPs) in this gene affect the enzyme-binding site for riboflavin, causing MTHFR to function more slowly. Those with "slow" variants of MTHFR can fix this by getting lots of riboflavin in their diet.[48] This allows MTHFR to function at a normal level and obviates the need for supplementation with L-methylfolate, which can have its own negative side effects.

How much riboflavin do we need to optimize methylation? No one knows for sure, but it appears to be on the order of 2-3 milligrams per day. This is an amount that is significantly greater than the currently recommended daily allowance (RDA), but good luck in getting this much bio-available riboflavin from plants! Spinach is the richest source of riboflavin in the plant world, but it has only 0.2 milligrams per 100 grams. You'd have to eat more than 3 pounds of spinach to get 3 milligrams of riboflavin! Can you imagine the gas you'd have after that or the amount of oxalates you'd be ingesting with such a mountain of this leafy green? Conversely, a savvy meat eater could obtain 3 milligrams of riboflavin in about 100 grams of liver or kidney!

In my personal experience as someone who is homozygous for the MTHFR 677 C->T polymorphism, my homocysteine levels have been as high as 13 μmol per liter during my vegan days and are now below 7 μmol per liter without L-methylfolate supplementation when I obtain adequate riboflavin from organ meats. I have observed similar patterns in my patients with MTHFR polymorphisms as well. There does not appear to be a need for supplemental L-methylfolate to obtain normalized homocysteine levels when there's enough riboflavin in the diet, but in terms of real food, we must obtain this from animal sources.

VITAMIN A

If we choose to get the majority of our food from plants, it is very likely that in addition to being depleted in minerals, we will also be short-changed in B vitamins, and the fat-soluble vitamins A and K2 as well.

"Vitamin A" from plants isn't really a vitamin at all. It's a precursor called beta-carotene that must be transformed by the enzyme BCMO into the form used in our biochemistry, known as retinol. The problem here is that this conversion isn't very efficient, and in some people with polymorphisms in BCMO, it's painfully slow.[49,50] Studies suggest that even without BCMO polymorphisms, twenty-one units of beta-carotene are needed to equal the biological value of one unit of retinol vitamin A (the form found in animal foods). Deficiencies of this nutrient are associated with night blindness, but the functions of this vitamin are numerous, and sub-optimal levels could contribute to a host of negative effects in the body.

Taking these conversion factors for beta-carotene to retinol into consideration, to obtain the recommended level of retinol in beta-carotene equivalents, 19,000 milligrams of this plant molecule would need to be consumed. That's almost a pound of oxalate-containing sweet potatoes—which are the richest source of beta-carotene—per day! Between a pound of sweet potatoes for vitamin A, and three pounds of spinach for riboflavin, how would you have time to eat anything else, much less any room in your stomach?

I hope you can see a pattern emerging here. With our human gastro-intestinal tract, it's basically impossible to consume enough plant foods to meet all of our nutritional needs, and if we try to do this, we are going to get *tons of toxins* in the process. Say it with me: "Plants are just survival foods!"

VITAMIN K

Vitamin K is another fat-soluble vitamin that exists in unique plant and animal forms. In plants, vitamin K occurs as K1 or phylloquinone. In animals, it's found as multiple menaquinones, which are named based on the length of their side chain and are collectively known as vitamin K2. You may have seen the various forms of K2 written as MK-4, MK-7, and MK-11. Menaquinones also occur in some rare fermented foods like natto, but in the West, consumption of these is quite rare.

Research on the biological activities of K1 vs. K2 reveal some intriguing differences between the plant and animal forms of this vitamin. Like beta-carotene, there are no known unique biological roles in humans for vitamin K1. Some texts claim that vitamin K1 is used in the formation of clotting factors, but vitamin K2 can serve this role as well.[51] Vitamin K2, in contrast, is known to have many distinctly important roles in our physiology, including management of proper calcium storage, bone density, and arterial health. Research comparing the health benefits of vitamin K1 vs. K2 have repeatedly demonstrated that those consuming higher levels of the latter have lower levels of heart disease and cardiovascular complications while showing no similar benefit from vitamin K1 consumption.

A well-known epidemiological investigation known as The Rotterdam Study followed 4,807 subjects and surveyed their intake of K1 and K2 for ten years.[52] The researchers recorded the incidence of several cardiovascular outcomes, including deaths due to coronary heart disease and aortic calcification. The results were striking:

> *"The relative risk of coronary heart disease mortality was reduced in the mid and upper tertiles of dietary [vitamin K2] compared to the lower tertile.* **Intake of vitamin K2 was also inversely related to all-cause mortality, and severe aortic calcification. Vitamin K1 intake was not related to any of the outcomes.** *These findings suggest that an adequate intake of menaquinone could be important for coronary heart disease prevention."*

These findings are illustrated in the visuals on the next page. As you can see from the first graphic, as levels of K2 increase in each of the three groups, death rates related to heart disease declined. Notably, levels of K2 intake in the highest tertile were still modest at 32 micrograms per day. Eating a nose-to-tail carnivore diet, one could easily obtain more than 100 micrograms of vitamin K2 daily. It would have been interesting to see how the levels of coronary heart disease death might decline even further with more robust K2 intakes like this.

CORONARY HEART DISEASE MORTALITY

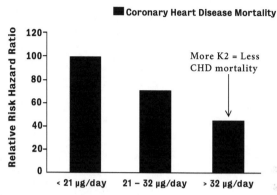

Geleijnse, JM. et al., (2004). Dietary intake of menaquinone is associated with a reduced risk of coronary heart disease: the Rotterdam Study. Journal of Nutrition, 134(11): 3100-5.

In the second graphic, the decline in levels of aortic valve calcification with increasing levels of vitamin K2 is depicted. Again, the trend is clear, showing higher levels of vitamin K2 strongly correlating with lower levels of aortic calcification and improved outcomes.

AORTIC VALVE SEVERE CALCIFICATION

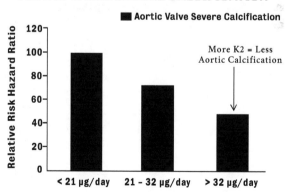

Geleijnse, JM. et al., (2004). Dietary intake of menaquinone is associated with a reduced risk of coronary heart disease: the Rotterdam Study. Journal of Nutrition, 134(11): 3100-5.

As the authors of this study point out, intake of vitamin K1 was not protective for any of the endpoints studied, suggesting that we don't convert this plant form of vitamin K into the useable form of vitamin K2 in any appreciable amount. Plant fail!

Another study of over 16,000 women who were followed for eight years showed similar results when cardiac events were compared with intake of vitamin K2:

> *"After adjustment for traditional risk factors and dietary factors, we observed an inverse association between vitamin K2 and risk of heart disease with a Hazard Ratio of 0.91 per 10 microgram per day of vitamin K2 intake. **This association was mainly due to vitamin K2 subtypes MK-7, MK-8 and MK-9. Vitamin K1 intake was not significantly related to heart diseae**...A high intake of menaquinones, especially MK-7, MK-8 and MK-9, could protect against heart disease."* [53]

What types of food were those people eating in these studies? Animal foods! Based on this data, every 10 micrograms of vitamin K2 consumed daily resulted in a 10 percent decline in the risk of heart disease. A single egg yolk or an ounce of liver has almost twice this amount. In Chapter Eleven, we'll thoroughly debunk the notion that animal foods contribute to heart disease, but these studies stand as a strong testament to the fact that consumption of animal foods is often associated with *lower* rates of cardiovascular disease, and *consumption of nutrients uniquely present in these foods is crucial for optimal health of our arteries.*

Sadly, we'll have to look hard to find resources showing the vitamin K2 content in foods, because for some crazy reason, the USDA has only ever measured vitamin K1. Animals, like humans, use K2 preferentially, and the richest sources of this nutrient are animal meats, organs, and eggs. Foods like liver are a particularly rich source. Natto is a dish made from fermented soybeans that has a good amount of vitamin K2, but in light of the numerous downsides to soy, I believe animal foods are much better sources of this vitamin. In Chapter Twelve, we'll talk all about what to eat on a carnivore diet and how to get a substantial amount of vitamin K2 in animal foods.

PROTEIN

No discussion of the relative nutritional value of plant vs. animal foods would be complete without consideration of protein. Though proponents of plant-based diets will claim that we can get enough protein by eating only vegetables, these claims don't hold water when examined carefully.

The best measure of protein quality is a score called the **digestible indispensable amino acid score,** or the DIAAS. This index gives us a sense of how much of protein in a food can actually be used. When comparing the DIAAS scores of animal and plant products, as depicted in the following graph, it's quickly evident that plant protein is a weakling!

BIOAVAILABILITY OF PROTEIN

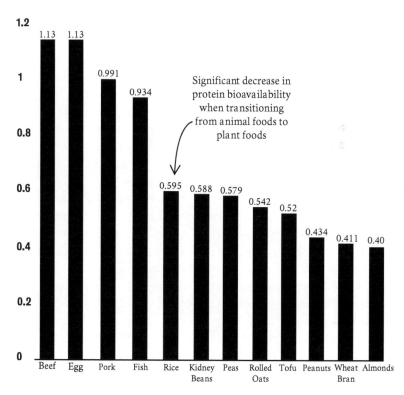

Mathai, J., Liu, Y., & Stein, H. (2017). Values for digestible indispensable amino acid scores (DIAAS) for some dairy and plant proteins may better describe protein quality than values calculated using the concept for protein digestibility-corrected amino acid scores (PDCAAS). *British Journal of Nutrition,* 117(4), 490-499. doi:10.1017/S0007114517000125

It's not only about how much protein is in a food, it's also about how bioavailable this protein is, and plant-derived protein is nowhere near as useable as animal protein on a gram-per-gram basis. If we want to avoid osteoporosis and maintain the muscle mass that is critical for insulin sensitivity throughout our life, high-quality animal protein is a crucial component of our diet. There are examples of heavily-muscled body builders who don't consume animal foods, but in order to maintain this physique, they must ingest tons of highly processed plant protein powders, with all of their heavy metal contaminants, lectins, oxalates, and other anti-nutrients. These vegan proteins are less effective at stimulating muscle growth and repair due to their lower leucine content, and they also use much more water to grow ingredients than an equivalent amount of protein from beef. Whether we are trying to look good at the beach or maintain the muscle we have for optimal longevity, animal protein is clearly superior to plant protein in every way. End of story.

OMEGA-3 FATTY ACIDS

There's a lot of buzz about omega-3s these days, and for good reason. For starters, they've got a really cool name. Doesn't "omega-3" sound like an Avengers superhero? In many ways, these essential fats *are* superheroes. Because we can't synthesize them from scratch, we must obtain them from our diets, and they play vital roles in the membrane of every cell in our body. Omega-3 fatty acids are especially enriched in our brains, with DHA making up 90 percent of this lipid pool. Deficiencies have been associated with depression, memory and attention deficits, fatigue, and infertility.[54,55,56-59]

Plants do contain omega-3 fatty acids, but much like the case of beta-carotene and vitamin K, these essential nutrients are found only in their precursor form in these foods. Humans don't use the plant form of omega-3—alpha linolenic acid (ALA)—in their biochemistry, but must convert it to the usable omega-3 fatty acids eicosapentaenoic acid (EPA), docosapentaenoic acid (DPA), and docosahexaenoic acid (DHA). Yes, vegetarian and vegans are also known to have suboptimal levels of omega-3 fatty acids.[60]

The problem with trying to obtain omega-3 fatty acids from plants is that this conversion of ALA to EPA and DHA is exceedingly poor. In one study that involved the feeding of 30 grams of ALA-rich flax seeds, or 6 grams of pure ALA, to healthy subjects, there was zero increase in EPA and DHA levels. Zero increase! The authors did note, however, that all those flax seeds caused some serious GI upset. Lignans from flax are also known to be endocrine disruptors, and I'd be willing to bet that if these researchers had looked at hormone levels, they would have seen negative changes in both men and women:

> *"No significant increase was detected in plasma eicosapentaenoic acid (EPA) or docosahexaenoic acid (DHA) levels in any of the flax-fed groups...Subjects in all of the groups exhibited some symptoms of gastro-intestinal discomfort during the early stages of the study...compliance was a problem in the whole flaxseed group."*

The best way to ensure optimal levels of omega-3 fatty acids is to obtain pre-formed EPA, DPA, and DHA from animal foods. In Chapter Twelve, we'll talk all about what animal foods I recommend to obtain highly bioavailable sources of these omega-3 fatty acids. Hint: it's not fish oil pills; these are likely to be highly oxidized!

To summarize this whole discussion regarding the relative nutritional content of plant vs. animal foods, I've included a graphic comparing examples of each. I think that by glancing at this chart, it quickly becomes evident what the real superfoods are!

PER 100 g	Blueberries	Kale	Ribeye	Beef Liver	Fish Roe	Egg Yolk
Vitamin A Retinol	0	0	5 mcg	4968 mcg	90 mcg	191 mcg
Thiamin (B1)	trace	0.1 mg	0.1 mg	0.2 mg	0.3 mg	0.2 mg
Riboflavin (B2)	trace	0.3 mg	0.2 mg	2.8 mg	0.7 mg	0.5 mg
Niacin (B3)	0.4 mg	1.2 mg	3.6 mg	13.2 mcg	1.8 mg	0.02 mg
Vitamin B6	0.05 mg	0.1 mg	0.4 mg	1.1 mg	0.2 mg	0.4 mg
Biotin (B7)	0.5 mg	0	trace	42 mcg	100 mcg	55 mcg
Folate (B9)	6 mcg	62 mcg	3 mcg	290 mcg	80 mcg	146 mcg
Vitamin B12	0 mcg	0 mcg	3 mcg	59.3 mcg	10 mcg	2 mcg
Vitamin C*	9.7 mg	93 mg	3.5 mg	25 mg	16 mg	0
Vitamin D	0	0	4 IU	49 IU	484 IU	218 IU
Vitamin E (mg)	0.6 mg	0.7 mg	0.1 mg	0.4 mg	7 mg	2.6 mg
Vitamin K2	0	0	15 mcg	263 mcg	1 mcg	34 mcg
Calcium	6 mg	254 mg	6 mg	5 mg	22 mg	129 mg
Choline	6 mg	0.4 mg	57 mg	333 mg	335 mg	820 mg
Copper	0.05 mg	0.15 mg	0.1 mg	9.8 mg	0.1 mg	0.1 mg
Iron	0.3 mg	1.6 mg	2.6 mg	4.9 mg	0.6 mg	2.7 mg
Magnesium	6 mg	33 mg	24 mg	18 mg	20 mg	5 mg
Phosphorous	12 mg	55 mg	210 mg	387 mg	402 mg	390 mg
Potassium	77 mg	348 mg	357 mg	313 mg	221 mg	109 mg
Selenium	0.1 mcg	0.9 mcg	24 mcg	40 mcg	40 mcg	56 mcg
Zinc	0.2 mg	0.4 mg	7.8 mg	4 mg	1 mg	2.3 mg

This chart does not take nutrient bioavailability into consideration. Studies show that b-complex vitamins and minerals have lower bioavailability in plant foods.

Murphy, Suzanne P., et al., (2003). Nutritional Importance of Animal Source Foods. *The Journal of Nutrition*, 133(11), 3932S-3935S.
Descalzo, AM, et al., (2007). Antioxidant status and odour profile in fresh beef from pasture or grain-fed cattle. *Meat Science*, 75(2): 299-307.

WHY DO VEGAN DIETS HELP SOME PEOPLE?

This is probably a great time for a bit of full authenticity and honesty on my part. Are you guys ready for a bomb? I used to be a vegan! And not just any vegan—a raw vegan! Go big or go home, right? I, too, was seduced by plant-based propaganda. It was a long time ago, fifteen years to be exact, and it didn't work well for me at all. I lost twenty-five pounds of muscle over the six-month period that I ate nothing but raw fruits and vegetables, and I looked like a skeleton. People would gently tell me I was too skinny all the time, but I was too entrenched in the ideology to hear these warnings. I also had horrible GI side effects, including bad gas and constant bloating. Laughably, some vegan proponents today argue that we should embrace the increased flatulence that invariably accompanies plant-based diets. The poor souls I shared an office with during my raw vegan days would beg to differ, as would many who have experienced the gas and bloating that often comes with plant-based or high-fiber diets.

It is important to acknowledge, however, that vegan diets do appear to help some people, at least in the short term. One key feature that both a vegan diet and the carnivore diet share is *elimination* of certain foods, and it is this elimination which can be incredibly powerful. The mistake in judgment that is often made with regard to plant-based diets, however, is that it is the elimination of animal meat that produces the positive changes. Thousands of stories of those finding vastly improved health on strict carnivore diets, or paleo and ketogenic diets that include meat, argue strongly against this supposition. In an overzealous attempt to demonize animal foods, many overlook the fact that a vegan diet often excludes mainstream dairy and processed foods. We can't go blaming meat for the damage that the bread, sugar, and junk food have done!

At our core, we are humans who became what we are today because we have been eating animals for 3 million years. Access to large amounts of animals foods allowed our brains to grow and our species to thrive over the last 2 million years. From an evolutionary perspective, it makes absolutely zero sense that animal foods would suddenly become bad for us, or bad for some people but not for others. Plant-based diets work in the short term for select people because they have eliminated some foods that were triggering their immune system. In the long term, however, plant-based diets fail due to lack of bioavailable nutrients or because of the activation of the immune system by many of the plant toxins discussed in the first section of this book.

Plant-based diets may also help with diabetes and weight loss in some people because they are so calorically diluted. When eating only fruits and vegetables, it's difficult to get enough calories to meet our basic metabolic needs. Primates must spend nearly all of their waking hours chewing plant matter and must ingest kilogram-quantities of it on a daily basis. A caloric deficit may sound like a good thing for someone who is overweight, but for those who are looking to maintain or gain lean muscle mass, plant-based diets are a nightmare, as I found out first hand. Long term calorie-limited diets also invariably result in disruption of hormonal balance, and due to the poor bioavailability of protein in plant foods, many of those who use these diets lose valuable lean muscle mass in the process as well.

Independent of the foods used, creating a caloric deficit in humans turns on genes that improve insulin sensitivity and inflammation subsequently decreases.[61] Mark Haub, a professor at Kansas State University, used a calorie-deficient diet composed entirely of Twinkies to lose twenty-seven pounds over a ten-week period; but would anyone argue that this is a viable long-term strategy or a healthy way to lose weight? Clearly, this type of diet would result in a myriad of nutrient deficiencies and a catastrophic collapse in health if followed over an extended period of time. All too often, this is the pattern that is observed with plant-based diets unless extensive supplementation is used. Many of those who try vegan diets notice improvements in the first few months to years, likely due to the elimination of processed foods and sugars. But down the road, they are afflicted with significant health issues, malnutrition, and hormonal disturbances.

The other question that often arises is why some people appear to be thriving on plant-based diets. The media would have us believe that jettisoning animal foods has helped athletes achieve better performance, but these claims are incredibly misleading. Stories of improvements in athletic performance when going plant-based often fail to highlight the fact that, prior to this transition, most of these athletes were eating diets full of processed food. Any intentional dietary choice is going to be better than a standard American diet loaded with junk food!

Many professional sports players claim to be following a diet that is "more plant-based," but it's difficult to know exactly what they are eating. The rates of injury among vegan athletes appear to be significantly greater than those that still eat meat. In just this past year, many of the athletes originally lauded for adopting plant-based diets have *returned to eating meat, while others had season-ending injuries.* These include tennis star Novak Djokovic; basketball players Kyrie Irving, Demarcus Cousins, and Lauri Markkannen; football quarterbacks Andrew Luck and Cam Newton; English freerunner Tim Shieff; and baseball pitcher CC

Sabathia. Tom Brady is often championed as being "plant-based," but he has clearly stated that he wisely includes meat in his diet. There are also many examples of elite athletes going vegan only to see their performance decline markedly, often leading them to early retirement. At the highest levels of competition, plant-based diets simply do not allow for optimal performance or durability in athletes. Case closed.

So, why do plant-based diets work for some people? It's not because of omitting meat from their diets, but because of the other junk they leave out. And long term, these diets simply do not work for humans.

THE PROBLEM WITH THE NOTION OF BIO-INDIVIDUALITY

Another manner in which some seek to reconcile the evidence that people appear to improve on both plant-based and animal-based diets is with appeals to bio-individuality. This is the idea that, because we are all genetically unique, vegan diets work for some people and carnivore, ketogenic, or paleo diets work for others. Though I won't dismiss the concept of bio-individuality outright, I believe this notion has been overly generalized and incorrectly applied. When we examine the genetic variation across humans, we discover that we're all actually much more similar than we are different. Let me explain.

There are two pieces to the bio-individuality equation: biochemistry and immune tolerance. Let's talk about biochemistry first. At our core, all humans share essentially the same biochemistry. We all need the same vitamins and minerals to help our internal machinery run optimally. We can think of human biochemistry like the inside of an old-fashioned watch, full of little gears, levers, and springs working elegantly together. If any of these parts are missing, the system begins to break down, and the machine slows down or stops working entirely. This is essentially what happens when one of the micronutrients we need is missing or is present in inadequate amounts. The gears, levers, and springs of our biochemistry start to turn slower, or can't turn at all, and our cellular processes function sub-optimally. Though there appears to be some variation between humans in terms of how much of any micronutrient we need to function well, these differences are quite small, and most of us need about the same amounts of vitamins, minerals, and fatty acids to allow our beautiful internal workings to flow smoothly. Plants simply don't match up to animals when it comes to providing the nutrients our inner machine needs to run optimally, and there is zero evidence that certain people are better adapted to receiving the nutrients they need from plants. Across the board, for all humans, animals are simply the best source of what we need to crush life day-in and day-out.

The second piece of this equation is immune tolerance, and this does appear to be quite variable between individuals, but not in the way most people imagine. In the last chapter, we discussed the plinko concept of inflammation and chronic disease. I suggested it is our individual genetic susceptibilities that determine how we get sick when inflammation arises. We all have our unique Achilles' heel, and these are brought to light when the immune system is triggered. I believe that a nose-to-tail carnivore diet is our fundamental ancestral diet, and that the vast majority of humans on the planet will thrive eating this way. I also believe that some people will be able to tolerate more plant foods than others, and that different plant foods will be triggering for different people. For those with autoimmune illness or another chronic disease, a full carnivore diet might be the best option, but for those who don't seem to be triggered by some less-toxic plant foods, these might be included in the diet from time to time. This latter type of diet could be thought of as carnivore-ish. We'll discuss all of the nuances of both carnivore and carnivore-ish type diets in Chapter Twelve, where you can also find my take on the spectrum of plant toxicity.

OUR BRAINS DON'T LIE—ANIMAL VS. PLANT FOODS

We've talked about a ton of studies in this chapter, but there's one more that just must be shared. In this experiment, researchers showed images of animal foods like meat and fish to vegetarians and meat eaters.[62] They then assayed both with subjective measures like the desire to eat, and objective measures like neural responses in the brain. The latter is done by measuring event-related potentials, or ERP's. I know, it's a lot of scientific jargon, but it basically can be thought of this way: when you see something that interests you, like food you want to eat, an attractive person, or a piece of art you appreciate, your brain responds positively, and this can be measured by looking at ERP's. Here's what they found:

*"In vegetarians, meat and fish dishes elicited lower desire to eat, pleasantness, and arousal during each condition as compared to both omnivores and vegetarian food. In contrast with the subjective data, **no group differences were observed in any of the ERP measures**, suggesting that similar neural processing of food-cues occurred in vegetarians and omnivores both during passive viewing and cognitive reappraisal... Overall, our findings suggest that, in vegetarians, aversion towards non-vegetarian food prevails at the subjective level and is consistent with their*

personal beliefs. ***In contrast, at the neural level, the intrinsic motivational salience of this type of food is preserved.***"

Basically, these investigators found that, while vegetarians have an aversion to meat at a subjective level, their brains still love it and respond positively at a more primal level. I find this to be pretty irrefutable proof that at a fundamental level, humans are programmed to eat meat! Though we can construct narratives around this and tell ourselves that we don't like meat or that it's not good for us, our brains and bodies still know it's incredibly valuable and respond to it positively.

WRAPPING UP

This chapter has been a doozie! I hope it's now clear that animal foods are the true superfoods in every way. They contain many nutrients vital for human health that don't occur in substantial amounts in plant foods, and they are much better sources of minerals, B vitamins, fat-soluble vitamins, omega-3 fatty acids, and protein—a clean sweep! As we've seen repeatedly throughout this chapter, those that rely on plant foods to obtain the majority of their nutrition often develop multiple nutritional deficiencies, unless they are supplementing heavily with synthetic vitamins and processed proteins. I've said it before, and I'll keep saying it: plant foods are survival foods at best. The more high-quality animal foods we eat, the more bioavailable nutrients we will receive, the fewer plant toxins we ingest, and the more we will thrive. In other words, animal foods win by knockout!

In the next chapter, we'll continue on our debunking crusade and directly attack the notion that we need fiber or plant foods for a healthy gut. Things are about to get even more interesting!

CHAPTER NINE

MYTH II
FIBER IS NECESSARY FOR A HEALTHY GUT

In the last chapter, we witnessed a one-sided battle between animal and plant foods for the throne of nutritional superiority, and animal foods won by knockout. The next series of chapters will continue to address many of the unfounded criticisms leveled at animal foods in a veritable buffet of myth busting. This chapter will focus on myths surrounding the gut, including fiber, short-chain fatty acids, and the microbiome. Prepare for the fallacies to crumble before our eyes.

The first question I usually get when I tell people that I don't eat any plants is "How do you ever poop without fiber?" I'll save you all the photographic proof of the heavenly quality of my daily bowel movements; you'll just have to take my word for it. You could also listen to the thousands of reports from other carnivores who have experienced improvements in gastrointestinal function with this way of eating. You don't need fiber to poop or to have a healthy gut, trust me. At a recent talk I gave, I asked more than 250 people there who had tried the carnivore diet if they had experienced any improvements in their bowel habits. Ninety-nine percent of the hands in the audience went up!

Though it seems to have nearly become canon within the medical world, the notion that humans need fiber from plants to have healthy bowel function is simply false. Examination of the literature regarding fiber and constipation quickly illustrates that plant fiber does not lead to better outcomes in patients with this condition.

When looking at these studies, it's important to understand that constipation is more than just infrequent bowel movements. Though this is one of its symptoms, constipation is also characterized by hard stools, which can be painful and difficult to pass and is often associated with the need for laxative use. Though studies with fiber may show an increase in stool frequency or volume, which often leads to even greater pain, they do **not** show any benefits in stool consistency, ease of passage, bleeding, the use of laxatives, or discomfort when having a bowel movement. Eating fiber causes those with constipation to have larger bowel movements because there's more material to excrete, but it does not improve any of the unpleasant symptoms of constipation. In fact, it often worsens them. Ouch!

If our stools are painful and difficult to pass, why would we want to increase the frequency and volume? What we really want are bowel movements that are easier to pass, less painful, and require no use of laxatives, and fiber has never been proven to achieve this.[1]

A review of five studies encompassing 195 patients demonstrated the lack of benefit for fiber in relieving pain or other symptoms of constipation:

> *"Dietary fiber intake can obviously increase stool frequency in patients with constipation.* **It does not obviously improve stool consistency, treatment success, laxative use and painful defecation symptoms were reported by several studies.** *Because data was presented by different methods, only painful defecation was analyzed, and results showed that there was* **no significant difference between dietary fiber and placebo groups.***"* [2]

Do we really want to give people with painful stools more of them? That doesn't sound like a good intervention to me. Studies with fiber supplementation in children have shown a similar lack of improvement in the symptoms of constipation, and in one study investigators compared high- and low-fiber groups concluding:

> *"Follow-up at six and twelve months showed…no significant benefit in terms of a reduction in laxative use or increased stool frequency associated with additional fiber intake."* [3]

These studies fly in the face of conventional wisdom, but they are only the beginning. Not only has the addition of plant fiber been shown to have no benefit in constipation, *removal of fiber* has been shown to *improve* constipation. Yes, you read that correctly, research has shown that kicking fiber to the curb can lead to complete resolution of constipation.

In an interventional study, people with constipation were divided into three separate groups who ingested high, low, and zero fiber diets. After a period of both one and six months, each group was examined for stool frequency, difficulty in the evacuation of stools, anal bleeding, abdominal bloating, and abdominal pain. The results were striking:

> *"Forty one patients who completely stopped fiber intake had their bowel frequency increased from one motion in 3.75 d ($\pm$ 1.59 d) to one motion in 1.0 d ($\pm$ 0.00 d) (P < 0.001)...There was no change in the frequency of bowel movement for patients who continued with high dietary fiber intake...There was also a difference between the groups in the proportion of patients with associated symptoms. For symptoms of bloating, all of those on a high-fiber diet continued to be symptomatic, while only 31.3% in the reduced fiber group and none of the no fiber group had symptoms (0%, P < 0.001). With regards to straining, all those on a no fiber diet no longer had to strain to pass stools. Symptoms of abdominal pain only improved in patients who stopped fiber completely while those who continued on a high-fiber diet or reduced-fiber diet did not show any improvement. In addition, those on a no-dietary-fiber diet no longer had symptoms of anal bleeding."* [4]

The results of this study showed that when fiber was completely eliminated, 100 percent of those with constipation *had a complete resolution of all of their symptoms*. How anyone can claim that plant fiber benefits constipation is beyond me. Because of this study and many others like it, I would go even further to suggest that plant fiber is worsening constipation in many individuals. Someone please hand me a microphone because I need to drop it right now!

SMALL INTESTINAL BACTERIAL OVERGROWTH (SIBO)

There are multiple mechanisms by which fiber might worsen constipation, but in many people with imbalances in the gastrointestinal microbiome, fiber appears to promote overgrowth of the wrong types of bacteria in the small intestine. This is a condition known as small intestinal bacterial overgrowth (SIBO). This disorder is often associated with constipation, gas, bloating, intermittent diarrhea, and painful stools, and in clinical practice, the most efficacious intervention for SIBO is often a removal of fiber from the diet. Other diets, like low FODMAP or the specific carbohydrate diet (SCD), can help but are not as effective as eliminating all fiber. Antibiotics and anti-bacterial herbs are often tried for this condition, but these fail most of the time, with relapse rates for SIBO being greater than 75 percent unless dietary changes are implemented.

At its root, SIBO appears to be a problem with gut motility. Normally, peristaltic waves pass through the length of our small bowel and sweep down towards the colon, preventing overgrowth of bacteria in the upper portions of our digestive tract. These waves are known as the **migrating motor complex** and occur every 45–180 minutes between meals. In patients with SIBO, the migrating motor complex appears to be hypoactive, allowing the populations of bacteria in the colon to move up into the small intestine, leading to an imbalance and a loss of diversity there.[5]

When these invading bacteria overgrow in the small bowel, they can ferment the plant fibers we eat, which causes painful gas and bloating. We can attempt to combat this dysbiosis with antibiotics, but the high relapse rates for SIBO suggest that until we fix the motility issues, overgrowth will return again within a few weeks.

In SIBO, removing plant fiber from the diet is a powerful first step for treating this condition. By not providing the overgrown bugs in the small bowel with fiber, they may gradually recede back to the colon where they belong, and the dysbiosis observed in this condition appears to improve. There's still much to learn about SIBO, but avoiding plant fiber can definitely provide symptomatic improvement.

Since you've made it this far in the book and are now a keen medical detective, I know you are already asking the two most important questions with regard to SIBO: "what has caused the underlying motility issue and how can we correct this?" No one really knows the answers here, but I believe that at its core, SIBO is an autoimmune condition in which the nerves responsible for the migrating motor complex become damaged.

As we've discussed previously, I believe that most autoimmune disease begins with damage to the gut and subsequent triggering of the large collection of immune cells there. We know that many things can damage the gut and initiate this process, but I think food, and specifically plants, are the main offenders. From our previous discussions of lectins, we also know that there is compelling evidence that plant toxins can affect the nervous system in a negative fashion, and it seems quite plausible that these compounds could lead to impairment of the migrating motor complex.

I believe plants are triggering most of the autoimmune illness we see today, including SIBO, psychiatric disease, and even skin issues like eczema and psoriasis. From this perspective, the fundamental way to treat SIBO is to remove the foods that are damaging the gut—which will allow it to heal and will allow the immune system to gradually calm down.

WHY YOU DON'T WANT A WEAK COLON WALL

So far, we've seen that the research does not support a beneficial role for fiber in constipation and that *removal of plant fiber clearly benefits those with this issue.* Another condition for which fiber is sometimes touted as beneficial is diverticulosis, but as we'll see, this is yet another illness where the mainstream thinking is very wrong. Diverticulosis is the pathological process that occurs when the innermost layer of the colon (the submucosa) protrudes through the outer muscular layer, forming small pockets that pouch out from the large bowel.

Diverticulosis is quite common in Western societies, occurring in more than half of the population in the United States and Canada by the sixth decade of life.[6] It increases the risk of gastrointestinal bleeding, which can be a life threatening issue. Diverticuli can also become infected and occluded, causing *diverticulitis.* Such a condition can lead to rupturing of the colon with resulting sepsis or more severe complications and, thereby, require the need for bowel resection. Basically, diverticulosis is not something you want, and it is not a normal part of healthy aging.

We can thank Dr. Denis Burkitt for many of the mainstream misconceptions about fiber and its role in diverticulosis. In the 1970s, he suggested that the high rates of this disease in Western populations were due to lack of fiber in the diet—based on his observation that rates of this condition were much lower in the high-fiber-consuming peoples of rural Africa.[7] As we know, *it's quite dangerous to infer causation from observed correlation,* but this notion gained widespread acceptance for many years—and to this day remains entrenched in the minds of many clinicians and patients alike. When controlled studies were later done examining this relationship, fiber did not demonstrate a protective role in the occurrence of diverticulosis. Furthermore, as with constipation, some studies suggested possible harm.

Studies of diverticulosis incidence are often done by surveying those who are undergoing a colonoscopy. They are questioned in regard to what they eat, and their responses are correlated with evidence of diverticular disease when the inside of the colon is visualized. In two such investigations, the results of colonoscopy from a total of 3,950 patients in Asia showed no benefit to consuming a higher level of fiber—or fruits and vegetables—in regard to the incidence of diverticulosis.[8,9] Even more striking were the results of a similar study on 2,014 patients, which showed an *increased* degree of diverticulosis when patients were eating more fiber:

> "High intake of fiber **did not** reduce the prevalence of diverticulosis. Instead, **the quartile with the highest fiber intake had a greater prevalence of diverticulosis than the lowest.** Risk increased when calculated based on intake of total fiber, fiber from grains, soluble fiber, and insoluble fiber. Constipation was not a risk factor. Compared to individuals with <7 bowel movements per week, individuals with > 15 bowel movements per week had a 70% greater risk for diverticulosis. **Neither physical inactivity nor intake of fat or red meat was associated with diverticulosis… A high-fiber diet and increased frequency of bowel movements are associated with greater, rather than lower, prevalence of diverticulosis.** Hypotheses regarding risk factors for asymptomatic diverticulosis should be reconsidered."[10,11]

It's interesting to see here that having more bowel movements, presumably associated with more fiber in the diet, was also associated with a greater incidence of diverticulosis, and that neither fat nor red meat consumption increased risk. This is an epidemiological study, so we can't infer causation between fiber and diverticulosis, but it's quite clear that fiber doesn't protect against this condition.

If it's not a lack of fiber or constipation driving diverticulosis, then what is causing this pathology? Some have hypothesized that increased pressure in the colon might cause this illness, but this seems unlikely as diverticuli can be found on the right side of the colon, which is low in pressure. The most compelling theory of diverticulosis suggests that it may actually be *inflammatory* in nature:

> "There is some evidence that low-grade chronic inflammation is present in subjects with diverticula, which is the forerunner of acute diverticulitis. This hypothesis is strengthened by early reports that anti-inflammatory mucosal agents such as mesalamine and immune process regulators such as probiotics may improve diverticulitis."[12]

If diverticulosis is inflammatory in nature, what could be causing the inflammation? Wouldn't it be intriguing, and a bit scary, if the reason plant fiber has been associated with higher rates of diverticulosis is because of inflammation associated with the consumption of plants? As we've seen, diverticulosis is incredibly common and increases in incidence with age. There must be some trigger that many are exposed to which is leading to the gut inflammation that precedes this condition. My money is on this trigger being plants with the many ways that they can damage our gastrointestinal tracts, as we've discussed previously.

Before we move on to the next section, I'll add that although there is some evidence that fiber may be beneficial for diverticul*itis*, the evidence is quite mixed.[13] The authors of a recent meta-analysis examine this data and summarize their findings as follows:

> *"High-quality evidence for a high-fibre diet in the treatment of diverticular disease is lacking, and most recommendations are based on inconsistent evidence."*[13]

Diverticulitis is also a completely different entity from diverticulosis, with the former being an acute infectious process and the latter appearing to be related to chronic inflammation. It's also clear that the absolute best way to avoid diverticulitis is to not get diverticulosis. At the end of the day, however, if you already have diverticulosis, there's no clear evidence that fiber is going to decrease your risk of progressing to diverticulitis, and certainly no evidence that eliminating plant fiber increases this risk.

FIBER AND COLON CANCER

So fiber doesn't help with diverticulosis or constipation, and it may actually worsen these conditions in some people. But there must be some evidence for benefits from fiber in other diseases, right? Well, I wouldn't hold your breath here.

Perhaps the other most common misconception about fiber is that it lowers the risk of colon cancer. Sadly, this has *been repeatedly proven to not be the case*. Some studies have even suggested an increased risk of pre-cancerous growths, known as adenomas, when fiber supplements are used. When thinking about the research that has been done on fiber and cancer, we must be careful to not be fooled once again by epidemiology. What we will quickly see when comparing types of research is that while observational trials may show an association between fiber intake and better outcomes, this is likely due to healthy user bias, and interventional trials paint a very different picture.

In 1999–2000 there were two such landmark interventional trials published in the very prestigious *New England Journal of Medicine* that looked at the effect of fiber on the incidence of pre-cancerous adenoma growth. In the first of these, 1,905 men and women with a known history of recently diagnosed colonic adenomas, also known as polyps, were divided into two groups. One group followed a low-fat, high-fiber diet with at least 18 grams of fiber per 1,000 calories eaten, and three-and-a-half servings of fruits and vegetables daily. The other group continued on their standard lower-fiber diet. Both groups were re-assessed for the recurrence of colonic adenomas at their next colonoscopy, which occurred within the following one to four years. I imagine researchers were sure they would see a difference between the two groups, but their findings were quite the opposite. They concluded:

> *"The rate of recurrence of large adenomas (with a maximal diameter of at least 1 cm) and advanced adenomas did not differ significantly between the two groups. Adopting a diet that is low in fat and high in fiber, fruits, and vegetables* **does not influence the risk of recurrence of colorectal adenomas***."*[14]

As these investigators were left scratching their heads, another group of researchers tried a similar experiment with 1,429 men and women who also had a recent history of colorectal adenomas. Half of the participants in this study received a high-dose fiber supplement containing 13.5 grams per day of wheat bran, and the other half received a lower 2 grams per day dose, with monitoring for adenoma recurrence by colonoscopy after about three years. The results were similarly dismal for fiber and provided no evidence of any difference between these two groups.[15] Strike two for fiber in pre-cancerous polyp prevention!

As if these two studies weren't convincing enough, researchers seemed determined to show that higher fiber diets could be beneficial for colon cancer prevention, and in 2007, a third study was published with similar design.[16] This study divided about 2,000 men and women with recently diagnosed colorectal polyps into either a low-fat, high-fiber diet group (18g fiber per 1000cal daily; 3.5 servings fruits and vegetables daily) or a standard diet group and followed them for four years. When there was no evidence displaying benefits from fiber at the end of this time, the investigators chose to follow both groups for another four years—with the hope that the findings would be different. However, after *eight years* of higher-fiber intervention, the results still did not reveal any benefit of fiber in colon cancer prevention:

"There were no significant intervention-control group differences in the relative risk for recurrence of an advanced adenoma or multiple adenomas… This study failed to show any effect of a low-fat, high-fiber, high-fruit and -vegetable eating pattern on adenoma recurrence even with 8 years of follow-up."

Strike three! Fiber is out of the colon cancer prevention game!

Before we move on to fiber's other disappointing showings, there's one more trial I want to tell you about. This one actually showed that fiber supplements might worsen colonic adenoma recurrence![17] This study also looked at people with a history of polyps, but it had three groups. The first group used a fiber supplement with 2.5 grams of isphagula (similar to psyllium husks or Metamucil), the second group was given 2 grams of calcium, and the third group was a control group given a placebo. In the isphagula group, there was actually a significant **increase** in the recurrence of adenomas. Still think that psyllium in your cabinet is a good idea?

TYPES OF FIBER

Let's take a moment to learn some fiber terminology that will make many of our discussions in this chapter a bit easier to understand. At a molecular level, plant fibers are chains of sugar molecules (polysaccharides) that can't be broken down by our digestion and don't have any nutritional value to humans directly. They pass through our stomach and end up in our small intestines intact. Then they are either broken down by bacteria or pass through us and out in the stool unchanged. Technically, plant fiber is composed of both soluble and insoluble molecules. These terms refer to the ability of the polysaccharide molecules to be dissolved in water. Soluble fibers—like pectin, beta-glucan, and gums—dissolve in water, while insoluble fibers—like cellulose, hemicellulose, and lignans—do not. Psyllium and isphagula are examples of soluble fiber, and wheat bran is a commonly used insoluble fiber.

Both soluble and insoluble fiber can be used by the bacteria living in our gastrointestinal tract to produce short-chain fatty acids (SCFAs), which are used as an energy source by colonic epithelial cells. The best known short-chain fatty acid is butyrate, but many others including acetate, isobutyrate, isovalerate, and propionate are also produced by our gut bacteria. Later on in this chapter, we'll debunk the common notion that plant fiber is the only way we can make butyrate or other short-chain fatty acids.

FIBER CONTINUES TO STRIKE OUT

Surely fiber has been shown to improve other measures of health like blood sugar control, right? Yet again, fiber's performance here is lackluster when put to the test in interventional studies. In the OptiFit Trial, 180 men and women with diabetes and pre-diabetes were given either 15 grams of insoluble fiber with a high-fiber diet or a placebo with a standard diet for one year. At the end of this time, multiple measurements of blood sugar control and diabetes severity were checked. Though HgbA1c was slightly lower in the fiber group, there were no significant differences noted in all the other measures of glucose sensitivity and glucose control, leading the authors to conclude that there was "no evidence for a beneficial effect of insoluble fiber on glucose metabolism."[18]

Plant fiber also usually comes as a package deal with more carbohydrates, which are almost certain to result in worse glycemic control. Stuffing diabetics full of fiber supplements doesn't seem to accomplish much, especially when the real issue is correctable by simply lowering overall carbohydrate intake. To make matters worse, fiber has also been shown to interfere with both hormonal metabolism (testosterone, estrogen, progesterone, LH, FSH) and nutrient absorption, so adding lots of fiber supplements or increasing plant fiber in the diet will likely have other negative health consequences.

Remember phytic acid from the last chapter? Foods rich in plant fiber are full of it, and numerous studies have demonstrated that plant-based diets often lead to deficiency due to decreased absorption of minerals. In a review article examining the effects of dietary fiber and phytic acid on mineral bioavailability, the authors state:

> "The capacity of dietary fiber to bind polyvalent mineral ions [Zn, Ca, Mg, Se, Fe] may also impart a **negative effect on the bioavailability of some nutrients....** In effect, the capacity of different fiber-rich vegetables to bind and hold metal ions on their surfaces and, thus, modify the balance of these cations can be attributed to some of the substances that make up their dietary fiber." [19]

Within this review, the author cites many studies which show that both soluble and insoluble fiber, as well as phytic acid, bind to minerals and negatively affect their absorption.[20,21,22-25]

In another epidemiological study of healthy and diabetic women, there was a strong correlation between fiber intake and lower blood levels of zinc, a mineral crucial for proper hormonal balance and the functioning of hundreds of enzymes in the human body. The researchers who conducted this study stated:

> "*Healthy and diabetic women consume phytic acid in amounts that are **likely to decrease the bioavailability of dietary zinc.** Recommendations to consume greater amounts of dietary fiber, much of which is associated with phytate, **increase the risk of zinc deficiency.**"*[26]

Fiber and associated plant compounds are robbing us of valuable minerals. Doesn't this cast a shadow on the mainstream recommendations to consume fiber liberally?

The downsides of fiber don't stop there, however. Increased consumption has also been associated with negative changes in hormone levels in women, possibly leading to an *increased risk of infertility*. These associations were investigated in a cohort study that followed 250 women for two menstrual cycles and examined their intakes of fiber during this time period. The researchers found that higher intake of fiber was associated with lower levels of multiple sex hormones, including estrogen, progesterone, and the hormones that signal the ovaries to make these (FSH and LH). Fiber intake was also correlated with an increased chance of not ovulating during a menstrual cycle—a 1.78 times greater risk of anovulation for every 5 grams per day increase in total fiber. The authors of this study concluded:

> "*These findings suggest that a diet high in fiber is significantly associated with **decreased hormone concentrations and a higher probability of anovulation.** Further study of the effect of fiber on reproductive health and of the effect of these intakes in reproductive-aged women is warranted.*"[27]

This is an epidemiology study so we cannot make causal conclusions, but the hypothesis that *increased amounts of fiber could negatively alter hormonal levels in reproductive women* is quite plausible. Fiber is known to bind to estrogen in the gut, decreasing its levels by interrupting the normal reabsorption of this hormone.[28,29] Decreased levels of estrogen could, in turn, imbalance progesterone levels, leading to menstrual irregularities. LH and FSH levels also appear to be negatively effected by increased intakes of fiber, independent of estrogen levels, further disrupting the delicate hormonal balance.

FIBER FOR FAT LOSS?

Weight loss and appetite control are other suggested benefits of dietary plant fiber, but yet again, the research isn't supportive of this. One of my good friends, who is an army ranger, told me that during his intense initiation period, he was put through prolonged periods of food deprivation. During this time, many in his group resorted to eating toilet paper—thinking that by filling their stomachs with something, they would suppress their appetites. This is essentially what we are doing by eating fiber and hoping for appetite suppression. The hormonal signals that control appetite and satiety are complex, and feeling full is more nuanced than simply filling the stomach with material that has no nutritional value. Carbohydrates that accompany plant fiber are also likely to cause spikes of insulin and other satiety impairing hormones, like GLP-1, leading to *augmentation of hunger cues* rather than decreasing them.

In controlled studies with fiber, neither soluble nor insoluble fiber has been found to be beneficial for weight loss or reduction of body fat. The authors of a study examining the use of pectin, beta-glucan, or methycellulose for three-week intervals concluded the following:

> *"Use of neither [soluble] nor [insoluble fiber] preparations was associated with body weight or fat loss. These pilot results suggest no role for short-term use of fiber supplements in promoting weight loss in humans."*[80]

Another review paper considering forty-nine studies came to the similar conclusion that there was no consistent evidence for a benefit of dietary fiber with regard to appetite.[31] I don't think these findings should be surprising to us. Appetite, satiety, and loss of fat are much more complex than simply filling our stomachs with non-nutritive plant fibers. In order to effectively create satiety signals, we need to provide our body with a nutrient-rich diet that does not promote massive swings in blood glucose or an excessive release of hunger-promoting hormones. If only someone would write a book about such a diet. Oh wait! You are holding it in your hands!

A nose-to-tail carnivore diet is known to be associated with greatly improved satiety and weight loss. These results are likely due to the nutrient richness, potential for ketosis, and increased insulin sensitivity attained when we return to eating like our ancestors by adopting the carnivore diet.

The Jungle Inside of You

So far, we've discussed how fiber has failed to show any benefit for constipation, diverticulosis, colon cancer prevention, diabetes, and weight loss. In some cases, there's even evidence that fiber could be worsening these conditions, and there's certainly evidence that many types of fiber and accompanying phytic acid decrease mineral bioavailability. The last bastion of hope that many who champion fiber cling to is the notion that it's necessary for a "healthy" gastrointestinal microbiome.

The immediate problem with this assertion is that our understanding of the gut microbiome is still in its infancy. Anyone who claims to know what the ideal looks like is simply spouting conjecture based on personal opinion rather than ideas based on solid science. We have some sense of what might make up a healthy microbiome, and we know which bacteria are generally bad actors, but at a granular level—our knowledge is far from complete.

In discussions of the microbiome, many claim that plant fiber is necessary for a healthy gut mucus layer, microbial diversity, and the formation of short-chain fatty acids like butyrate. Let's examine each of these concepts individually.

Microbial Diversity

Fiber advocates often claim that we must consume plants in order to have a diverse array of organisms living in our guts, but they only cite epidemiology comparing rural and urban individuals. They would argue, also, that low diversity has been found in conditions like Type II diabetes and inflammatory bowel disease, and then conclude that by not consuming plant fiber, we increase our risk of these conditions.[32,33] These arguments quickly fall apart when we examine them closely, however.

For starters, there's no scientific evidence that we need plant fiber in order to achieve a robust level of diversity in our microbiome. There are studies suggesting that a Western diet is associated with a lower microbial diversity, generally referred to as **alpha diversity**, but claims that *this is causally related to the low-fiber aspect of such a way of eating* are premature.[34] As we have shown, there are many inflammatory components in the standard American diet that could be damaging the gut and negatively altering microbial populations. Who's to say it's the lack of fiber doing this and not sugars, oxidized vegetable oils, or the many plant toxins we've already discussed?

Diets high in fructose and glucose have clearly demonstrated an ability to negatively alter the microbiome, and are much more likely to be some of the culprits in the decline of alpha diversity seen in those eating a Western diet.[35] Let's also not forget about the data we saw in Chapter Seven on lectins suggesting that these plant toxins can also decrease alpha diversity by allowing overgrowth of facultative aerobes like *E. coli*.

Furthermore, interventional trials with increased fiber *do not reveal increased* alpha diversity,[36] and trials with a zero-plant-fiber carnivore diet *do not show decreased alpha diversity*.[37] Low-fiber ketogenic diets have also been shown to not decrease diversity scores.[38] In a trial following patients with multiple sclerosis for six months, the alpha diversity actually *increased* in those eating a ketogenic diet during this time.[39]

Many of those eating carnivorous diets, including myself, have done microbiome testing and found robust diversity scores, suggesting that it is entirely possible to have a healthy, diverse microbiome without eating *any* plant fiber. In summary, fiber doesn't increase alpha diversity, and animal-based diets don't decrease alpha diversity. Examination of the microbiota of those eating a carnivore diet show robust diversity coupled with improvements in previous gastrointestinal symptoms. I'd say we can put the notion that *plant fiber is needed for a diverse microbiome* to rest.

Short-Chain Fatty Acids: More Than Just Butyrate

There's good evidence that short-chain fatty acids play an important role in the large bowel by acting as a fuel for colonic epithelial cells.[40,41,42] The false conventional notion here is that butyrate is the only short-chain fatty acid utilized by these cells, and that in order to obtain this, we must feed the bacteria in our gut with plant fiber. If we listen to many of the health pundits today, they'll tell us that more fiber is better and that if we just keep increasing fiber intake, surely all of our gut issues will be healed. Sadly, they appear deaf and blind to the thousands of people who are experiencing significant gas, bloating, constipation, diarrhea, and pain with increased amounts of plant fiber in the diet.

The truth of the matter is that many different short-chain fatty acids can be used by the colonic epithelium, as can ketones like beta hydroxybutyrate from within the circulation when eating low-carbohydrate diets. In addition to butyrate, propionate, isobutyrate, isolvalerate, and acetate are all short-chain fatty acids produced by bacterial fermentation of protein.[37] In a study examining changes in gut flora with plant-based versus animal-based diets, researchers noted a shift from predominantly *butyrate and acetate on a plant-based diet* to *isobutyrate and isovalerate on a carnivore diet*. The authors of this study make an interesting observation regarding the flexibility of the human gut microbiome, and even they suggest that plant foods might simply be survival foods:

> *"Our findings that the human gut microbiome can rapidly switch between herbivorous and carnivorous functional profiles may reflect past selective pressures during human evolution. Consumption of animal foods by our ancestors was likely volatile, depending on season and stochastic foraging success, with plant foods offering a **fallback** source of calories and nutrients. Microbial communities that could quickly, and appropriately, shift their functional repertoire in response to diet change would have subsequently enhanced human dietary flexibility."*

It's also notable that although the diets in this study were isocaloric, the animal-based diet resulted in significant weight loss over five days, while the plant-based diet did not. There was also no change in the alpha diversity between these two groups, again showing that plant fiber is not necessary for a diverse microbiome.

Discussions of short-chain fatty acids in the gut quickly become complex, and there are some nuances here that I'd like to clarify. Short-chain fatty acids are formed within the lumen of the gastrointestinal tract and can be taken up by the epithelial cells of the colon for energy. Within these cells, they go through a series of chemical reactions transforming them into beta-hydroxy butyrate, a molecule you may recognize as one of the major ketones produced in our body when we are in a state of ketosis. Thus, when we choose to eat a ketogenic diet, our colonic epithelial cells can also use the beta-hydroxy butyrate present in our circulation for fuel, lessening the need for short-chain fatty acids from the lumen of the gut.

This detail of our physiology is quite important. Overgrowth of the wrong type of organisms within our gastrointestinal tract can impair the oxidation of short-chain fatty acids that is necessary for them to be taken up by epithelial cells. If we already have dysbiosis, eating more fiber is only going to work against us as the butyrate formed can't be taken up by the cells of the colon and they begin to starve, creating inflammation and leaky gut.[43] In this situation, the delivery of ketones through the bloodstream to these starving cells can be very helpful, and not surprisingly, ketogenic diets have been found to be beneficial in cases of dysbiosis and inflammatory bowel disease.[44,45]

In addition to being energy substrates, short-chain fatty acids also serve signaling roles within the gut, and butyrate is known to bind to multiple receptors on cells of the gastrointestinal tract. Isobutyrate and other short-chain fatty acids have also been shown to bind to these receptors, often with greater efficacy than butyrate.[46,47] The data here is pretty clear: butyrate isn't the only game in town when it comes to short-chain fatty acids, and eating an animal-based diet provides fuel for colonic epithelial cells in the form of other short-chain fatty acids and ketones within the blood.

Within this conversation, there's another wrinkle that is quite fascinating. It appears that animals and humans can ferment collagenous tissues from animal meat into short-chain fatty acids. Collagen is the protein that composes most of the connective tissue in our body, including bones, ligaments, tendons, and cartilage. A study done on cheetahs, examining the ability of their microbiota to ferment these connective tissues into short-chain fatty acids, found the following conclusion:

> *"Collagen induced an acetate production comparable with [plant fiber] and a markedly high acetate-to-propionate ratio (8.41:1) compared with all other substrates…This study provides the first insight into the potential of animal tissues to influence large intestinal fermentation in a strict carnivore,* **and indicates that animal tissues have potentially similar functions as soluble or insoluble plant fibers.** *"*[48]

A nose-to-tail carnivore diet provides ample amounts of collagen for the production of short-chain fatty acids, so the next time someone asks you about fiber, just tell them you get all the "animal fiber" you need from eating meat and connective tissue!

MAGICAL MUCUS

We discussed the mucus layer in the gut previously in Chapter Seven when we learned about the microscopic anatomy of the gastrointestinal epithelium and the goblet cells that produce the polysaccharides necessary to compose this protective covering. There is evidence that this layer is dysfunctional in inflammatory bowel diseases, as well as in diabetics.[49,50] In animal models, when mice are fed a "low-fiber, Western diet" that contains oxidized vegetable oils and simple sugars, there is also evidence of breakdown of the mucus layer.[51] The assumption in many of these cases has traditionally been that it's the "low-fiber" part of this equation that's the problem. Just like the story of alpha diversity, however, I fear that most in the nutritional world are making "Burkitt's big mistake" again here—seeming all too eager to repeatedly blame all of our ills on a lack of fiber without examining other, more compelling causes of gastrointestinal dysfunction present in the standard American way of eating.

As we've spoken about previously, there are many components of a Western diet that are quite inflammatory to the gut, and these are likely the real factors driving degradation of the mucus layer. Recall from our discussions in Chapter Seven that dysfunction of this layer and decreased microbial diversity occur together when lectins are introduced in animal models. These two conditions are also often observed to co-occur when studied in humans. It's unclear which comes first, but from these studies, a compelling hypothesis appears to be that lectins are interacting with goblet cells to decrease mucus production—leading to an overgrowth of certain luminal bacterial populations and decreased alpha diversity.[52,53] This is a complex area of research where more study is needed to disentangle cause and effect, but the suggestion that low-fiber diets lead to mucus layer dysfunction is simply not supported by hard science and overlooks so many other potentially damaging factors within the Western diet.

Further confirmation that lack of fiber is not to blame here comes from the striking clinical evidence of the thousands of people eating a carnivore diet who experience significant improvement in gastrointestinal issues. There are hundreds of recorded stories of improved gut health with a carnivore diet shared at *MeatHeals.com,* and multiple published case reports in medical literature describing resolution of severe gastrointestinal issues like Crohn's disease. A nose-to-tail carnivore diet has also been used in the treatment of autoimmune issues and cancer with impressive results. We'll discuss this further in Chapter 12.

WRAPPING UP OUR FIBER-DEBUNKING ADVENTURES

Despite mountains of evidence that fiber is just not good for us, our teenage crush on it remains strong. What began with "Burkitt's big mistake," and the notion that a lack of plant fiber is behind the ills of Western society, has become a part of our collective consciousness—much to the detriment of our guts and the unnecessary production of copious flatulence. As we've seen in this chapter, however, study after study has clearly demonstrated that plant fiber is not beneficial for constipation, diverticulosis, diabetes, weight loss, appetite, or colon cancer. Nor is it necessary for a healthy gastrointestinal tract or a diverse microbiome, and as we will see in Chapter Twelve, implementing a carnivore diet while eliminating plant fiber has demonstrated unprecedented efficacy in reversing autoimmune and inflammatory conditions.

None of this should come as a surprise. Eating animals made us human and has been a central part of our story as humans for millions of years. A carnivore diet is written into our book of life as the most fundamental diet that humans can thrive on. Plants have always been "fallback" foods and can be quite triggering to some people, leading to activation of the immune system, inflammation, leaky gut, and autoimmune disease. In the next chapter, we'll continue on our parade of debunking and will address the notion that red meat might lead to cancer or decrease our longevity. Under scrutiny, these big myths will continue to fall like Goliath. Finally, from an intuitive perspective, consider this question: Why would foods that have been at the center of our human evolution do such evolutionarily inconsistent things?

CHAPTER TEN

MYTH III
RED MEAT WILL SHORTEN YOUR LIFE

In the last chapter, we thoroughly examined plant fiber and discovered that it's definitely not all it's cracked up to be. We also found that the protein and collagen in meat can act like "animal fiber" in our large intestine and provide short-chain fatty acids for the epithelial cells there. But for many, the concept of eating a diet rich in animal foods conjures up thoughts of colon cancer and shortened lifespans. As we continue on our myth-busting adventure, let's address these faulty notions. Onward, there's further truth to be found and flawed reasoning to be swiftly dispatched!

Most of the misconceptions that red meat causes cancer comes from a report by the World Health Organization's International Agency for Research on Cancer (IARC) that was released in 2015. Sounds like a really fancy title doesn't it? Surely, something coming out of an organization like that would be reliable and reputable, right? Sadly, this report has been wildly misinterpreted by mainstream media and is based on some very questionable interpretations of the science it claims to review.

The IARC report is a consensus statement from a group of twenty-two scientists from ten countries who met in France for two weeks in 2015. Their goal was to examine the research on the relationship between meat intake and cancer and to produce a summary statement about potential risks. After considering 800 studies, they came to the conclusion that for every 100 grams of red meat eaten per day, there was a 17 percent increase in colon cancer risk. They also concluded that for every 50 grams of processed red meat, there was a risk increase of 18 percent. They went on to classify red meat as probably carcinogenic to humans in a damning report that sent shockwaves through the media when it was released.

Sounds bad, right? But what were these statements actually based on? Examination of a more detailed 2018 report on their findings reveals that only 14 of the 800 studies were considered in their final conclusions—and every single study was **observational epidemiology.** Why the other 786 were excluded remains a mystery, and included in this group were many interventional studies in animals which clearly did not show a relationship between red meat and cancer.

Of the fourteen epidemiology studies that were included in the IARC report, eight showed no link between the consumption of meat and development of colon cancer. Yes, you read that correctly, the *majority* of the studies considered in this report did not show a correlation between consumption of red meat and colon cancer. Of the remaining six studies, only *one* showed a statistically significant correlation between meat and cancer. Within epidemiology research, in addition to looking for correlation between two things, we can look also for the strength of the correlation. When two things are correlated, but not to a level of statistical significance, it suggests this correlation is showing up by chance or because of errors in calculations. In medicine, when the correlation between two or more things does not reach statistical significance, we don't take it seriously. We know that more research is needed to clarify the relationship, and we certainly don't make a sweeping proclamation about something causing cancer if the correlation isn't statistically significant.

Thus, in the IARC report, only *one* of the fourteen studies considered showed a correlation between red meat and cancer that achieved statistical significance.[1] Interestingly, this was a study of Seventh Day Adventists in America—a religious group that advocates for a plant based diet. We will discuss a population of Seventh Day Adventists living in Loma Linda, California, later in this chapter when we debunk the notion of "Blue Zones," but for now, I'll mention that in this study, those who were eating red meat tended to engage in other unhealthy behaviors as well. This is an illustration of the concept we've referred to previously as unhealthy user bias, a confounder that often comes into play in studies of those eating red meat.

In cultures or religious groups—like the Adventists—where the narrative surrounding red meat is negative, those who choose to disregard these ideas generally tend to also do other rebellious and unhealthy things, like smoking, drinking alcohol, and exercising less. In studies of red meat and health outcomes, these "rebellious" behaviors can be particularly problematic and often skew results. If a member of a motorcycle gang smokes, drinks, doesn't exercise, is overweight, and likes to eat steak, how can we conclude that his or her increased risk of cancer, heart disease, or shorter life span is due to the steak and not one of the other behaviors? But this is exactly what epidemiology studies like this one attempt to do. In order to really get a sense of what's going on, we must look for interventional studies on humans or animals that establish mechanisms by which two things are *causally* related rather than just being *correlated* like in epidemiology studies.

In the study of the Adventists, the authors also note that the strongest correlation between red meat and colon cancer occurred in obese individuals with a *higher propensity for insulin resistance*. Since both obesity and diabetes/insulin resistance are known to be strong risk-factors for the development of cancer,[2,3] doesn't it seem much more likely that these factors were driving the increased cancer risk in this group of individuals rather than the red meat consumption? Epidemiology studies cannot answer this question, but when we consider the totality of the studies looked at in the IARC report, their recommendations start to look shadier than a winter afternoon in Seattle.

WHAT WAS LEFT OUT OF THE IARC REPORT

As we've just seen, a huge number of studies were omitted from consideration in the IARC report, including a large number of epidemiology studies that did not show correlation between red meat intake and adverse outcomes. We've previously discussed a large study of Asians, which included over 200,000 participants observed for an average of ten years, that showed *decreased* rates of cardiovascular mortality and cancer mortality in the men and women who ate the most meat, respectively.[4] Another large epidemiology study of over 60,000 vegetarians and non-vegetarians in the United Kingdom found that rates of colon cancer were actually *higher* in vegetarians.[5]

Also excluded from the IARC report were all of the interventional studies about meat consumption performed in animals that showed no increase in colon cancer risk. In one of these studies, rats were injected with an agent that induced colon cancer and fed a diet supplemented with bacon, chicken, beef, or their standard chow for 100 days. The researchers found *no increase* in occurrence of colon cancers with the addition of meat to the diet relative to the control group. They concluded:

> *"Thus the hypothesis that **colonic iron [from meat], bile acids, or total fatty acids can promote colon tumors** is **not supported by this study**. The results suggest that, in rats, **beef does not promote the growth of [colon cancer]** and chicken does not protect against colon carcinogenesis. A bacon-based diet appears to protect against carcinogenesis."*[6]

So bacon cures colon cancer? Wouldn't that be heavenly? We'll need a few more studies to fully prove that possibility, but many animal studies like this one similarly fail to support the hypothesis that meat of any kind contributes to increased rates of colon cancer.

We know that animal studies aren't as good as human studies, but there are no formal human interventional trials with red meat looking at cancer incidence. There are, however, interventional trials in humans looking at markers of oxidative stress and inflammation with red meat. Any guesses what they found? Nada, zilch, zero increase in these end points with the addition of red meat. In one of these trials, thirty-seven diabetics were divided into two groups for six weeks. One group ate a diet rich in animal protein (30 percent of their calorie intake), and the other group ate a diet rich in plant protein (also 30 percent of their calorie intake). At the end of this time, markers of systemic and gastrointestinal inflammation revealed no significant increases in inflammatory markers (including IL-6, and TNF-alpha) on the animal based diet.[7] On the other hand, calprotectin, a marker of gastrointestinal inflammation, showed a trend towards an increase with the plant protein-rich diet. Might this suggest gut inflammation from plant toxins? It certainly could, but more studies are needed here.

In another eight-week study, sixty participants were divided into two groups. One was a control group that ate their normal diet while the other lucky group replaced dietary carbohydrates from plants with an extra 8 ounces of red meat every day—an amount that the IARC claimed would increase colon cancer risk by 40 percent. At the end of the study, multiple markers of inflammation and oxidative stress were measured and the following findings were reported:

> *"The results of our study **suggest decreased rather than increased oxidative stress and inflammation when lean red meat intake is increased at the expense of dietary carbohydrate-rich foods...**"*

Our results do not support the suggestion that higher red meat intake leads to increased risk of heart disease and Type II diabetes via effects of iron to increase oxidative stress and inflammation."[8]

Let's just be clear on this. According to the IARC, red meat is a class 2A carcinogen. But participants in this study, who did their ancestors proud and jettisoned some plant-based carbohydrates in favor of red meat, saw improvements in inflammatory and oxidative stress markers. In other words, animal foods are the best foods on the planet, my friends. The more of them we include in our diet, the more we will thrive, and the IARC is just out to lunch with their recommendations.

Another study was recently published by a group of investigators who similarly questioned the work of the IARC, stating:

*"These [IARC] recommendations are, however, primarily based on observational studies that are at **high risk for confounding and thus are limited in establishing causal inferences**, nor do they report the absolute magnitude of any possible effects. Furthermore, the organizations that produce guidelines **did not conduct or access rigorous systematic reviews of the evidence**, were limited in addressing conflicts of interest, and did not explicitly address population values and preferences raising questions regarding adherence to guideline standards for trustworthiness."*[9]

These investigators felt that the IARC did not do their due diligence in examining studies and that their findings were at a high risk of possessing confounding variables. Basically, they're saying the IARC's suggestions aren't to be trusted, and they wanted to do their own rigorous analysis in which they found the following:

*"For our review of randomized trials on harms and benefits (12 unique trials enrolling 54,000 participants), we found low- to very low-certainty evidence that diets lower in unprocessed red meat may **have little or no effect on the risk for major cardiometabolic outcomes and cancer mortality and incidence…There is also evidence of possible health benefits of omnivorous versus vegetarian diets on such outcomes as muscle development and anemia…The panel suggests that adults continue current unprocessed red meat consumption."***

These findings are making headlines throughout the country as I am finishing the writing of this book in the fall of 2019. We already knew that red meat wasn't bad for us, but it's good to see the scientific community at large waking up to our ancestral truths as well.

THE MEAT AND CANCER MYTH DEBUNKED ONCE AND FOR ALL

At this point, we've thoroughly dismantled the IARC report from 2015, but it's still useful to examine the proposed mechanisms by which red meat is hypothesized to cause cancer, and in the process, to fully dispose of this farcical notion. These mechanisms include heme iron, n-nitroso compounds, and the heterocyclic amines that may be formed during the cooking process.

As we discussed in Chapter Eight, heme iron is a special form of iron found only in animal foods that is much more easily absorbed than the non-heme iron found in plants. There is absolutely zero evidence that this molecule is directly toxic to the gut and it is an incredibly valuable nutrient in human physiology. Studies with heme iron have only shown a potential to induce pre-cancerous lesions in calcium-deficient mouse and rat models.[10] When these animals are fed adequate amounts of calcium, heme iron does not appear damaging to the gut, as was previously demonstrated in the study of beef, bacon, and chicken in rats.[6,11] As we'll talk about in Chapter Twelve, a nose-to-tail carnivore diet includes sources of calcium, so contrived rodent models suggesting harm of heme iron are irrelevant.

Part of the proposed mechanism for heme iron is that it may promote the formation of n-nitroso compounds in the gastrointestinal tract. Generally speaking, these compounds are formed by the addition of an NO group to other molecules. There are many types of n-nitroso compounds, but the important thing to note here is that those associated with meat consumption have *not* been implicated in formation of colon cancers. In a paper examining the mechanistic evidence connecting red meat and cancer, the authors review all of the available interventional studies on this topic and come to the following conclusion:

> *"The evidence from [test tube] studies utilized conditions that are not necessarily relevant for a normal dietary intake and thus do not provide sufficient evidence that heme exposure from typical red meat consumption would increase the risk of colon cancer. Animal studies utilized models that tested promotion of preneoplastic conditions **utilizing diets low in calcium**, high in fat combined with exaggerations of heme exposure that in many instances represented intakes that were orders of magnitude above normal dietary consumption of red meat. Finally, clinical evidence suggests that the type of n-nitroso compounds found after ingestion of*

red meat in humans consists mainly of nitrosyl iron and nitrosothiols, **products that have profoundly different** *chemistries from certain n-nitroso species which have been shown to be tumorigenic through the formation of DNA adducts.* **In conclusion, the methodologies employed in current studies of heme have not provided sufficient documentation that the mechanisms studied would contribute to an increased risk of promotion of preneoplasia or colon cancer at usual dietary intakes of red meat in the context of a normal diet."[12]**

Thus, eating in a way that mimics our ancestors' diet has not been shown to increase the rates of colon cancer growth in test tubes, animals, or human experiments. Why are we not surprised?

It has also been suggested that heterocyclic amines (HCA) and polycyclic aromatic hydrocarbons (PAH) are mechanisms by which red meat may induce cancer growth in the gut. These can be formed when meat is cooked on a hot surface or exposed to smoke from a fire or a grill. I do think it is important to be aware of these compounds and to limit them from our diets as much as possible. Much like our old enemies, the isothiocyanates, these compounds activate the NRF2 system in the liver and must be detoxified, but our body appears to have plenty of mechanisms to deal with them in moderate quantities.[13]

The key word here is *moderate*. Epidemiology studies have suggested an increased risk of issues with these products of cooking only when they are consumed in very high quantities.[14,15] Think charred, burned, and massively overcooked meats. Yuck, and who cooks their meat that way, anyway? By choosing slow, low-temperature cooking methods, we can easily avoid significant amounts of these compounds in our diets. I'm going to break some hearts here, but I'm not a big fan of grilling and smoking meats for this reason. These are probably fine in moderation, but I think the majority of our food should be prepared with more gentle cooking methods. In Chapter Twelve, we'll talk in detail about my preferred methods of cooking meat and animal foods to moderate HCA/PAH exposure. It's also important to point out that whenever anything is cooked at high temperatures, be it coffee, grains, bread, or other foods, compounds are formed that have been implicated in possible cancer risk. Ultimately, we have to eat something, and I believe that it's much better to consume nutrient-rich animal products that are intentionally prepared than to shun these foods out of fear of minimal amounts of HCAs and PAHs.

Neu5Gc: Not a Cause for Concern

Speaking of things we really don't have to be that worried about, let's move on to talk about Neu5Gc, another molecule that some have suggested may contribute to colon cancer risk with red meat consumption. When we examine these claims closely, however, we again see that they simply don't hold any merit.

Neu5Gc belongs to a family of molecules known as sialic acids, all of which have an acidic nine-carbon backbone structure. These molecules are attached to glycoproteins on the surface of cells in our body, which are used for cell-to-cell signaling and binding to different tissues. We don't make Neu5Gc, due to a mutation in the enzyme that synthesizes it (known as CMAH), but humans do produce Neu5Ac, which differs by just one oxygen atom. The loss of function in this enzyme appears to have occurred 2–3 million years ago and is hypothesized to have been a protective adaptation to infectious insults, such as pathogens like bacteria, viruses, and parasites. Such pathogens use the sialic acids on the surface of our cells to attach and gain entry.

Some contend that because humans do not possess Neu5Gc, while ruminants like cows, deer, and lamb do, eating these animals could trigger an immune reaction. There is no evidence in humans to support this idea, however, and these claims are based on tenuously constructed animal models with limited relevance to us. We do appear to generate antibodies to Neu5Gc, but there is no research to suggest these antibodies lead to inflammation or damage, and there are studies that demonstrate the opposite.

As part of the process of kidney transplantation, many patients receive large doses of rabbit antibodies known as polyclonal IgG, which contain significant amounts of Neu5Gc. These patients are known to subsequently generate antibodies to this molecule and have higher levels of anti-Neu5Gc antibodies than the general population. In a very large study of kidney transplant recipients, no increase in colon cancer rates were seen in the 38,000 patients who received the polyclonal rabbit IgG compared to those in the control group who had not received it.[16] Those investigators stated:

> *"In summary, our findings obtained in a large cohort of over 200,000 kidney transplant patients…**do not support the hypothesis that long term over-exposure to anti-Neu5Gc antibodies, in our analysis as a result of [polyclonal IgG] treatment, triggers a malignancy in the colon.** Polyclonal IgG treated patients did not de-*

velop colon cancer at an increased rate even though their immune system was suppressed."

In addition to this data suggesting that elevated levels of anti-Neu5Gc antibodies do not elevate colon cancer risk, there's another interesting nuance about Neu5Gc that is often overlooked. Humans are not the only species to lack this sialic acid molecule. The Mustelids—ferrets, badgers, martens, weasels, etc.—are a family of carnivorous animals that also lack Neu5Gc but commonly consume other animals that do possess this molecule. This behavior mirrors the consumption of Neu5Gc in red meat by humans.[17] Since we don't see wild ferrets becoming extinct from rampant cancers, and since humans have done nothing but thrive for the last 3 million years eating Neu5Gc-containing animals, I think it's pretty safe to say that the notion of this molecule being connected with cancer is no less than a fairy tale and not something to worry about.

mTOR: The Molecular Growth Switch

Another concern some individuals in the scientific community have expressed about consumption of meat is over-activation of mTOR. Discussions in this sphere can quickly become complex, and in order to understand what mTOR is and how it functions, let's first discuss some cellular biology.

At a very basic level, the cells in our body receive inputs from the external environment communicating how they should behave. Sometimes they receive signals that tell them to repair or to perform organized cell death (apoptosis). At other times, like when nutrients are abundant or after exercise, our cells get the signal to proliferate and grow. These two opposing processes of cell-breakdown and cell-growth are respectively known as **catabolism** and **anabolism**, and both serve vitals roles throughout our lives as our bodies oscillate between periods of building and recycling of cellular components throughout the day. When we eat or exercise, we send anabolic signals to our cells to build and grow. During periods of fasting between meals, our cells receive signals that it's a good time to do some catabolic house cleaning, also known as **autophagy**.

Simply speaking, mTOR is part of a signaling pathway that tells cells to grow and divide. More specifically, mTOR is a kinase—a molecule that adds a phosphate group (PO_4) to other molecules. This process is known as **phosphorylation**, and it generally turns things like enzymes on. Throughout our lifespan, mTOR is active during periods of rapid growth, like childhood and puberty. During adulthood, it also serves an essential function in maintenance of muscle mass and is turned on in response to resistance exercise.

mTOR participates in the anabolic signaling process within our cells in response to four distinct signals. These include insulin-like growth factor-1 (IGF-1), insulin, protein (mostly mediated through the amino acid leucine), and exercise.[18] Insulin is released primarily in response to carbohydrates and protein, although the response to the latter occurs less intensely in the setting of a ketogenic metabolism. IGF-1 is produced in response to the growth hormone secretion that occurs with eating, sleep, and exercise. Leucine is an amino acid found in proteins and is especially rich in animal meat, but it is found in much lower amounts in plant-based proteins. While leucine appears to be able to diffuse across the cell membrane and activate mTOR directly, insulin and IGF-1 bind to cell surface receptors, initiating an intracellular cascade that activates mTOR.[19] Thus, resistance exercise, sleep, carbohydrates, and leucine can all increase mTOR signaling and lead to cellular growth.

On the flip side of anabolic mTOR signaling lies the AMP kinase (AMPK) pathway. This pathway generally serves a catabolic role in our cells and is triggered by the absence of nutrients or growth signals. In a simplified view of our cellular workings, we might think of a seesawing balance between mTOR and AMPK activation. When one is activated, it generally eclipses the other, though both serve vital roles, and in order to be optimally healthy, a balance is necessary with periods of growth as well as periods of cellular housecleaning.

If mTOR serves such vital roles in the human body, what's all the fuss about over-activating it these days? These concerns arise from studies which show that some cancers harbor mutations in mTOR associated pathways, leading to excessive cellular growth and proliferation.[20,21] It has also been noted that in people with **Laron syndrome**, who possess a defect in growth hormone signaling, there is a low incidence of cancers. This syndrome also comes at the cost of profound growth deficits, low blood sugar, and sleep disturbances. Experimental models of Laron syndrome suggest that in these individuals, mTOR signaling is altered due to low levels of IGF-1.

With these findings in mind, some scientists and physicians have suggested that minimizing mTOR signaling can help us deter cancer. The problems with this interpretation are immediately apparent, however, as it's quite evident that we need mTOR to be strong and healthy humans and to maintain muscle mass as we age. Nevertheless, those fearful of mTOR advocate for dietary limitation of things that might increase IGF-1 or activate mTOR directly, like the amino acid *leucine* or animal protein in general.

When the notion of an entirely animal-based diet, like the carnivore diet, is raised, these individuals fall out of their chairs in dismay. They exclaim that eating this much protein will surely cause mTOR to go into overdrive and increase the risk of cancer. To substantiate this, they can only point to poorly constructed epidemiology studies that *correlated* lower protein intake with improved outcomes in those less than sixty-five years of age.[22] What they don't tell you is that in this same study, in the above sixty-five age group, *higher* protein intakes were associated with a better lifespan and less cancer.

This study again illustrates the dangers of using epidemiology to make sweeping recommendations. How can higher levels of protein be bad for us when we are young but protective when we age? This makes absolutely no sense, and almost certainly reflects confounding and bias in this study. Furthermore, low-protein diets have been repeatedly associated with muscle wasting, a process known as **sarcopenia**, and are a known major risk-factor for mortality.[23,24]

Another often ignored part of the mTOR equation is that this anabolic pathway can be stimulated by *both* carbohydrates (through insulin) and protein. Studies comparing anabolic potential show that activation of mTOR by insulin is much more robust, and lasts three to four times as long as its activation by leucine.[25] The main trigger for insulin release is carbohydrates. Protein can also trigger the release of this hormone, but in the setting of a low-carbohydrate diet, the degree of this stimulation is much lower than when protein is eaten with carbohydrates.

To suggest that we can lower cancer risk or live longer by limiting animal protein suggests an incomplete understanding of mTOR signaling and ignores millions of years of evolutionary wisdom. Throughout our evolution, we've always had periods of abundance and periods of scarcity. During the times of plenty, our body receives signals to grow from the mTOR pathway, and during times of scarcity, the cellular housecleaning pathways directed by AMPK take over. We need both. mTOR isn't bad, and we shouldn't seek to completely abolish its actions. Nor should we fast all the time, which is really just starvation. There must be times of feasting on nutrient rich animal foods for our bodies to become as strong as they can be. In Chapter Twelve, we'll talk more about meal timing and fasting, and how to incorporate these strategies with eating to optimize our health.

Interventional studies with meat consumption and longevity would take a long time to do, but some of the longest lived people on the earth eat lots of meat. As we've already seen from conveniently ignored epidemiology studies in Asia, those who ate the most meat had the lowest rates of cancer mortality and cardiovascular disease mortality. Cancer is a complex topic, and our understanding of the mechanisms that underlie its development is far from complete. But to suggest that over-activation of mTOR with a nutrient-rich diet might trigger cancer is an unsupported intellectual leap that ignores the actions of insulin on this signaling pathway and incorrectly vilifies animal foods.

RED MEAT: NOT THE FOE OF BONES, KIDNEYS, OR BIG TOES

In addition to claims that red meat will shorten our life or cause cancer, many have heard that eating a significant amount of protein will harm their kidneys or lead to kidney stones.

There have been multiple studies in those consuming high protein diets, and invariably these have failed to find a detrimental effect on kidney function.[26,27] In one study, kidney function *improved,* and there was no increased risk of kidney stones over two years when obese adults were placed on a low-carbohydrate, high-protein diet. In another meta-analysis of twenty-eight studies looking at 1,358 participants, there was no evidence that a high-protein diet adversely affected kidney function.

As we've discussed previously in this book, the majority of kidney stones are formed from calcium oxalate, and increased intake of oxalate-containing plant foods appears to be the major risk factor here. Within the medical literature, there's just no clear evidence that higher protein diets are linked to kidney stones.

Another common criticism leveled at high-protein diets is that they may lead to lower bone density, or osteoporosis, due to a higher acid load. While it is true that protein in the diet represents an acidic input, this can be balanced by obtaining enough alkalinizing minerals, such as calcium, magnesium, and potassium.[28,29] In Chapter Twelve we will talk in detail about sources of these minerals on a nose-to-tail carnivore diet that will balance protein consumption from a pH perspective such as bone broth, bone meal, and bone marrow.

Furthermore, high protein diets have been shown to increase calcium absorption in the gastrointestinal tract and have been correlated with *increased* bone density and a lower risk of fractures.[30,31,32] A consensus statement by the International Osteoporosis Foundation stated the following:

> *"Adequate supplies of dietary protein are required for optimal bone growth and maintenance of healthy bone... In older people with osteopo-*

*rosis, higher protein intake (≥ 0.8 g/kg body weight/day, i.e., above the current RDA) **is associated with higher bone mineral density, a slower rate of bone loss, and reduced risk of hip fracture, provided that dietary calcium intakes are adequate.** Intervention with dietary protein supplements attenuate age-related bone mineral density decrease, and reduced bone turnover marker levels, together with an increase in IGF-I and a decrease in PTH. **There is no evidence that diet-derived acid load is deleterious for bone health. Thus, insufficient dietary protein intakes may be a more severe problem than protein excess in the elderly.*"*

If we want strong bones and muscles, a good amount of high-quality animal protein balanced with alkalinizing minerals in our diet is the answer.

The notion that red meat will cause gout is yet another unjust accusation thrown in the direction of animal foods. Gout is caused by the deposition of uric acid in joints of the body, and elevated levels in the blood appear to be a risk factor for this disease process. The mechanism by which uric acid crystallizes in joints is not fully understood, however, and elevated levels of uric acid in the blood do not appear to be enough to cause gout independently. Fasting can cause levels of uric acid to rise, possibly due to cell breakdown as part of the process of autophagy, but does not appear to result in gout flares. The strongest associations with gout appear to be things that cause insulin resistance, which negatively affects uric acid excretion and likely contribute to disease progression in other ways as well.[33]

Not surprisingly, the strong association between gout and diabetes is well known.[34]

But if meat doesn't cause insulin resistance, why does it get implicated in gout? Perhaps it is because purines in meat and shellfish are broken down into uric acid. Therefore, the common thinking is that eating lots of these foods will cause the amount of uric acid in our blood to rise. Looking at the medical literature reveals a very different story, however.

When we consume purines in meat, our body actually increases the excretion of uric acid and levels stay essentially the same.[35] *The real culprits in gout appear to be fructose and alcohol,* two substances that can create insulin resistance and *decrease* the excretion of uric acid by the kidneys. In a large review with over 125,000 subjects, there was a strong association between fructose consumption and the incidence of gout.[36]

Since this is epidemiology we cannot claim a causal relationship, but the mechanisms by which fructose and alcohol could cause gout are well established. The next time you hear someone say that meat caused a gout flare, ask them how much sugar or alcohol they had with it! Again, we must not fall into the trap of blaming meat for what some other damaging food eaten with it has done. If you or someone you know has gout, the best thing that can be done is to eliminate fructose, alcohol, and processed carbohydrates from the diet while enjoying a steak.

THE MYTH OF THE BLUE ZONES

The concept of Blue Zones was first suggested by Dan Buettner in a 2005 National Geographic article based on the work he had done with Michel Poulain and Gianni Pes. They described five regions of the world where people were observed to live longer than average and suggested reasons for this by looking at similarities in diet and lifestyle between these disparate peoples. The locations included were Okinawa; Sardinia; Loma Linda, California; the Nicoya region of Costa Rica; and Ikaria in Greece. According to Buettner, common to all of these regions were low rates of smoking, a focus on family, social engagement, constant moderate physical activity, and a plant-heavy diet. He subsequently published a book advocating for this lifestyle as a way to attain longevity and vitality. Sounds great, right? Here's the magic formula for the fountain of youth!

Sadly, it's not this simple and there are some real problems with his conclusions and the way in which this story was told. The first of these is that there are many regions of the world that demonstrate similar degrees of longevity that were left out of the Blue Zones. Hong Kong has one of the highest life expectancies in the world (85 years) and is also the world's third largest consumer of beef per capita, with an average consumption of almost 1.5 pounds of total meat per day. Furthermore, comparing life expectancy to the percentage of calories obtained from animal foods paints a very different picture from the one Buettner suggests with his Blue Zones.[37]

ANIMAL PROTEIN CONSUMPTION AND INCREASED LIFE EXPECTANCY

Animal PRO % Daily Kcal Percentile

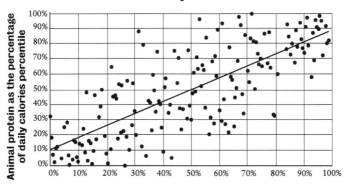

Life expectancy percentile at birth 2005

P. Grasgruber, M. Sebera, E. Hrazdíra, J. Cacek, T. Kalina. Major correlates of male height: A study of 105 countries, Economics & Human Biology, Volume 21, 2016, Pages 172-195, ISSN 1570-677X, https://doi.org/10.1016/j.ehb.2016.01.005 (http://www.sciencedirect.com/science/article/pii/S1570677X16300065)

As you can see from this FAO data, there's a clear correlation between increasing amounts of animal protein and longer life expectancies. This is epidemiology data, so as always we cannot draw a causal relationship here, but this correlation is strong. It is also true that, as the wealth of a country increases, the amount of meat consumed also increases, and wealth has been associated with greater life expectancy. It's possible that part of this trend is due to this association between affluence and meat consumption, but it's also very clear that populations of countries that eat more meat do not appear to be suffering shorter lives in connection with this.

Other epidemiology studies have also failed to demonstrate a negative correlation between meat consumption and longevity. In the NHANES III Project, a study of 17,611 individuals found that the consumption of white meat was associated with a decreased mortality rate in men, and there was no evidence that consumption of red meat worsened overall mortality.[38] Similarly, in a very large Australian cohort, there was no observed benefit to a plant-based diet on all-cause mortality:

> *"Among 243,096 participants....there was no significant difference in all-cause mortality for vegetarians versus non-vegetarians. There was also no significant difference in mortality risk between pesco-vegetarians ,or*

*semi-vegetarians versus regular meat eaters. **We found no evidence that following a vegetarian diet, semi-vegetarian diet or a pesco-vegetarian diet has an independent protective effect on all cause mortality.** "* [39]

Another large study comparing all-cause mortality between vegetarian and non-vegetarians in the United Kingdom also resulted in similar findings.[40] Thus, the epidemiology literature does not suggest a clear correlation between plant-based diets and longevity nor a detrimental effect of meat in the diet. In some studies, increased red meat is even associated with improved all-cause mortality. As previously mentioned, two studies in Asia demonstrated that intake of red meat was associated with decreased rates of cardiovascular mortality in men and decreased cancer mortality in women.[4] Because of their inherent limitations, epidemiology studies won't ever be the final word in this discussion, but they can help illustrate the inaccuracy of the notion that plant-heavy diets are universally associated with increased longevity or that meat consumption will lead to shorter lives.

In the world of longevity research, **telomeres** are a hot topic. Remember that DNA contains our genetic code and is wrapped around histone proteins and coiled into chromosomes. Like the tabs at the end of our shoelaces that prevent the ends from becoming frayed, the telomeres cap the ends of DNA helping to protect the edges of our genetic material from damage. These amazing structures are composed of a repeating series of nucleotide bases and can gradually shorten with every cell division. Investigators use the length of a cell's telomeres to get a sense of its biological age. Though these measurements aren't as precise as once thought, shorter telomeres generally signal an older cell closer to programmed cell death, and longer telomeres indicate a resplendent, youthful cell with an impressive six pack. It's well known that in addition to the process of aging, poor lifestyle choices can also shorten our telomeres prematurely. The good news is that on the flip side, healthy lifestyle choices can lengthen our telomeres.[41]

What sorts of things are associated with longer telomeres? For both vegetarians and non-vegetarians it is all the great lifestyle stuff we've previously discussed: exercise, adequate sleep, moderate sunlight exposure, finding meaning in our lives, and a tight-knit community. It's no surprise that Buettner found these as commonalities between his Blue Zones. But guess what? When it comes to food, there's only one thing that has been correlated with longer telomeres, and it's **not** plant foods. *It's red meat!*

In a three-year long observational study, a group of researchers looked at the length of telomeres in twenty-eight subjects and surveyed them to see what they ate. Here's what they found:

> *"Among nine food types (cereal, fruits, vegetables, dairy, red meat, poultry, fish, sweets and salty snacks) and eight beverages (juices, coffee, tea, mineral water, alcoholic and sweetened carbonated beverages)* **only intake of red meat was related to [telomere length]**. *Individuals with increased consumption of red meat had higher [telomere length] and the strongest significant differences were observed between consumer groups: 'never' and '1–2 daily' (p = 0.02)."* [42]

The authors of this study may have been surprised about the correlation between red meat and increased telomere length, but it's probably not a surprise for us at this point in our journey. By now, we know how valuable animal foods are in providing robust amounts of nutrients that allow us to achieve favorable antioxidant status and in protecting our cells from the oxidative stress that can lead to DNA damage and aging.

Another *big* problem with Buettner's Blue Zones and his claim that longevity is due to plant-focused diets is apparent when we closely examine the *actual* patterns of eating in these areas. The Nicoya region of Costa Rica is well known for exceptional longevity, but only for males. These lucky fellows are *seven-times more likely to live to the age of one hundred* than the general Costa Rican population, and they have life expectancy two years greater than Japanese males, another group well known to possess robust longevity. Compared to the general population in Costa Rica, this group of men have lower levels of cardiovascular risk markers, longer telomeres, and higher levels of male sex-hormones.[43] Sounds like a pretty hale and hearty group of older dudes, right? But guess what? They are also well known for their affinity for meat. The Nicoyans cook most of their foods in animal fat, eat more animal foods, and live longer than the general Costa Rican population. Clearly there's something else going on here! Seems like Buettner missed these inconvenient details.

Similarly, assessments of meat consumption in Sardinia and Okinawa in Buettner's work appear to have grossly underestimated the vital role of animal foods in the diets of individuals living in these locales. Anyone who has visited these regions of the world will know first hand that animal foods play very important roles in the diets of these peoples. Sardinia is well known for the "Sarda pig," a special type of swine raised on open range in the forests that is treasured by the people of this island. In a review of male longevity in Sardinia, the typical diet of a Sardinian shepherd is described as follows:

"The major discrepancy between the lowland areas, where peasants were the majority of the population, and the mountain areas, essentially pastoral, was the relatively superior consumption of animal-derived foods in the latter."[44]

Doesn't sound like a plant-based diet, does it?

As has been detailed in multiple surveys of their dietary habits, Okinawans are also known to consume more meat than the general Japanese population.[45] The authors of one paper looking at the diet of Okinawans stated:

"The food intake pattern in Okinawa has been different from that in other regions of Japan. The people there have never been influenced by Buddhism. Hence, there has been no taboo regarding eating habits. Eating meat was not stigmatized, and consumption of pork and goat was historically high. . . The intake of meat was higher in Okinawa... **Unexpectedly, we did not find any vegetarians among the centenarians."**

Well now, that's a quite a different picture regarding the diets of Okinawans than we have been led to believe, isn't it?

The story of misrepresentation of diet by Buettner also holds true for Ikaria, where meats like lamb and goat are a central part of the diet. In an epidemiology study of the Ikarian diet, none of the plant foods surveyed were associated with improved all-cause mortality, but those who ate the most calories appeared to live the longest.[46] It appears plausible that increased consumption of animal foods with their higher calorie content may have accounted for this discrepancy, though the authors of this study do not comment directly on this.

Unfortunately, it seems that the central nature of animal foods in the diets of Nicoyans, Sardinians, Okinawans, and Ikarians was ignored in the conceptualization of the Blue Zones. If you have any doubts about this fact, I urge you to visit these places and experience their rich culture, vitality, and zeal for animal foods first hand. Doctor's orders!

There's one more Blue Zone to consider, and this one demonstrates some very interesting trends further suggesting that plant based diets aren't all they are cracked up to be. Of the five so-called Blue Zones, Loma Linda represents a unique community. Located in Southern California, this location is home to a large population of Seventh Day Adventists, a religious group who advocate for a plant-based diet as well as abstinence from tobacco and alcohol. Surveys of Loma Linda residents suggest that about half of the population is lacto-ovo vegetarian, with a smaller percentage espousing a full vegan diet. Though some studies suggest that residents of Loma Linda live an average of seven years longer than the general population in California,[47] similar improvements in longevity have also been found in other religious groups in California, like Mormons, who also shun tobacco and alcohol but do not shy away from meat consumption.[48]

How can it be that the plant-focused diet is resulting in longevity in the Loma Linda community when similar longevity benefits are also seen in steak-loving Mormons in the same state?[49] It's much more likely that the avoidance of destructive behaviors is responsible for the longevity in Loma Linda rather than the increased consumption of plants, and decreased consumption of animal foods. Seems reasonable, right? If you smoke, drink, and don't have a great community of people who care about you, you're more likely to kick the bucket sooner.

Our investigation of Loma Linda doesn't stop there, however. Research on this highly plant-based population has even more to tell us about the potential downsides of choosing to make plant foods the mainstay of our diet. In a study done on 474 males in Loma Linda, researchers discovered some very striking differences in the sperm quality of vegans and lacto-ovo vegetarians versus those who consumed meat. Yes, I said sperm quality! This is actually a very useful measure for assessing the nutrient adequacy of a diet. Studies at Harvard show that men who consumed the most fruit and vegetables had the worst sperm quality.[50] These poor broccoli-munching fellows demonstrated both a lower number of sperm and sperm that seemed lackadaisical rather than the energetic critters they're supposed to be. The study of Loma Linda males echoed these findings:

> *"Lacto-ovo vegetarians had lower sperm concentration. Total motility was lower in the lacto-ovo and vegan groups versus non-vegetarians.* **Vegans had lowest hyperactive motility**...*The study showed that the* **vegetables-based food intake decreased sperm quality**. *In particular, a reduction in sperm quality in male factor patients would be clinically significant and would require review."*[51]

These were not small differences either. The vegans had the worst motility and sperm counts by far. Even the vegetarian's swimmers paled in comparison to those from the guys eating meat. Does Loma Linda still sound like Blue Zone to you?

In addition to healthy lifestyle behaviors, zones with higher than average lifespans appear to have *clustering of genes associated with improved longevity*. Studies of both Okinawans and a cohort of centenarians in

New England reveal that exceptional longevity appears to run in families.[52,53] This suggests a clustering of favorable gene polymorphisms that are involved in the inflammatory response, insulin sensitivity, and lipid metabolism. Individuals with these favorable genetics appear to experience diseases later in life, a phenomenon known as "compression of morbidity." If you've obtained an assessment of your genetics through commonly available programs, you can look for polymorphisms in genes like FOXO3, the sirtuins, or inflammatory cytokines like IL-6 and TNF-alpha to get a sense of your genetic "poker hand" when it comes to longevity. Remember, however, that epigenetics are much more important than genetics when it comes to overall quality of life and maintenance of health. Ultimately, the foods we eat and the radical or not so radical way in which we live our life will be the best predictors of how much butt we kick.

As we end our discussion of the so called Blue Zones, let's summarize what we've discovered when we put this notion to the test. Though people living in these locations do appear to live longer than their neighbors, there are many regions of the world with similarly exceptional longevity that were left out of consideration. If there's any magical formula to why people live longer lives, the most consistent commonalities appear to be *avoidance* of damaging habits like smoking and alcohol, *participation* in meaningful communities, and favorable genetics. Contrary to the narrative Buettner pitches about the Blue Zones, in many of these regions, as well as other parts of the world where life expectancies are long, meat is quite an important part of the culture and is consumed frequently. Life expectancies in Loma Linda may be better than the rest of California, but they are paralleled by other meat eating groups that also avoid the aforementioned vices and similarly value community and family. The outlook does not look good for the virility of males eating a plant-based diet in Loma Linda, either, raising the question of *exactly what part of this population is blue?* If we want to live lives that are as long and rich as possible, we should definitely include nutrient-rich animal foods, as well as creating time for community, family, and finding meaning on a day-to-day basis.

Let's move on from our debunking of the Blue Zones to address another common concern when considering animal-based diets. After I assure people that they will likely have the best health of their life eating a carnivore diet, the next question they usually ask me is:

Won't I Get Scurvy Eating Only Animal Foods?

Since Linus Pauling famously championed vitamin C fifty years ago, there has been a fascination with this molecule and the great hope that it would turn out to be a panacea. Numerous studies have been done in efforts to prove these hypotheses, and truckloads of vitamin C have been ingested. Sadly, this vitamin has not lived up to the hype.

Vitamin C, also known as ascorbic acid, is a compound we appear to have stopped synthesizing about 60 million years ago when the primate lineages known as Strepsirrhini and Haplorhini split, with the latter no longer producing vitamin C.[54] At first glance, this may appear to have been an evolutionary mistake, but natural selection doesn't really make mistakes, and when unfavorable mutations happen, they are quickly eliminated from the population.

The fact that our predecessors got along just fine for a very long time after the loss of the ability to synthesize vitamin C suggests that they consistently had access to ample amounts of this nutrient and, perhaps, that this genetic change was even favorable in some ways. In a moment, we'll discuss evidence regarding how much vitamin C we really need to function optimally, but it appears to be much less than we've previously thought. A loss in the ability to break down uric acid also occurred at approximately the same time as these changes in vitamin C synthesis, and some have hypothesized that this molecule may have taken over some of the antioxidant roles of vitamin C as well.[55,56]

I'm not debating that vitamin C serves important roles in our physiology. It's known to be involved in at least eight enzymatic reactions including the endogenous formation of carnitine and collagen.[54] In the synthesis of the latter, ascorbic acid is involved in reactions that add hydroxyl (OH) groups to single strands of collagen, allowing them to eventually wrap around each other in a triple-helix structure, forming a mature collagen molecule that can be used in our tissues. Without enough vitamin C, we can't make collagen properly and scurvy develops—with slow wound healing, bleeding gums, skin changes, brittle hair, and loose teeth. It's not a pretty picture!

Historical accounts, beginning with James Lind's 1747 report that scurvy in British Sailors could be cured with limes, have led us to believe that we must include plants in our diet to obtain enough vitamin C. But do you want to know something else that's incredible? Fresh meat and animal organs also cure scurvy, a historical fact that has been known for hundreds of years but recently seems forgotten. Contrary to popular belief, animal foods contain vitamin C. Muscle meat has been shown to have approximately 15 milligrams of vitamin C per pound. Organs such as kidney, liver, thymus, and brain are even better sources of this vitamin, possessing 30–40 milligrams per 100-gram serving. Similar to the case of vitamin K2, the issue here is that the USDA hasn't formally measured this nutrient in meat and organs, and as a result, it is often reported as being zero—but it certainly is not. Vitamin C also appears to be more heat-stable in animal foods than plant foods, so cooking meat and organs will likely not result in as much loss of this nutrient.[57]

Even though it's difficult to debate the presence of vitamin C in animal foods, critics of a carnivore diet might claim that we can't get enough of this nutrient eating only animals. Is there any scientific evidence to support this critique, and how much of this nutrient do we actually need to function optimally?

A series of experiments done on conscientious objectors in the 1940s give an indication of the amount of vitamin C needed to allow for proper collagen synthesis and to prevent scurvy. By completely withholding vitamin C in the diet, the first symptoms of scurvy developed within two months in these detainees. When doses of either 10, 30, or 70 milligrams of vitamin C were provided, all groups recovered in days with no notable clinical differences between them. This response illustrates that doses as low as 10 milligrams per day are enough to prevent scurvy and clinical signs of deficiency—much lower than the mega doses of vitamin C that we are often admonished to consume.

So 10 milligrams of vitamin C is enough to prevent scurvy, but surely there's evidence that larger doses are beneficial in other ways, right? The benefits of this vitamin have been extolled for decades, so one would think that there must be clear evidence that bigger doses improve antioxidant status or other biomarkers of health, but this just isn't the case! Though vitamin C does have roles in our body beyond enabling proper formation of collagen, it's unclear that doses beyond those that are known to correct scurvy are of any further benefit. Many of the misconceptions about the benefits of vitamin C are based on epidemiology studies, and yet again, interventional research tells a very different story.

Interventional studies with supplemental doses of vitamin C have repeatedly failed to show benefit on the endpoints of total mortality, cardiovascular disease, blood pressure, or incidence of the common cold.[58,59] Supplementation with vitamin C has also failed to result in changes in biomarkers of oxidative stress or DNA damage and does not protect against colorectal cancer, skin cancer, breast cancer, or non-Hodgkin's lymphoma.[60,61,62,63] This vitamin is not exactly the fountain of youth it's been touted to be!

To emphasize these points, let's examine one such interventional study in detail. In this randomized trial, nineteen men and twenty-six women eating less than 3 servings of fruit and vegetables per day were divided into two groups. For twelve weeks, one group continued eating their previous diet, and the other added a *pound* of fruit and vegetables and 300 milliliters of fruit juice per day. At the end of this study, blood levels of vitamin C, antioxidant capacity, and markers of DNA damage were obtained in both groups and compared to pre-intervention levels. Despite consuming a significantly increased amount of vitamin C in their diet (70mg vs. 250mg) and demonstrating elevated blood levels of this nutrient, **no improvements** in any of the markers assayed in the interventional group were seen! The investigators stated:

> *"While plasma vitamin C [increased by] 35%, there were no significant changes in antioxidant capacity, DNA damage and markers of vascular health. Conclusion: **A 12-week intervention [with increased fruits and vegetables] was not associated with effects on antioxidant status or lymphocyte DNA damage.** "*[64]

Previously in this book, we've examined research similar to this showing that increased consumption of fruit and vegetables does not improve markers of oxidative stress or DNA damage, findings that fundamentally call into question the notion that phytochemicals like polyphenols have any benefit in humans. What's even more striking about this study is that investigators measured vitamin C intake and blood levels pre and post intervention, and demonstrated that despite nearly quadrupling (70mg to 250mg), there were also no changes in antioxidant markers or DNA damage!

Vitamin C does appear to have some role in antioxidant defense, recycling glutathione and vitamin E in the human body, but interventional studies like this clearly demonstrate that moderate intakes of this nutrient are enough to fulfill these roles optimally, and that further dosing does not demonstrate clear benefits. Vitamin C amounts between 10–70 milligrams per day can easily be obtained eating fresh animal foods by consuming organ meats in addition to muscle meat, as our ancestors always have. We'll go into detail about how to do this nose-to-tail eating in Chapter Twelve where I break down how to eat a carnivore diet.

Contrary to what Linus Pauling and plant-based advocates would have you believe, there's also evidence that too much vitamin C can be harmful in humans with reports of an increased incidence of oxalate kidney stones, nausea, bloating, acid reflux, B_{12} deficiency, and even increased oxidative stress.[65,66] When given in large doses, vitamin C appears to turn into a pro-oxidant in our bodies, and even moderate doses of vitamin C found in common supplements (500mg to 1000mg) have been linked with increased rates of kidney stones.[54,67]

One of the biggest challenges when looking at nutrient needs and utilization in humans is that almost every study done is on populations that are likely insulin resistant and consuming a very poor diet. This metabolic dysfunction appears to lead to less absorption and utilization of vitamin C, and a large study demonstrated that despite similar intakes of vitamin C between those with and without diabetes, the latter group had lower blood levels of this nutrient.[68]

Thus, in those with greater insulin sensitivity, it's possible that more of the vitamin C we consume is able to be absorbed and utilized. Furthermore, flavonoids have been shown to compete with vitamin C for absorption,[69] and the absence of these compounds on a carnivore diet would likely further enhance our body's ability to efficiently assimilate this nutrient. Among thousands of people following a nose-to-tail carnivore diet for a period of several months to over twenty years, there have also been no reported cases of scurvy or its symptoms.

On a personal note, I'll add that my surfing wounds heal just fine these day, and there's no evidence of increased oxidative stress in my blood work. For the geeks out there, I've looked at this in detail in myself, measuring blood markers like lipid peroxides, 8-OH-2-deoxyguanosine, GGT, hsCRP, fibrinogen, myeloperoxidase, and many others with no evidence of issues.

So, how much vitamin C do we really need? It's pretty clear that we need enough to prevent scurvy, which has been established as 10 milligrams daily. It doesn't look like daily consumption of 30–100 milligrams per day in our foods is going to be harmful for us, but there's no evidence that we need to supplement with more than this in order to achieve optimal health. Current RDA's for vitamin C are 60–80 milligrams per day for men and women, an amount that appears to lead to saturation of most cells with ascorbic acid and is easily obtainable from animal foods if we include organs in our diet.

The takeaway from this discussion is that nature didn't make a mistake when our genetics changed and we stopped making vitamin C. Because we can easily obtain a more than adequate amount of this nutrient by eating fresh plant or *animal* foods, it's unlikely that vitamin C has been a limiting nutrient during our evolutionary history. Contrary to the prevailing thinking, I believe that, throughout this time, our main sources of vitamin C would have been from animal foods, since plant sources would have been scarce at times, depending on the time of year and the latitude. With regard to supplementation, there is not a shred of evidence that mega-dosing with vitamin C from supplements is helpful, and it may be harmful. The next time you want to reach for that orange for vitamin C, remember that you could also eat some liver, kidney, or steak!

SUMMING IT UP

We have decades of bad observational epidemiology studies to thank for the incorrect notions that red meat will cause cancer or shorten our lives. Thankfully, there's plenty of evidence, which we've reviewed, that exposes these assertions as blatantly false and not based on sound science. It is also immediately apparent from an ancestral perspective that red meat or animal foods causing cancer or shortening our lives is evolutionarily inconsistent. These are the foods that made us human, and the foundational foods that our diets have been based on for the last 2 million years. Eating these foods has allowed us to grow much larger brains and to become a smarter, stronger, and more resourceful species.

In the next chapter, we will directly attack the misconception that red meat and animal foods will lead to cardiovascular disease. This is yet another evolutionarily absurd idea based almost entirely on misleading epidemiology. Onward, courageous warriors, there's still more ground to cover and untruths to slay.

CHAPTER ELEVEN

MYTH IV
RED MEAT CAUSES THE HEART TO EXPLODE

We've covered many miles so far, my courageous companions, and we are nearing the end of our journey to understand our ancestral roots and fully discover what is written in our user manual. But before we conclude our sojourn through treacherous lands, there's one more beast to slay, and it's a big one. Few things conjure more fear in the hearts and minds of the general population than the big, bad cholesterol monster and the associated trepidation that red meat will cause our arteries to become filled with plaque. After all, we've been told by cardiac surgeons that when they scoop plaque out of the arteries in our heart or neck, it looks just like animal fat, eggs, or butter. *Surely, the only way to avoid atherosclerosis is to eat benign plants. By doing that, we'll live long prosperous lives that are free from vascular disease, right?* No way. Nothing could be further from the truth!

In this chapter, we'll debunk the notion that eating animal meat, fat, or organs is bad for our heart and blood vessels and slay this final beast once and for all. We'll see that these false notions have been based on more misleading epidemiological literature and how interventional and mechanistic studies tell a very different story. Come, brave adventurers, our destiny of discarding unfounded ideologies and reclaiming the vibrant health of our ancestors awaits!

THE BASICS OF LIPOPROTEINS AND CHOLESTEROL

Cholesterol and lipids are a complex topic. In order to really understand why meat is not bad for our hearts, we'll need to understand all of the dramatis personae in the elegant system of lipid metabolism. The word "cholesterol" is often used colloquially to refer to all of the lipoproteins in our blood, but technically, cholesterol is a steroid backbone type of molecule that is used to make all sorts of vital compounds in human physiology.

Our body makes around 1,200 milligrams of cholesterol every day for many important purposes, including the proper formation of all of our cell membranes. Without cholesterol these would fall apart instantly, and we'd melt into a pile of mush on the floor. The cholesterol molecule is also used as a precursor for *all* of the steroid hormones in our body. These include estrogen, testosterone, cortisol, progesterone, and aldosterone—hormones that are kind of a big deal when it comes to kicking lots of butt. The bile acids used to help digest fats are made from cholesterol as well; without them we would quickly become malnourished and deficient in fat-soluble vitamins like A, K2, and E. When our skin is exposed to sunlight, cholesterol is also a precursor for the formation of vitamin D and cholesterol sulfate, a molecule hypothesized to play a role in preventing atherosclerosis.[1,2]

Because cholesterol isn't soluble in the water-based (aqueous) environment of our bloodstream, our body uses a lipoprotein transportation system to shuttle it between the liver and the various tissues where it is needed to perform the aforementioned functions. Lipoproteins have a phospholipid membrane composed of both fat-soluble (hydrophobic) and water-soluble (hydrophilic) regions. They are able to package fat-soluble cholesterol and triglycerides within them, but remain soluble in the aqueous compartment of the blood. This is the "lipid" part of "lipoprotein." The "protein" portion of these molecules refers to specific proteins, know as **apolipoproteins**, inserted into the lipid membrane. There are multiple types of lipoproteins in the human body that we'll need to be familiar with, all of which are identified according to the unique apolipoproteins present in their membranes.

The fat we eat is absorbed from our intestines and packaged as triglycerides with dietary cholesterol into a type of lipoprotein known as **chylomicrons**, marked with apolipoprotein B48. These particles circulate in the blood stream, dropping off their contents to cells of the body before becoming chylomicron remnants and being taken up by the liver. The liver can then use the remaining triglycerides and cholesterol in these particles or repackage them into another type of lipoprotein known as **VLDL** (very low-density lipoprotein). VLDL particles are sent out into the peripheral circulation delivering cholesterol and triglycerides to peripheral cells. As triglycerides are extracted from VLDL, these lipoproteins contain a higher percentage of cholesterol and increase in density, becoming intermediate- and then low-density lipoproteins (IDL & LDL).

LDL particles therefore contain both triglycerides and cholesterol as they circulate through our bloodstream and are identified by an important apolipoprotein known as **APOB100**. They continue to drop triglycerides and cholesterol off to cells in need of them, and then eventually make their way back to the liver where they are reabsorbed. High-density lipoproteins (HDL) are also made in the liver and in the gut and are marked by the apolipoprotein **APOA1**. These particles are a bit different from the others we've discussed. When they are created, they are essentially empty and become filled with cholesterol and triglycerides from chylomicrons, VLDL, IDL, and LDL within the bloodstream as well as from peripheral cells of the body. The main role of HDL is to take extra cholesterol back to the liver in a process known as **reverse cholesterol transport**, but as we'll see later, HDL and other lipoproteins also serve vital roles in the immune response.

We might think of this whole process of the movement of cholesterol and triglycerides throughout the body as a bus system with various routes and different buses carrying passengers throughout these. Buses carrying dietary fat and cholesterol called chylomicrons depart from the intestines to the liver, which is basically the central bus station. Here, passengers get off the chylomicron bus and can get on the departing VLDL buses where they are joined by new passengers from the liver. The VLDL bus makes stops throughout the body and eventually has many less passengers. Along the way, it becomes the LDL bus, which continues on its routes before eventually returning to the liver. The HDL bus starts empty in the liver or intestines and picks up passengers from cells of the body or other buses, taking them back to the central liver bus station. This is an oversimplification, of course, and the lipoproteins in our bodies do much more than simply shuttle fat and cholesterol around our body, but at a basic level, this model describes how the lipoprotein particles move and interact.

In medicine, the term "total cholesterol" refers to the sum of all the cholesterol molecules in the blood and is usually measured directly in laboratory tests. In order to know how much of this cholesterol resides in the different lipoproteins, these must be measured individually. Most current lipid testing measures HDL, LDL, VLDL, and triglycerides directly, but older assays measure only some of these and must calculate LDL, which you may see written as LDL-C. For this reason, many previous research studies have looked at total cholesterol levels rather than LDL. Historically, elevated levels of total cholesterol have been assumed to correlate with elevated levels of LDL, and unless triglycerides are extremely elevated, this is generally a reasonable assumption. In the studies we'll discuss in this chapter, I'll specifically note whether investigators measured total cholesterol levels or LDL levels. I'll also mention that the words coronary artery disease, atherosclerosis, heart disease, and cardiovascular disease all generally refer to the process of plaque formation in the arterial wall, and I'll use them interchangeably in this chapter.

THE VITAL ROLE OF LDL IN OUR BODY

Most of the cells of our body can make a bit of cholesterol from scratch, but they also rely heavily on the delivered supply of this molecule to build membranes and hormones. In the ovaries and testicles, for instance, cholesterol delivered by LDL is necessary to make the lovely sex hormones estrogen and testosterone, which are crucial for libido and reproductive function. Without LDL, these and many other steroid hormones wouldn't be made effectively. Wait, haven't we been told that LDL is "bad cholesterol" and that the lower it is, the better? I'm sad to say that we've been led astray with regard to the true character of LDL, which is much more of a superhero than a supervillain.

In addition to its vital role transporting building blocks and nutrients, LDL also serves important roles within the immune system. Yes, you read that correctly, LDL plays a valuable part in our response to assault by infectious invaders, as do many of the lipoproteins, including HDL. When gram-negative bacteria seek to invade our body, they release a cell wall component known as **endotoxin**, which is quite inflammatory and can strongly trigger the immune system. But don't worry, friendly neighborhood LDL is around to bind-up this toxin and prevent things from getting out of hand. LDL also binds the alpha toxins produced by the gram-positive organism *Staph aureus*, which has antibiotic resistant strains known as MRSA.[3,4,5]

Bacteria attempting to besiege us also secrete molecules telling each other when it's a good time to divide and go on the attack. This communication system is known as **quorum sensing**, and it's bad news for our immune system. But LDL can again fight in this battle by binding up these molecules and helping to disable such lines of bacterial communication. Mice with experimentally increased levels of LDL are eight times more resistant to endotoxin. As a result, they have significantly delayed mortality when directly injected with gram negative bacteria.[6] Conversely, rats bred to have decreased levels of LDL had much higher mortality rates and levels of inflammation when injected with endotoxin—deficits that could be remedied by providing them with exogenous supplemental LDL.[7]

Let's take a moment to let all of that sink in. In both humans and animals, lipoproteins and LDL are known to serve invaluable roles in immune function. Increasing the amount of LDL in the bloodstream, something that 99 percent of physicians now fear in humans, resulted in profoundly increased survival when animals were challenged with virulent bacteria. Having a low LDL resulted in mice dropping like flies when exposed to bacteria, but the problem was immediately fixed by giving these poor critters some LDL back. Paralleling LDL depletion studies in mice, there is a known human condition (Smith-Lemli-Optiz syndrome) in which total cholesterol is very low due to a genetic mutation in the cholesterol synthesis pathway. Children born with this mutation are often stillborn, but those who do survive suffer frequent and severe infections that are remedied with a dietary supplementation of cholesterol, leading to higher levels of LDL in the bloodstream.[8]

COULD MORE LDL BE PROTECTIVE?

But what about in humans? Is there evidence that higher levels of LDL could be protective against infection in us? You bet there is! There are *many* studies that show elevated levels of LDL are *not* a risk factor for increased all-cause mortality or cardiovascular mortality in the elderly.[9] Furthermore, there are many studies suggesting that *higher* levels of LDL are protective as we age, which is most likely connected with its role in immune function.[10,11,12-20]

Highlighting a few of these studies will help to clearly illustrate this point. In a sample of 347 individuals over the age of sixty-five, those with low total cholesterol had a significantly higher risk of dying by non-vascular causes, while those with elevated total cholesterol had half the risk of the reference population.[10] Another study of 105 individuals over the age of eighty living in Iceland found that those with the highest total cholesterol level had less than half the all-cause mortality of those with lower levels.[21] An even larger investigation called the Leiden 85-plus study had even more striking results. This study included 724 elderly individuals living in the Netherlands in whom the correlation between total cholesterol and all-cause mortality was measured for ten years. The authors found that for every 38 milligrams per deciliter increase in the total cholesterol, there was a corresponding 15 percent *decrease* in the risk of dying over this time period. They concluded:

> *"Mortality from cancer and infection was significantly lower among the participants in the highest total cholesterol* category *than in the other categories, which largely explained the lower all-cause mortality in this category. In people older than 85 years, high total cholesterol concentrations are associated with longevity owing to lower mortality from cancer and infection.'*[22]

The sheer magnitude of studies showing this association between high levels of total cholesterol and longevity in elderly individuals is strong evidence of LDL's protective role in humans. Some have claimed, however, that this correlation reflects an artifact related to a known drop in lipid levels that occurs prior to death in many people with cancer. Thus, they assert that the association of low levels of cholesterol with worse outcomes may reflect these diseased people in the population. However, in the majority of these studies, researchers excluded people who died within two years of sampling from their analyses, essentially removing the possibility of this confounder. In many of these studies, it was also shown that rates of cancer death were lower in people with higher levels of total cholesterol. Taking this into consideration, along with the large number of studies that show this trend, it seems pretty safe to say this association is real and that LDL appears to be quite protective as we age.

There's also a large body of literature regarding total cholesterol levels and infectious disease, which lends further support to the notion that LDL is a superhero rather than a supervillain. A large meta analysis of 68,406 individuals found an inverse correlation between levels of total cholesterol and death by respiratory and gastrointestinal diseases, most of which are infectious in etiology.[23] That is, those with the highest levels of total cholesterol experienced the smallest number of deaths from these types of illnesses. Similarly, in a fifteen-year study of over 120,000 patients, those with the highest total cholesterol levels had the *lowest* risk of being admitted to the hospital for an infectious disease.[24] In this study, statistically significant inverse associations were found between total cholesterol and multiple types of infections, including urinary tract, viral, musculoskeletal, skin, respiratory, and gastrointestinal. These findings were replicated in another fifteen-year study of over 100,000 patients, which showed an *inverse* association between total cholesterol and hospital admission for pneumonia or the flu.[25] In studies of HIV-infected patients, there is also evidence of an inverse association between total cholesterol levels and AIDS mortality.[26] Still think LDL deserves the ignominious moniker of "bad cholesterol"?

LDL in Heart Disease: Criminal or Firefighter?

Clearly, LDL is a valuable particle in our blood and serves many indispensable roles. Doesn't it seem a bit incongruous that nature would have designed something that is so valuable but also damages our arteries and causes atherosclerosis? How can LDL be both protective and harmful? This doesn't seem to make any sense! The answer is that LDL itself is **not** harmful, but in certain situations, it can be involved in the process of responding to injury and inflammation—making it look like it's a bad actor when it's merely present at the scene of the crime. Let's explore the evidence used by those who believe that LDL is causing atherosclerosis to promote their claims. In doing so, it will become clear that LDL is not a double-agent but has been wrongfully pegged as a criminal when there's something much more sinister behind the scenes that is actually driving heart disease.

Some observational epidemiology studies do show an association between levels of total cholesterol, or LDL, and cardiovascular disease. Since you've come this far with me on our epic journey, you'll already know that epidemiology doesn't tell the whole story and that we must look deeper into this association to see what's really going on here. The Framingham Study is one of the most commonly referenced epidemiological investigations by those looking at the relationship between total cholesterol levels and the incidence of cardiovascular disease. In this study, 5,129 subjects living in Framingham, Massachusetts, were followed for fourteen years and had levels of their cholesterol checked twice per year while they were monitored for the onset of coronary artery disease. In this population, researchers noted that as LDL levels rose, there was indeed an increase in the incidence of heart disease.[27]

Their sentiments were strengthened by microscopic studies showing that LDL is present in atherosclerotic plaques, often having been ingested by immune cells known as macrophages within the arterial wall.[28] Considered together with epidemiology studies showing a correlation between LDL and cardiovascular disease, this finding has led many to believe that elevated levels of LDL are to blame for the initiation and progression of atherosclerosis. If we examine plaque formation in detail, however, we'll see that it's far from proven that the LDL molecule is intrinsically damaging to our arteries or is enough to initiate plaque formation within the arterial wall on its own.

As we continue our quest to understand the true roots of atherosclerosis, we need to pause a moment to take a detailed look at the anatomy of our blood vessels and the processes occurring there during plaque formation.

The walls of both veins and arteries are composed of multiple layers. The single cell layer closest to circulating blood is known as the endothelium—below which lie the cells of the intima—and then a layer of smooth muscle cells. Interestingly, just like the gastrointestinal epithelium, the endothelium in our blood vessels also possesses a glycocalyx composed of glycoproteins protruding from its surface. In order to move into the vessel wall, lipoproteins like LDL must pass among the "forest" of this glycocalyx, through the endothelial cell layer, and into the cells of the intima, which lie in the subendothelial space. After dropping off some of its contents, LDL then appears to move back out into the circulation, but it can also get stuck to the proteoglycan scaffolding within the deepest layers of the intima.[29,30] There is a region of the APOB100 molecule in the LDL membrane that is known to bind to proteoglycans, and when this binding site is removed from the APOB gene of mice, it prevents the progression of atherosclerosis in animal models of this disease.[31] LDL may also arrive at the subendothelial space through the blood stream in perforating capillaries that supply the deep intimal and muscular layers of the artery wall.[32,33]

The currently accepted paradigm of plaque formation is known as the **response-to-retention hypothesis**. According to this theory, LDL in our bloodstream passes through the endothelium of the artery wall, and can become retained ("stuck") in the intimal cell layer below. When LDL gets stuck in the arterial wall, it may become oxidized, altering the structure of the APOB100 molecules in its membrane and triggering an immune response in which macrophages within the intima ingest LDL and become lipid ladened "foam cells." This is thought to be the beginning of an atherosclerotic plaque.[34]

Therefore, according to the response-to-retention theory, the greater the amount of LDL in circulation, the greater the risk that it will be retained in the subendothelial space and lead to plaque formation. Thus, anything that raises LDL throws most physicians into a tizzy and sends them running to the medicine cabinet with strong suggestions of statins and other cholesterol-lowering agents to their patients. The problem here is that *this key portion of the theory has not been proven*. There is exactly zero research that conclusively shows that the amount of LDL retained is directly linked to the amount of LDL in the circulation, and there are many studies that suggest exactly *the opposite*.

In the elderly, higher levels of LDL appear to be protective and are associated with greater longevity. Epidemiology studies of women, Canadian and Russian men, Maoris, and Asians do *not* show associations between total cholesterol or LDL levels and incidence of heart disease or all-cause mortality.[23,35,36-38] Why would LDL behave differently throughout the lifespan, between men and women, or across the globe? *If the process of atherosclerosis were really as simple as "more LDL in the circulation leading to more plaque formation," this correlation would be present across all age groups, sexes, and cultures.*

Vegetarians are also far from immune to atherosclerosis. They, too, display rates equivalent to the general population despite lower average levels of LDL.[39] Furthermore, in statin trials, there is not a true dose-response relationship between levels of LDL and the degree of plaque formation.[40,41,42] In studies with both statins and PCSK9 inhibitors (which lower LDL levels below 40 milligrams per deciliter), the majority of patients continue to suffer progression of cardiovascular disease despite extremely low levels of LDL.[43] Clearly, there's much more to this equation than we have been led to believe, and the progression of atherosclerosis depends on more than simply the amount of LDL in the bloodstream.

Data from the Framingham Study provides us with key insights into how the response-to-retention hypothesis is flawed.[44] If we look at a graph comparing total cholesterol levels to the incidence of cardiovascular disease across all participants within this study, we get a graph that looks like the following:

THE FRAMINGHAM STUDY
CAD RISK BY LDL

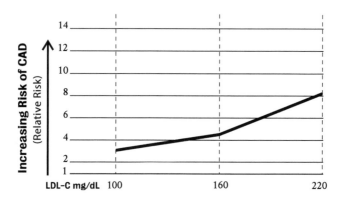

Gordon, T. et al., (1977). High density lipoprotein as a protective factor against coronary heart disease: The Framingham study. *The American Journal of Medicine*, 62(5): 707-714.

We can see why researchers might look at this and believe that there's a direct relationship between the amount of LDL in the blood and cardiovascular disease: the more total cholesterol and LDL, the more people from this study had cardiovascular events. But a very interesting thing happens to this graph when we separate all of the people studied into groups based on their levels of HDL.

Up to this point we've spoken about HDL only briefly when we discussed its role in reverse cholesterol transport. Another very interesting thing about HDL is that its level correlates directly with insulin sensitivity.[45,46,47] In those with insulin resistance, HDL levels fall and triglyceride levels rise, a change in blood parameters known as metabolic dyslipidemia.[48] Thus, those with the lowest levels of HDL are much more likely to have insulin resistance than those with higher levels of this lipoprotein.[49,50] Looking at the graph that follows, it's immediately apparent that differences in HDL make a huge difference in cardiovascular disease risk. Keep in mind that this is exactly the same data from the Framingham Study depicted in the previous graph, but participants have been split into groups based on their HDL levels.

THE FRAMINGHAM STUDY
CAD RISK BY LDL AND HDL

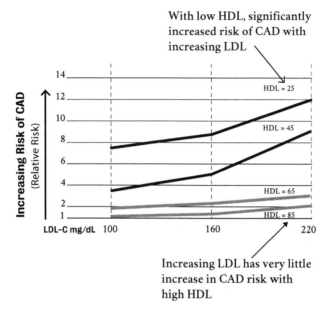

With low HDL, significantly increased risk of CAD with increasing LDL

Increasing LDL has very little increase in CAD risk with high HDL

Gordon, T. et al., (1977). High density lipoprotein as a protective factor against coronary heart disease: The Framingham study. *The American Journal of Medicine*, 62(5): 707-714.

What we quickly notice looking at this graph is that with low HDL (less than 45 milligrams per deciliter), there is a clear correlation between total cholesterol and heart disease, but in those with higher levels of HDL, *this correlation vanishes almost entirely*. What we see here is exactly what proponents of the response-to-retention hypothesis are missing. Atherosclerosis is about much more than just total cholesterol or LDL. **In those who are insulin sensitive, rising LDL levels do not correlate with increased rates of heart disease.**

Thinking about LDL levels within a vacuum is a critical mistake and a dangerously myopic perspective. When it comes to total cholesterol and LDL, context is everything! If we are insulin resistant, higher levels of LDL may very well contribute to plaque formation and progression, but if we are insulin sensitive, higher levels of LDL are not associated with increased atherosclerosis and are likely protective.

These findings help us explain the discordance in the epidemiology data regarding LDL and heart disease. It's not just about LDL, it's about insulin resistance. When thinking about heart disease risk and lipids, we must consider the overall health of the individual rather than looking only at LDL. And yet the vast majority of the time, if LDL is elevated, clinicians become overly focused on this, disregarding the HDL and triglycerides and very rarely taking into consideration other blood-markers reflective of insulin sensitivity, such as fasting insulin.

ATHEROSCLEROSIS—IT'S ALL ABOUT THE STICKINESS!

So far, we've seen that if LDL gets stuck within the intima, it can become oxidized, triggering an immune reaction and leading to macrophage engulfment.[51] Binding of LDL to proteoglycans with subsequent oxidization appears to be a key step in this process because "native" or non-oxidized LDL does not contribute to the progression of coronary artery disease.[52]

If it's only the LDL that gets "stuck" in our artery walls that contributes to atherosclerosis, could a higher amount of LDL in our blood stream lead to more LDL in the subendothelial space and the progression of this phenomenon? At first glance, one might think so, and this is indeed what advocates of the response-to-retention hypothesis believe. But as we've seen based on the Framingham data, levels of LDL in the blood do not consistently correlate with the progression of coronary artery disease in the absence of insulin resistance. With a little more examination of the amount of LDL in our body and plaque formation, we'll see why the notion that more LDL equals more atherosclerosis is clearly unfounded.

There are more than a quintillion (1,000,000,000,000,000,000—or—1×10^{18}) particles of LDL floating around in our bloodstream. That's 1,000 times more LDL particles than there are cells in our whole body. If every LDL particle that entered the subendothelial space in our arteries led to the formation of a plaque, we'd be deader than a doornail long before our first birthday. Every second of every day, lipoproteins like LDL are moving in and out of the walls of both veins and arteries, delivering nutrients to the cells there for energy and the construction of membranes. Clearly, there must be another part of this equation that leads to retention of some of these LDL particles within the arterial wall.

Interestingly, HDL particles are smaller and ten times more numerous than LDL. They carry more cholesterol in our blood stream, but these particles do not participate in the formation of atherosclerotic lesions. Why not? Because they do not get stuck in the subendothelial space. Within the arterial wall, it appears that only particles containing the APOB molecule are able to bind to the proteoglycans within the intima and be retained.[53] *It's not the size of the particle, or the number of particles moving into the vessel wall that's important, it's how likely a lipoprotein is to be retained that determines whether or not it contributes to the process of plaque formation.*

If you were to throw tennis balls at a wall, unless both were coated in velcro, they would not stick. It would not matter how many times you threw them. Similarly, it appears that unless LDL and the intimal space are sticky, no matter how many LDL particles we have floating around our bodies, the LDL "balls" only get stuck to the intimal "walls" when both are coated in a "molecular velcro" that makes them sticky. *LDL is not enough to initiate atherosclerosis on its own, it has to get stuck in the arterial wall to participate in this process.*

What determines how sticky the LDL particle and the intimal space are? Ah, my friends, this is truly the million-dollar question! The good news is that I believe we've already got a million-dollar answer, and that we already know what it is from our analysis of the Framingham data. There's very good evidence that during the states of insulin resistance and inflammation, *both* the LDL particle and the intimal space get coated in "molecular velcro" and become more sticky.[54,55,56-58] Specifically, studies looking at the arteries of diabetics and arterial wall injury have shown changes in the proteoglycan matrix that increase its affinity for LDL.[59] Additional research reveals that the LDL particle becomes more likely to be bound to proteoglycans in the intimal space when it is enriched with apolipoprotein ApoC III—a process that occurs during states of insulin resistance—making for a dangerous combination that strongly predisposes to plaque formation. The risk of atherosclerosis is so high in diabetics that rates of heart attack are elevated in this population even with low levels of LDL.[60]

At this point, you may be saying, "Sure, I believe you on this, but doesn't atherosclerosis occur in people without diabetes or pre-diabetes? How common is this scenario of insulin resistance?" Fantastic question! If I could give you an enthusiastic high five right now, I would! You've hit the nail on the head with this one, and the answer might surprise you: though diabetes and pre-diabetes are diagnosed in 35 percent of the American population, there's strong evidence that insulin resistance is *much* more common than this!

As we've discussed previously, there is evidence that **a whopping 88 percent of the American population has some degree of metabolic dysfunction**.[61] If the vast majority of people around us have insulin resistance, is it any wonder that some studies have shown a correlation between LDL levels and cardiovascular disease? Almost the entire population of the U.S. has velcro on their lipoproteins and within their arteries, and the tennis balls are getting stuck to the wall! So to answer the previous question, there's good evidence that when atherosclerosis does occur, it is almost always in the setting of insulin resistance and metabolic dysfunction.

One of the biggest mistakes Western medicine makes is to extrapolate these pathologies to the 12 percent of us who are *not* insulin resistant and *not* inflamed, warning us that certain cardiovascular disease will swiftly follow with an elevated LDL.

Those of us with good insulin sensitivity are essentially a different breed, and there are many striking stories of plaque *regression* among insulin-sensitive individuals with "elevated LDL" eating carnivore or ketogenic diets. In the absence of insulin resistance and inflammation, higher levels of LDL are probably protective because of their roles with the immune response. Want to live a long time? Eat in a manner that allows for insulin sensitivity, decreases inflammation, and leads to a robust amount of valuable LDL particles. Carnivore diet, anyone?

FURTHER DOWN THE LDL RABBIT HOLE

Although LDL is found in atherosclerotic plaques, it has not been shown to be able to initiate plaque formation on its own. Just because a fireman shows up to a house on fire—or a policeman arrives at the scene of a crime—does not mean that they caused the mayhem. In the case of atherosclerosis, the compelling alternative hypothesis is that *although LDL is present in an atherosclerotic plaque, it's probably not performing as the criminal who started the fire, but rather, as the fireman arriving at the scene to quell the blaze.* There's good evidence to believe that LDL is not causing atherosclerosis but may be involved in plaques as part of a repair process in response to injury to the vessel wall.

If the presence of LDL in the arterial lesion is the main indictment of its guilt, what evidence do we have of its possible innocence in this pathological process? Consider this: If LDL alone were enough to cause atherosclerosis, why is it that plaque formation is only observed in arteries and not veins? The amount of LDL circulating through our blood vessels is the same throughout our body, be it in the higher pressure arterial system leading from the heart to organs and extremities, or in the lower pressure venous system that returns blood from these distal regions back to the good old ticker. Our blood vessels form a continuous loop with a consistent amount of lipoproteins evenly distributed throughout it. The endothelium of our veins is exposed to exactly the same amount of LDL as the endothelium of our arteries—and yet, only the latter display atherosclerotic lesions.

A clue as to why this occurs is found in the common location of plaque build-up at arterial branch points, where turbulent blood flow can damage the lining of our arteries.[62] It appears that atherosclerotic plaques occur in locations where the endothelium has become damaged. This damage can occur as a result of turbulent blood flow, inflammation, insulin resistance, or other causes.[63,64] Intriguingly, when veins are subjected to the higher pressures of the arterial vascular tree, in cases such as cardiac bypass surgery, *they quickly develop aggressive atherosclerotic lesions.* Similarly, in animal models, arteries transplanted into the venous circulation do not develop atherosclerosis.[65] These findings suggest that it's not something about the veins themselves that protects them from plaque formation, but rather, the higher pressure system of the arterial circulation that predisposes the endothelium of arteries to injury.

We've covered a heck of a lot so far on this complex topic; let's tie all of this together to present a complete picture of what's probably happening in the development of atherosclerotic plaque. We know that LDL and other lipoproteins serve vital roles in the body—delivering nutrients to all of our cells—and without them, we wouldn't be alive. The intimal cells of our arterial walls need these nutrients to function properly, just like all of the other cells of our body, and they receive them through the diffusion of lipoproteins within the bloodstream into the subendothelial space.[32] When everything is copasetic, these lipoproteins move into the intimal cell layer and then move back out into the circulation, continuing their journey and eventually ending up back at the liver. But when the arterial wall is damaged by states of insulin resistance, inflammation, oxidative stress, hyperglycemia, or arterial turbulence, it displays increased levels of proteoglycan molecules and becomes "stickier." This traps the circulating lipoproteins that may also be coated in "molecular velcro." Once stuck in the deepest layers of the intima, LDL is more likely to become oxidized and engulfed by the macrophages there, leading to the beginnings of atherosclerosis.[33]

Within this framework, the accumulation of lipoproteins within the arterial wall might be viewed as a molecular repair mechanism. This can progress to atherosclerosis when it gets out of control and is driven by pathophysiological states like insulin resistance and inflammation. From this perspective, LDL is probably just like the firemen who arrive at the scene of the fire. They didn't set the fire, but if the blaze gets out of control, a whole lot of them show up to fight it. In the case of atherosclerosis, when a whole lot of LDL firemen start showing up and get stuck, subendothelial plaque can form. This process of arterial repair from micro-injury is always happening in our arterial walls, but when it gets out of hand, it can lead to atherosclerosis and eventually heart disease. It's not the LDL that initiates plaque formation, it's injury to the arterial wall. The notion that LDL deposition may in fact be part of an arterial repair mechanism is strengthened by the fact that all placental mammals, including herbivores, omnivores, and carnivores, are known to demonstrate LDL deposition in the arterial wall.[66,67,68,69]

Maybe we should send a card to LDL apologizing for badmouthing it over the last sixty years when it was just trying to help. On second thought, LDL would probably appreciate a few steaks and liver more.

THE SKINNY (AND NOT SO SKINNY) ON INSULIN RESISTANCE

At this point in our adventure, we've seen that insulin resistance is quite sinister, making both LDL and our arteries much more sticky. But what causes insulin resistance in the first place, and how do we stay in the 12 percent with slick "balls and walls" who are insulin sensitive? Let's dig into what we know about this pathological process and how to avoid its damaging clutches.

Although there's no formal characterization of insulin resistance, it's generally defined as a diminished response to the actions of insulin by all of the tissues of the body. Insulin is a peptide hormone secreted by the beta cells of the pancreas in response to protein or carbohydrate intake, but more so with the latter. It signals the peripheral tissues to take up glucose from the bloodstream and to proliferate. When cells of the body become resistant to insulin, more is needed to achieve the previous effect, and blood levels begin to rise. Insulin resistance is essentially synonymous with pre-diabetes, but because the manifestations are subtle, this condition is often missed. The need for higher levels of insulin puts stress on the pancreas, but initially it is able to meet the increased demand. If nothing changes, insulin resistance gradually worsens, and by the time we develop full-blown diabetes, our poor pancreas has been overproducing insulin for a long time and can barely keep up. Type II diabetics often end up needing supplemental insulin when the pancreas can no longer respond adequately to the increasing needs of the peripheral tissues, and blood glucose levels begin to rise significantly.

Most of the evidence points to the roots of insulin resistance being within the mitochondria, the organelles that are our cellular power plants. It is within these incredible energy factories that the protein, fat, and carbohydrates we eat are ultimately converted into energy in the form of ATP. In states of insulin resistance, mitochondria send out signals to the rest of the cell in the form of reactive oxygen species (ROS), telling them that they are overloaded with energy, usually from excess calorie consumption.[70,71,72] These reactive oxygen species cause the cell to refuse the signals from insulin to take up glucose and other nutrients, and insulin resistance develops.

In this situation, the main issue is usually excessive food consumption, especially excess carbohydrates combined with fat. Intriguingly, overfeeding with each of these macronutrients *individually* does not appear to lead to insulin resistance or weight gain, but when they are consumed together in excess, it appears to cause negative metabolic consequences in our body.[73] If we are consuming natural sources of carbohydrates and fat, our satiety mechanisms usually kick in at the proper time to prevent this, but the consumption of *processed food or a pre-existing metabolic dysfunction* (88 percent of Americans) can impair these processes and lead to problems. In situations of insulin resistance, one of the most effective therapeutic interventions is to significantly limit either carbohydrates or fat from our diet until we have lost excess weight and *regained proper insulin sensitivity.*

Since this is a book about the carnivore diet, you might be able to guess that I favor a high-fat, low-carbohydrate approach to insulin resistance related to obesity, but a high-carbohydrate, low-fat approach may also work for some people. The latter approach does not have the neuroprotective or satiety benefits of a ketogenic metabolism (a metabolism based on burning primarily fat rather than carbohydrates),[74] and many people find a high-fat/low-carb strategy easier to maintain long term for weight loss and body composition.

Within the natural world, the combination of both carbohydrates and fat is rare, and these macronutrients almost never occur together other than in breast milk, a uniquely valuable food in infancy. This combination appears to have less of an effect on our satiety signals than either of these macronutrients individually, something that has been leveraged to an extreme degree by junk food manufacturers. In a sinister recapitulation of the unique evolutionary combination of fat and carbohydrates in breast milk, candy bars, ice cream, and many other junk foods similarly function to *short-circuit* normal mechanisms of satiety and induce rapid weight gain and insulin resistance when eaten as part of a caloric surplus.

Our ancestors would have sought out the fattiest animals, but it's unlikely that they always had a lot of fat in their diet unless their hunts were successful. Carbohydrates are similarly scarce within the natural world.

Depending on latitude and time of year, a small amount of fruit may have been available occasionally, but this was likely rare. It's also interesting to note that fructose, the five-carbon sugar prevalent in fruit, has been shown to promote both insulin and leptin (a satiety hormone) resistance when consumed in excess.[75,76] We'll talk more about this in Chapter Twelve, but overconsumption of fruit is probably a bad idea in terms of both metabolic and dental health.

Throughout our evolution, we might have occasionally found carbohydrates in the form of tubers, but many of these contain toxic compounds like cyanogenic glycosides and oxalates. Most of the tubers we see in the grocery store today also look nothing like those that could have been eaten by our ancestors, which would have been much smaller, more fibrous, and probably tasted pretty horrible. Survival foods to be sure. Remember that the lack of the amylase gene duplication in Neanderthals and Denisovans also suggests that we have not been eating significant amounts of tubers for the majority of our evolution.

The takeaway here is that in the case of obesity, *insulin resistance usually results from excess calorie consumption in the form of carbohydrates combined with fat*, leading to mitochondrial dysfunction with signaling through increased reactive oxygen species. The clear way to correct this is to make efforts toward weight loss by not consuming excess calories, by avoiding processed food, and by limiting either fat or carbohydrate intake.

OTHER CAUSES OF INSULIN RESISTANCE

Though overfeeding is the first thing we usually think of with regard to obesity and insulin resistance, there are other things that can also cause this metabolic derangement, including infections, inflammation, and lifestyle factors such as stress and lack of sleep.

Experiments in humans show that intravenous infusion of endotoxin from gram-negative bacteria results in immune activation and metabolic dysfunction with insulin resistance.[77] At first, this may sound like a bad thing, and in situations of chronic inflammation, it can be. But there's evidence that transient insulin resistance might actually be a part of our body's normal response to infectious insults. Concentrations of lipoproteins are also known to change during acute infection, resulting in increased levels of VLDL and LDL observed in the circulation, likely related to the roles these particles play in the immune response.[78]

Insulin resistance can also be caused by systemic inflammation and is observed in many chronic autoimmune conditions, including rheumatoid arthritis, lupus, ankylosing spondylitis, polymyalgia rheumatica, depression, and schizophrenia.[79] If you are surprised to see depression in that list, remember that many psychiatric diseases appear to be inflammatory in nature. Not surprisingly, rates of heart disease are also greatly increased relative to the general population in people with these inflammatory conditions.[80]

As previously mentioned, damage to the gastrointestinal epithelium can lead to systemic inflammation, so it will come as no surprise that leaky gut can also cause insulin resistance and has been strongly linked to diabetes.[81] Via this mechanism, it's plausible that plant toxins, which are known to open tight junctions in the gastrointestinal tract,[82] could also be contributing to insulin resistance in some individuals. Not only might nightshades be making our joints hurt, they might also be causing leaky gut and metabolic dysfunction. Do we still think tomatoes are a health food?

The stress we encounter on a day-to-day basis is much greater and of a different quality than that which our ancestors traditionally bore. They might have had short periods of increased stress when fighting for survival or weathering a storm, but the unrelenting moderate level of stress we experience as humans today is something new for us. Our sleep environments are also significantly different from the past. We now have much more blue light at night, which disrupts the circadian rhythm. Managing stress and prioritizing good quality sleep are mandatory lifestyle modifications we need to make if we hope to be as insulin sensitive as possible.

The best metrics of health will be our energy, overall mood, sleep quality, libido, and body composition, but laboratory markers can be a useful adjunct to these. Within the bloodwork section of the Appendix, I have included tests that give us a sense of insulin sensitivity. These include *fasting glucose, fasting insulin, c-peptide, fructosamine, and fasting leptin.* Though fasting glucose is commonly ordered, the others are rarely looked at but are some of the most valuable data points we can gather.

Triglyceride and HDL levels also give a good indication of insulin sensitivity. I prefer to see triglycerides less than 75 milligrams per deciliter and view a triglyceride/HDL ratio of less than one as a good indicator that someone is likely insulin sensitive. LDL particle size has traditionally been used as a proxy for this as well, with less than 22 nanometers being a possible indicator of insulin resistance, though this is a less specific measurement.

You may notice that I've left hemoglobin A1c off this list. This marker looks at the percent of hemoglobin with attached sugar molecules and is meant to be a measure of the average blood glucose over the last one hundred days, which is the approximate life span of a red blood cell. I have found hemoglobin A1c to be somewhat inaccurate, however. The best way to get a sense of our average blood sugar is to use a continuous glucose monitor (CGM). These monitors are quite valuable as they can also show us how blood glucose levels change postprandially (after eating) and throughout the day and night. When postprandial glucose levels are elevated, it is a signal that some degree of insulin resistance or metabolic dysregulation is occurring in response to specific foods. Research suggests that glucose excursions from baseline should not be more than 50 milligrams per deciliter, and that less than 30 milligrams per deciliter is probably ideal. Furthermore, there should be a return to baseline within one to two hours.[83,84]

What happens in our body when our blood sugar spikes after meals? There's good evidence that these high levels of glucose can damage the endothelium of our blood vessels, leading to inflammation within the vessel wall and atherosclerosis.[85,86] Similarly, elevated blood sugar has been found to directly damage the gastrointestinal epithelium, the endothelium in the kidneys, and the blood-brain barrier.[87,88,89] **Elevated blood glucose levels appear to make all of the tissues of our body leaky,** which is not good and should be avoided if we hope to live radical lives.

What does a continuous blood glucose monitor reading look like from someone eating a nose-to-tail carnivore diet? If you take a look at the readings from multiple days below, you'll see that it's just about the most boring thing ever, but that is a very good thing. These readings are from a client of mine who gave me permission to share them. As you'll see, the average blood glucose sits right around 80 milligrams per deciliter, and there is essentially no change when he eats. On a carnivore diet, his meals are protein and fat with essentially zero carbohydrates, and this doesn't change his blood glucose at all. Contrast this with the reading from the day that he consumed carbohydrates and you'll see his glucose rise after eating and stay elevated for hours. As we've seen, this probably isn't the best thing for the endothelial lining of his blood vessels.

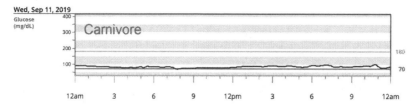

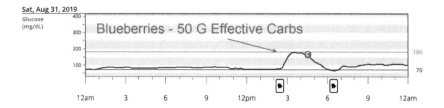

I'm not saying that all carbohydrates are bad. Certainly, at times throughout our evolution, we would have eaten some fruit or tubers if we needed to, but I do not believe these made up a significant proportion of our diets. There are indigenous peoples who eat significant amounts of carbohydrates and maintain good health,[90,91] but there are also examples of groups like the Pima Indians in whom a high-carbohydrate diet has led to an enormous rate of diabetes (greater than 80 percent) with profound negative health consequences.[92,93] It appears that we all have a genetic set point regarding how many carbohydrates we can handle, with the type of carbohydrate and consumption with fat being relevant. Processed carbohydrates like breads, pasta, flours, and sugars appear to be universally detrimental, but some people may be able to tolerate reasonable amounts of non-processed carbohydrates without apparent negative metabolic consequences. For other people, however, moderate amounts of many carbohydrates appear to contribute to weight gain, difficulty with appetite control, and worsening of disease symptoms like brain fog, fatigue, depression, and anxiety.

The big takeaways from this discussion of insulin resistance are that it appears to be driving atherosclerosis by making both LDL and arterial walls sticky. Insulin resistance is pervasive and skews much of the way research is interpreted. Many things can cause it, including chronic inflammation, infections, leaky gut, excess carbohydrates or fructose in susceptible individuals, chronic stress, and poor sleep. We definitely don't want insulin resistance, and it appears to be **the single greatest driver of chronic illness in Western populations living today,** but the good news here is that it's fairly easy to detect, and it's completely avoidable if we pay some attention to our diet and lifestyle.

Let's move on to talk about a few more aspects of lipoproteins as we dig into the biochemical basis of rising LDL levels on a ketogenic diet—and why this isn't something to be concerned about.

WHY DOES LDL RISE ON A KETOGENIC DIET?

When we think about LDL with an antiquated framework, elevations of this lipoprotein can look scary. As we've seen in this chapter, however, it's high time that we revise the LDL paradigm and stop incorrectly vilifying this crucial component of our healthy physiology. Elevated LDL is only a problem in the presence of insulin resistance, and if we don't have "sticky" LDL molecules and arterial walls, more is probably a good thing! Nevertheless, it's interesting to examine the mechanisms by which LDL rises during ketosis in order to explain this biological phenomenon and to allay further fears.

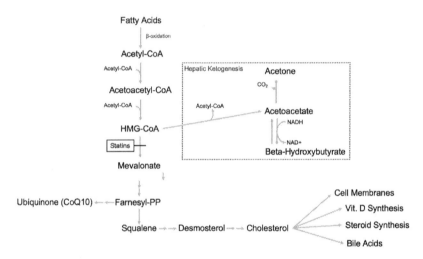

Examining the diagram of cholesterol synthesis above, which is known as the **mevalonate pathway**, we see that during ketosis, our body naturally breaks down fatty acid molecules into **Acetyl-CoA**. Acetyl-CoA can be used directly for energy in the mitochondria through the Krebs cycle. It can also be made into HMG-CoA and, subsequently, into cholesterol, or it can be made into ketones like **beta-hydroxybutyrate** (BHB). Mechanisms by which ketosis could be increasing cholesterol synthesis are complex and not fully understood, but it appears that since ketones and cholesterol share this common pathway, when more Acetyl-CoA is made into HMG-CoA for ketone synthesis, some of this could also form cholesterol. Strengthening this hypothesis is the observation that other cholesterol precursor molecules like **desmosterol** are also increased on a ketogenic diet.[94] Ketones are also known to provide the substrate required for the massive synthesis of cholesterol in the rapidly growing brains of infants and children through this synthesis pathway.[95]

Furthermore, both VLDL and LDL increase during fasting, which is most likely connected with this ketogenic physiology and a coupled increase in cholesterol synthesis.[96,97] Throughout our evolution, it is certain that our ancestors experienced prolonged periods of calorie deficits or complete caloric deprivation when hunts were not successful and there were few plant fallback foods available. Does it make even an iota of sense that our bodies would have evolved a system in which a molecule that is *bad* for us, like so many claim LDL to be, would increase significantly during such times? No way! Intentional fasting is now practiced by millions around the globe with resulting weight loss, improvements in diabetes, and other metabolic derangements. Are people simultaneously getting healthier and developing atherosclerosis? Of course not! In this chapter, we've already talked in great detail about the hard science suggesting that LDL does not cause atherosclerosis, and from an evolutionary perspective, this possibility also appears illogical.

As we observed previously in our discussion of the Framingham Study, elevated LDL on its own does not appear to be contributing to the progression of atherosclerosis. Similarly, LDL that rises in the setting of ketogenic physiology is very unlikely to contribute to plaque progression and isn't something to be concerned about.

There's another situation of elevated LDL that we should touch on briefly here, known as **familial hypercholesterolemia** (FH). There are more than 2,000 polymorphisms in lipoprotein metabolism that can cause FH. Those with this condition often show levels of LDL that climb above 200 milligrams per deciliter. Proponents of the response-to-retention hypothesis will often point to genome-wide association studies or mendelian randomization studies of those with FH showing a correlation between LDL and heart disease. But there's a problem here. FH does not represent normal human physiology, and these polymorphisms often occur in conjunction with a propensity toward forming excess blood clots.[98,99,100,101] Hmmm, let's think about this for a moment. Might this coexisting hypercoagulability confound things just a bit in these studies? I'd say so! We must not be fooled by this sort of data when thinking about the relationship between LDL and heart disease. For this reason, FH is clearly not a good model system for predicting the effect of elevated LDL in the setting of a ketogenic diet.

SHOULD YOU TAKE A STATIN FOR AN ELEVATED LDL?

If we choose to begin a ketogenic diet like most versions of the carnivore diet, it's certainly possible that our LDL levels will rise. At this point in our journey, we know that this probably isn't a big deal and is likely protective, but those thinking about lipids in the traditional way might believe that such a change would require the immediate need for a statin. It's important to address these medications briefly and to take a look at their limited pros and abundant cons.

At a fundamental level, we know that cholesterol is a precious molecule in our body and serves many, absolutely essential roles. Intuitively, wouldn't it seem that interrupting the synthesis of such a valuable compound would be a very bad idea? Surely we wouldn't want to do such a misguided thing. But this is exactly what millions of people throughout the world do every day when they take statin drugs. These pharmaceuticals significantly impair our body's ability to produce cholesterol by inhibiting the enzyme HMG-CoA reductase, one of the key steps in the mevalonate pathway.

As you can see from the previous graphic depicting this pathway, throwing a monkey wrench into the workings of this crucial enzyme won't just inhibit the formation of cholesterol, it will also inhibit everything else that is made downstream. This includes valuable compounds like CoQ10, which plays a vital role in proper functioning of mitochondria. We've talked about the mitochondria previously, but these cellular powerhouses are particularly dense in the heart and other muscles, and they play a critical role in insulin sensitivity. Wait, did I just suggest that by damaging mitochondria, statins could lead to insulin resistance? That's exactly what I am saying here! Depleting CoQ10 can lead to mitochondrial dysfunction, and not surprisingly, the use of statins has been associated with lower levels of this molecule, increased rates of heart failure, and diabetes.[102,103] Use of statins has also been associated with increased rates of cognitive impairment because the synthesis of cholesterol needed by the brain is hindered by these drugs.[104] In large trials with these medications, rates of death by violent crime rise and mood worsens.[105,106,107,108] As it turns out, depriving the brain of a vital nutrient like cholesterol makes people unhappy and angry.

Are these drugs really something that should be "in the water" as so many proponents of the response-to-retention theory have claimed?[109] In trials like Fourier and 4S, the use of statins decreases the incidence of heart attacks by a small percentage.[43,110] I'm not saying that statins do not decrease cardiovascular mortality. They certainly have been shown to do this, but it's not happening by lowering LDL. As we've discussed earlier in this chapter, there is no dose-response relationship between LDL lowering with statins and improved outcomes, and many other drugs not in the statin class of medications that also lower LDL have repeatedly failed to show any benefits in terms of cardiovascular outcomes. Statins have other pleiotropic effects, including being anti-inflammatory and immunomodulatory, which likely account for the small, but significant, improvements in cardiovascular endpoints observed in studies.

At the end of the day, I'm not a huge fan of statins. I don't believe that we should be focused on LDL lowering, but rather, correction of the insulin resistance and inflammation that are really driving atherosclerosis. The risks of these medications outweigh their benefits in most people, and diet and lifestyle modifications are a much more effective way to positively change the course of our cardiovascular health.

TMAO: The Sheep in Wolf's Clothing

Another common criticism of eating red meat is that it will elevate the level of TMAO, or trimethylamine n-oxide, in our body. This mouthful of a compound is made within our liver from its precursor TMA, which is produced by certain bacteria in our gut when we ingest choline and carnitine. These are two of the substances I spoke about in Chapter Eight as uniquely beneficial and present only in animal foods. What's going on here? Have I led us astray? Not a chance, I'd never do such a thing! As we'll soon see, just like LDL, TMAO has gotten a bad rap and has been unjustly criminalized.

We should recall that choline is critical for making the membranes of every cell in our body along with the neurotransmitter *acetylcholine*, and it plays a role in the methylation cycle at the center of our biochemistry. Deficiencies of this nutrient are associated with fatty liver disease, and the best food sources are egg yolks and organ meats.[111] Carnitine in meat plays a vital role in the redox balance within the body, acting as an antioxidant and lowering levels of advanced glycation end products. Clearly, choline and carnitine are very valuable.

In order for the argument that choline and carnitine in animal foods should be avoided to hold water, wouldn't it seem reasonable to show that TMAO is damaging to humans? One would certainly think so, but this has never been demonstrated. Claims that TMAO is bad for us are based entirely on observational epidemiology.[112,113] There are studies that show a correlation between elevated levels of TMAO and increased rates of diabetes and cardiovascular disease—but as we know all too well, correlation does not equal causation.

The first hint that there's something suspicious about the TMAO story comes from the fact that many species of fish contain pre-formed TMAO in levels greater than what would be formed by eating a similar amount of red meat, yet fish have never been associated with higher rates of cardiovascular disease or diabetes.[114] TMAO can also be produced by the bacteria living within the gastrointestinal tract when we eat vegetables, but this little nugget of information is never discussed by those who claim it's harmful for us.[115,116] Higher levels of TMAO have also been observed in humans eating fish and vegetables than in those eating meat.[117] In rats, doses of TMAO at four to five times normal levels have shown *benefit,* leading to improvement in models of hypertension, and displaying no harmful effects on the circulatory system.[118] Something about the claims that *red meat is bad for us because of TMAO production* doesn't add up.

This all begins to make a bit more sense when we look at the liver's normal production of TMAO by an enzyme called FMO3. The thing about FMO3 is that its activity can be upregulated by insulin. When there's more insulin around, FMO3 is going to crank out more TMAO in the liver from TMA produced in the gut. Do we know any common conditions in which insulin levels might be increased? Are insulin levels increased in diabetes and in those with cardiovascular disease who have underlying insulin resistance? Yup! So in the 88 percent of the population with some degree of insulin resistance, it's very likely that elevated levels of insulin are driving up levels of TMAO production by the liver.

The fundamental flaw of epidemiology studies looking at TMAO levels and cardiovascular disease is that although they might show correlation, they are blind in knowing what direction the arrow of causality might go. That is, epidemiology studies that show a correlation between TMAO and these diseases can't show us if TMAO is causing diabetes and cardiovascular disease, or if it's the other way around. In this case, based on the dependence of FMO3 on insulin, it's much more likely that rising insulin levels are driving the production of TMAO rather than TMAO leading to disease. A recent statistical analysis of the research done with TMAO came to exactly the same conclusion:

> *"Our findings support that T2DM and kidney disease increase TMAO levels and observational evidence for cardiovascular diseases may be due to confounding or reverse causality."* [119]

Well, doesn't that just drive a big old stake into the vampire heart of the TMAO myth? The notion that something formed in our gut from vital nutrients was harmful sounded suspicious from the very beginning, and research now points to the idea of TMAO causing cardiovascular disease or diabetes being nothing more than a red herring. We shouldn't worry about carnitine and choline in red meat. These nutrients are incredibly valuable and should not be avoided due to concerns regarding the mythical monster TMAO.

SATURATED FAT: WHY VEGETABLE OIL COMPANIES SAY IT'S BAD

No chapter on animal foods and heart health would be complete without a discussion of saturated fat. Recall that we name fats as saturated or unsaturated when we are referring to the absence or presence of double bonds between the carbons that form the backbone of these molecules. Fats are termed saturated when they do not possess any double bonds. A molecule with one double bond is known as a monounsaturated fat, and polyunsaturated fats possess multiple double bonds. Although saturated fat is generally associated with fat from animals, in reality, most animal fat is composed of almost equal proportions of monounsaturated and saturated fat and a small amount of polyunsaturated fat. Although many plant foods contain some amount of saturated fat, the highest concentrations of saturated fat from plants are found in coconut oil and palm oil, both of which contain significantly more of this type of fat than animal foods.

If we peruse the interwebs looking for information about which foods are healthy and which aren't, we quickly encounter the notion that saturated fat is bad for us. Any guesses where this comes from? More misinterpreted, poorly done epidemiology. Specifically, the notion that saturated fat is bad for us originated in the early 1960s with the work of Ancel Keys, who published the now-infamous Seven Countries Study looking at the relationship between diet and heart disease in cohorts of people living in the U.S., Japan, Yugoslavia, Greece, Italy, the Netherlands, and Finland. This observational study showed a correlation between *the amount of saturated fat consumed in the diet with blood cholesterol levels* and *the incidence of heart disease*. This gave rise to the "Diet-Heart" hypothesis, which postulated that saturated fat in our diet raises cholesterol levels and leads to heart disease. This theory was quickly espoused by the American Heart Association (AHA) in the 1960s and became deeply engrained in our collective health consciousness—despite the fact that *a lack of association* between blood cholesterol levels and the degree of atherosclerosis was noted as early as the 1930s.[120]

We now know that there were multiple flaws in Keys' research, including his exclusion of many countries that did not fit his theory, a type of bias known as "cherry picking." To make matters worse, there was also a more nefarious, unseen political agenda driving the formulation of the dietary guidelines in the 1960s. Millions of dollars were donated to the AHA by companies within the food industry who produced vegetable oils and low-fat, grain-based foods. At the expense of the declining health of the general population, these companies profited enormously from the recommendations of the AHA. We were all told to use canola oil and to eat grains while our waistlines ballooned and heart disease rates rose sharply during the seventies, eighties, and nineties.

Thankfully, more people are beginning to wake up to the fact that saturated fat is not the outlaw it's been labeled as. We've been eating animal foods with saturated fat in them for the entirety of our evolution as humans. This has led us to become the extremely intelligent, large-brained, strong, and adaptable people we are today. Science has also recently begun to support the things we already knew to be true, and studies have shown that high-fat ketogenic diets containing plenty of saturated fat *reverse* diabetes and insulin resistance.[121,122] They also lead to weight loss and improvements in inflammatory markers, as well as a reduction in hypertension, dementia, polycystic ovarian syndrome, and a host of other conditions.[123,124,125-131] Animal studies show that saturated fat does not induce leaky gut, but polyunsaturated vegetable oils, like corn oil, do open tight junctions and damage the gut lining.[132] It has also been demonstrated that when saturated fat in the diet is decreased, and polyunsaturated fat increased, levels of oxidized LDL *increase*.[133] As we've seen previously, this process of LDL oxidation has been associated with the progression of atherosclerosis and is not something we want to fuel. There is simply no interventional evidence that saturated fat is damaging to humans, and studies like this suggest that it serves valuable roles in our body.

Many recent epidemiology studies have also been done showing no link between saturated fat and cardiovascular disease, calling into question previous results that suggested such a connection. A large meta analysis of forty-three studies, published in 2019, found no correlation between total fat or saturated fat intake and cardiovascular disease.[134] Not surprisingly, this study found a linear relationship between processed trans fat in vegetable oils and heart attack risk. This suggests that the exact type of fats pushed upon us for the last sixty years by the AHA are one of the real culprits in the current heart disease epidemic. Imagine that!

Another large trial of forty-two countries in Europe, published in 2016, echoed these findings and came to the following conclusions:

> *"The most significant dietary correlate of* **low cardiovascular disease (CVD) risk was high total fat and animal protein consumption**...*The major correlate of* **high CVD risk was the proportion**

of energy from carbohydrates and alcohol, or from potato and cereal carbohydrates...Our results do not support the association between CVDs and saturated fat, which is still contained in official dietary guidelines. Instead, they agree with data accumulated from recent studies that link CVD risk with the high glycemic index/load of carbohydrate-based diets. In the absence of any scientific evidence connecting saturated fat with CVDs, these findings show that current dietary recommendations regarding CVDs should be seriously reconsidered." [135]

This study found that the *more* animal fat and protein people ate, the *less* cardiovascular disease they experienced, while those who ate the most carbohydrates had the highest rates of this pathology. As always, all of the usual epidemiology caveats apply here, but these results fly in the face of those touted by the mainstream media for the last sixty years and cannot be ignored. It warms my little carnivore heart that the authors also went as far as suggesting that the current dietary recommendations regarding cardiovascular disease are basically malarkey and should be reformulated. Hopefully, this time we can keep agribusiness interests out of this process. It's not saturated fat or animal meat that are causing heart disease, it's processed vegetable oils and processed carbohydrates that are the real malefactors here!

THE EDGE OF ZION

We saved the best for last, didn't we? In this chapter we've traversed some rocky country, but at the end of it all, we've arrived at the edge of Shangri-La unscathed and much better for all of our efforts. Though many in the mainstream equate LDL with "bad cholesterol" and shudder at the thought of elevated levels of this lipoprotein, we now know that the opposite is true. Not only does LDL serve indispensable roles in the body, but in the absence of insulin resistance, elevated levels of this cholesterol-carrying particle are probably protective against infectious disease and are associated with robust longevity in the elderly. This is far from the scary bedtime story we've been told, and for so long, we've been led astray by observational epidemiology. We must not continue to make this mistake if we truly hope to find the optimal health we all deserve.

In the final sections of this book, we'll talk about how to eat like our ancestors did. We'll discuss how to eat a nose-to-tail carnivore diet in detail and outline a clear plan for us to follow in our daily life. Some of these concepts, like eating organ meats, may seem foreign at first, but the premise remains simple: if we eat animals like our ancestors did and use plant foods only as survival foods, we will thrive.

SECTION IV

CHAPTER TWELVE

WHAT TO EAT ON A NOSE-TO-TAIL CARNIVORE DIET

Ah, my friends, what a journey it has been. At long last, we have arrived in the Promised Land. As we stand on a coastline with some decent looking surf, we find that we are surrounded by verdant pastures on which healthy ruminants graze under the warm sun and drink from clean, flowing streams. Before we take up the bow and head off hunting or go rambling to the ocean to collect some shellfish, let's rest for a moment on the grass and reflect on our journey thus far.

At the beginning of our adventures to find the lost user manual, we saw that stable isotope analyses of fossils strongly suggests our ancestors were high-level carnivores. They ate mostly large animals and displayed higher levels of δ15 nitrogen than those of contemporary carnivores, like hyenas. We also dug into the data regarding duplications in the salivary amylase gene and discussed *why* the fact that only *Homo sapiens* possess this suggests strongly that we have not had many starchy foods in our diet for the majority of our evolution. An examination of the size of the human brain revealed the striking finding that, about 2 million years ago, our noggins started increasing in size dramatically, right when we began hunting animals and using stone tools and weapons. This trend continued up until about 40,000 years ago. No one knows why our brains have been shrinking since then, but it's intriguing to note that this point in our history correlates with the advent of agriculture and a decrease in our access to B_{12} and other nutrients vital for brain health found predominantly in animal foods.

When we consider the sharp decline in human health observed with changes in the human diet at the time of the Neolithic Revolution, "the worst mistake in human history" might just be an accurate characterization of our decision to join the cult of the seed. In the final chapter of this book, we'll talk more about the impact mono-crop agriculture has had on our environment, but it's not pretty. In contrast to the way that this type of farming depletes the land of precious nutrients and leads to erosion of topsoil, the grazing of ruminant animals in a manner consistent with their evolutionary place within grassland ecosystems *enriches* the land and increases the carbon-carrying capacity of the soil.[1]

After exploring our human origins as hunters and remembering that hunting and eating animals made us into the amazing beings we are today, we journeyed through the dangerous lands of plant toxins. Roaming in the isothiocyanate jungle, we saw that these compounds aren't our friends after all but are just out to harm our thyroid glands and damage our DNA. Within the hinterlands, the true nature of polyphenols was revealed to us. We discovered that these plant defense molecules were little more than toxins that benefit only plants and supplement manufacturers. Across the oxalate desert we bravely traveled, learning a myriad of ways in which this molecule can harm our joints and kidneys and how it can become deposited in soft tissues, causing unnecessary pain and suffering. After crossing the rough seas of plant lectins and observing how these molecules can damage our gut, we finally arrived on the shores of the next phase of our journey.

We fought on with unbroken spirits, quickly learning of the incredible nutritional density of animal foods and of the many misleading fables told to us about the nutritional value of plants. The next leg of our quest saw us undergo a series of challenging trials as we thoroughly debunked the pernicious notions that plant fiber is necessary or beneficial for humans and that red meat will cause cancer or shorten our life. In a display of formidable prowess, we then slayed the biggest dragon of them all as we dispatched the incorrect notions that eating animals will cause heart disease and that LDL is something to be feared. With thuds that shook the earth, these giants fell after careful examination of the scientific evidence and consideration of our evolutionary past.

As I said at the outset of our adventures, this book is going to ruffle a whole lot of feathers. There will be many detractors, and I look forward to answering their criticisms as we continue on this path to positively impact as many lives as possible. Ultimately, the true test of the information I have shared within this book will be improvements in our personal health as we shift to a nose-to-tail carnivore diet. In this chapter, I'll break down how to do this so that we have all of the tools needed to eat like our ancestors did. In return, all that I ask is this: if you find benefit in this way of eating and this way of life, do not remain silent about it. Share your experience with your tribe and those who may benefit from this diet as well. The world needs to know what we have learned. They need to know that although we've lost the way and are being led astray, we can regain our vitality by remembering where we came from.

Is It Ethical to Eat Animals?

As we explore details of how to eat a carnivore diet, let's first address the ethics of eating animals. Vegans often deride the act of killing and eating animals as cruel, but nothing could be further from the truth. Few things in my life have been as moving as hunting an animal in nature. Stalking deer with my bow required me to be in the wilderness for long periods of time, something that changes any human who experiences such a communion with the natural world. When killing an incredibly beautiful deer, I felt an immediate *responsibility* to honor the life of that animal by being the best human I could be. I was reminded of this every time I ate the meat and organs that I had procured for myself.

Sadly, I don't get the opportunity to hunt as much of my food as I'd like. Ideally, all of my food would come from animals that had been respectfully hunted, but for now I obtain some meat and organs from a butcher or a grocery store. When I do this, I am struck by how separated I feel from the animals that nourish my body and soul and am reminded of how different it felt to hunt my own food. By understanding where our food comes from, we realize that in order for something to live, something else must die. This is the way of life. By being a participant within this beautiful cycle of death and life, we all bear the responsibility to live a compassionate and kind life that comes with it.

Eating animals isn't cruel. It is something that we must do in order to live healthy lives. Furthermore, notions that vegan or vegetarian diets result in less death are woefully myopic and misinformed. The large number of animals killed in the process of harvesting plants (with large machines that kill small animals like rabbits, mice, and other rodents) far outweighs the loss of life when we consume animals directly. The disruption of ecosystems with mono-crop agriculture also disrupts an even greater number of organisms on a long-term basis. Not only do plant-based diets that require mono-crop farming result in greater loss of life and ecosystem disruption, they also rob us of our vitality and prevent us from living as abundantly as possible.

How to Eat a Nose-to-Tail Carnivore Diet

This is what we have been waiting for!

Now that we've journeyed so far together, I consider each and every one of you to be a part of my tribe. Maybe we'll even get to hunt together one day. When our ancestors hunted with their tribe, they always appreciated that every part of the animal possessed unique nutrients, and they wasted nothing. Indigenous groups were known to eat the animals they killed in their entirety, from "nose-to-tail." Not only did this provide them with a complete array of nutrients and more calories, it also showed respect to the animal whose life they had taken to nourish their own. Mirroring their history, eating animals from nose-to-tail provides us with optimal human nutrition and is one of the best ways we can honor these animal's lives and properly occupy our position within the cycle of life and death.

Any intentional change we choose to make to our diet that includes a good amount of animal products and eliminates some plants will result in significant improvements to our health. I realize that the way I eat isn't going to be the best fit for everyone reading this book. So, in an effort to make the carnivore diet as accessible at it can be, I've created five tiers of carnivore eating. The diets that I describe within *all* of these tiers are amazing in my eyes. My advice is to find what works best for you and to begin your personal journey there. In this way, you can progress according to your own needs and goals. Later this year, I'll also be releasing *The Carnivore Code Cookbook* with my friends Ashley and Sarah Armstrong, which will have 150 nose-to-tail carnivore recipes to expand your ancestral palate. Let's begin our discussion with Tier 1, the most basic version of a carnivore diet.

Tier 1: The Carnivore-*ish* Diet

Yes, it is totally possible to eat a carnivore-type diet and still eat some plant foods. I call this a carnivore-*ish* diet, and it's a great place for many people to start who are looking to lose weight or improve their overall health. If you have autoimmune disease, significant gut issues, or evidence of inflammation, I would recommend starting with at least a Tier 2 carnivore diet or, preferably, Tier 3.

A Tier 1 carnivore diet emphasizes animal food consumption as the majority of the diet, but it also allows some room for the least toxic plant foods. Because animal foods represent the most nutrient-rich sources of bio-available vitamins and minerals, they form the majority of the diet. Approximately 80–90 percent of the diet will be animal foods and might include beef, bison, lamb, poultry, and fish. It could also include eggs and certain dairy items. In addition to these foods, "low toxicity" plant foods may be included for flavor, preference, texture, or color. I will reiterate here that I see plant foods as *survival foods* and don't believe they provide unique nutrients for humans that are not available in animal foods. More importantly, remember that plants do not want to be eaten and contain toxins that can irritate the gut and the immune system.

If we do decide to include some plants while making animal foods the majority of our diet, which would be least toxic and less likely to trigger our immune system? In the following graphic, you'll find what I consider to be a spectrum of plant toxicity. I generally think of the least offensive plant foods as non-sweet fruits, including things like winter/summer squash, avocados, cucumbers (without skin or seeds), and olives, as well as seasonal berries. Squash, in particular, contains higher amounts of carbohydrates and will impede efforts toward ketosis if that's a goal. On the flip side, for those interested in incorporating carbohydrates into their diets prior to long, intense athletic efforts, squash might be a good option. Removal of skin and seeds from both squash and cucumbers decreases lectins significantly.

SPECTRUM OF PLANT TOXICITY

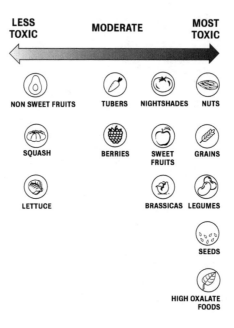

What about more toxic foods? At the opposite end of the spectrum are seeds, grains, nuts, and beans. These are all plant seeds, and they are all very heavily defended by plant toxins. As we've discussed previously, seeds contain lectins, digestive enzyme inhibitors, and high amounts of phytic acid. Plants don't want to get eaten, and they certainly don't want their seed babies to get eaten either, so these are often their most toxic parts. Even nuts like almonds and walnuts, and seeds like chia or flax, that are widely regarded as health promoting can disrupt healthy digestion and put the immune system on high alert. For this reason, I am not a fan of the many nut flours that are so common on traditional ketogenic diets. I'm sorry to be the bearer of bad news, but keto cookies made with almond flour just aren't doing us any favors.

ARTIFICIAL SWEETENERS AND SPICES

While we are talking about keto junk food, we should discuss stevia and artificial sweeteners. I am not a fan of these at all. The stevia plant is used by indigenous tribes of the Amazon as a form of birth control. It has been shown to reduce fertility and negatively affect hormonal balance in animal models.[2,3] High rates of allergy and anaphylaxis to stevia have also been found in children with a history of eczema and allergies.[4] There is further evidence that artificial sweeteners like sucralose and saccharin can alter the composition of our gut flora and predispose us to obesity: [5,6,7]

> *"Data in both animal models and humans suggest that the effects of artificial sweeteners may contribute to metabolic syndrome and the obesity epidemic. Artificial sweeteners appear to change the* **host microbiome, lead to decreased satiety, and alter glucose homeostasis, and are associated with increased caloric consumption and weight gain.** *Artificial sweeteners are marketed as a healthy alternative to sugar and as a tool for weight loss. Data however suggests that the intended effects do not correlate with what is seen in clinical practice."* [8]

The take-home message here is that artificial sweeteners of both plant and synthetic origin have no place in a healthy diet and are probably going to sabotage our efforts at weight loss, satiety, and overall improved health. If you absolutely need a sweet taste in your foods or beverages, I'd recommend the amino acid glycine, but ultimately, any molecule that is sweet can cause release of incretin, hormones which negatively affect satiety.[9] If weight loss is our focus, breaking up with sweet flavors—at least temporarily—can significantly help us reach that goal.

Many spices are also made from the seeds of plants and are best avoided on any type of carnivore diet. These include black and white pepper, coriander, cumin, cardamom, nutmeg, cloves, mustard, and caraway. Cinnamon is made from the bark of a tree and can also cause immune reactions in some people. Spices made from plant leaves are often referred to as herbs and might be more tolerable than seed-based spices, depending on the individual. These include oregano, basil, rosemary, parsley, dill, sage, and mint, all of which might be a part of a carnivore-*ish* diet for flavor or variety, but I don't believe they have any unique benefit.

In terms of flavoring for food, the best place for most people to start is a good sea salt. I personally prefer Redmond Real Salt, which is mined from an underground inland deposit in Utah. Sadly, many sea salts derived from ocean waters are contaminated with microplastics and other environmental pollutants. When transitioning to a ketogenic diet, or fasting, it is important to keep an eye on salt intake, and most people feel best when they are getting 6–10 grams of salt per day. We'll talk more about this in the next chapter on potential pitfalls.

In addition to plant seeds, high-oxalate foods are at the furthest reaches of the plant toxicity spectrum and are best fully avoided. In

Chapter Seven, we discussed oxalates in detail and described ways in which they can contribute to kidney stones, chronic pain, and many other negative effects in the body. You may want to refer back to that chapter for a chart showing some of the highest oxalate-containing foods, but the worst offenders are spinach, turmeric, almonds, potatoes, navy beans, and beets.

The nightshade family also resides on the toxic end of the spectrum and is known to be a common immune trigger. This family of vegetables includes tomatoes, eggplants, white potatoes, goji berries, bell peppers, paprika, and chili peppers. As we've seen previously, foods from this group have been shown to open tight junctions in the gastrointestinal tract, creating leaky gut.[10] Give these a pass.

Based on their content of isothiocyanates, I'd also place *Brassica* vegetables far to the right on the spectrum of plant toxicity. Remember, kale doesn't love us back, and it's not doing great things for our thyroid or the cell membranes in our body. If for some reason we are still on the sulforaphane bandwagon, we should refer back to the in-depth discussion of this in Chapter Four and recall that we don't need this molecule to achieve optimal antioxidant status.

DIDN'T OUR ANCESTORS EAT FRUIT?

It may come as a surprise that I've placed most fruit on the bad side of the plant toxicity spectrum. In this graphic, "sweet fruit" is basically all of the fruit we traditionally think of except berries, which we'll discuss a bit later. This includes things like apples, pears, grapes, mangoes, and so on. At first glance, these types of fruit seem like something our ancestors would have eaten when they were available, and they probably did from time to time. But they did so only for very limited portions of the year and in very specific parts of the world. Think about the forests, deserts, plains, and other wild spaces near where we live. How often do we see fruit growing out in the wild? Rarely!

Closer to the equator, fruit is more available, but still occurs seasonally. The vast array of fruit that we see in grocery stores every day of the year is an incredibly inaccurate representation of the availability of these foods in the natural world. There's nowhere on the planet that things like melon, mango, berries, apples, and citrus fruit all grow wild in the same place or year round, and the ancestral versions of many of these fruits are nothing like what we find on the aisles of grocery stores today. Over the last hundred years, through hybridization practices, most of the fruit we eat has been made much sweeter and larger than its wild cousins.

When thinking about eating fruit, we also need to ask ourselves what nutritional benefit we might derive from such a practice. We've previously discussed the fallacious notion that polyphenolic pigments in fruit provide any real benefit to humans. We also don't need to be eating five oranges a day to get an adequate amount of vitamin C, nor would this have been something that our ancestors could have done across various latitudes. There's good evidence that even a modest amount of this nutrient is enough to satisfy our needs, and that beyond this amount, the benefits of vitamin C are highly questionable. So if it's not for polyphenols or vitamin C, what the heck are we eating fruit for in the first place?

Aside from the lack of beneficial effects, there are also concerns that fructose and glucose in fruit might be bad for us. Excess consumption of both of these sugar molecules have been shown to have all sorts of harmful effects in the human body: increased advanced glycation end product formation, insulin resistance, metabolic syndrome, hypertension, cardiovascular disease, leptin resistance, mitochondrial dysfunction, and obesity.[11,12,13-20] Furthermore, fructose and glucose are also known to negatively affect the gut microbiome.[7,21]

Overindulgence in fruit is also linked with changes in pH of the mouth, which can lead to tooth decay; anywhere there's someone who eats a lot of fruit, a dentist with job security isn't far behind. Conversely, the dental benefits of a low-carbohydrate diet, like the carnivore diet, are well documented, with studies showing reductions in tooth decay and types of gingivitis-promoting bacteria like *P gingivalis* that have been linked to Alzheimer's disease.[22,23,24,25] There are also numerous reports from those eating a carnivore diet of reversal of gingival disease and recession of the gums—further evidence that when constructed correctly, this way of eating provides an adequate amount of vitamin C.

Fruit generally benefits plants more than the animals who eat it. Plants are pretty crafty creatures, and with fruit, they discovered an ingenious way to get animals to help in spreading their seeds. By coating their seeds with natural candy, plants entice animals to eat them and poop them out in another location right in the middle of a pile of fertilizer. And as we've seen, plants also contain toxic substances in the seeds of these fruit to discourage animals from chomping on this precious cargo. Fruit is like a pin-up girl dressed in bright colors that plants place front and center to entice us, but ultimately, they just want to use us rather than be in a long-term, mutually beneficial relationship. Beyond sheer calories, fruit doesn't have much redeeming nutritional value. It's just a plant's way of getting us to do it a favor and move its seeds around to fertile locations. Perhaps there was a time in our evolutionary past when it served a role in the human diet by providing calories for survival, but far fewer people in the Western world are in danger of calorie deficiency these days.

Honey is another fructose-rich food that probably should not make up a significant proportion of any healthy diet. Evidence of tooth decay in avid honey eaters within certain African tribes and Pacific islanders stands as further testament of the potential dental downsides to over-consumption of such sugar-rich food.[26,27] Occasionally, small amounts of honey are a better sweetener than table sugar, stevia, or other artificial sweeteners, but for most of us, working to eliminate sweet flavors from our diet for at least the first few months of transition to a carnivore diet will be very helpful.

TUBERS AND BERRIES

In the middle of the spectrum of plant toxicity, we find tubers and berries. Though berries are technically a fruit, due to their lower sugar content I'd consider them to be a bit less likely to cause issues than the "sweet fruit" we discussed in the last section. Polyphenols in berries probably aren't that good for us and are really just plant pigments, but if we are going to consume fruit, berries are better than other, sweeter types.

In regard to tubers, although our ancestors may have eaten them, they don't appear to have made up a significant proportion of their diets and were almost certainly "fallback" foods. Have you ever eaten a wild carrot? They are about half the size of your pinky finger! Expending energy looking for food like this would have been a very bad use of time if other more nutrient and calorie-rich foods were available. It's also important to remember that both tubers and berries contain significant amounts of oxalates and many wild tubers contain toxic cyanogenic glycosides.[28] If we are going to include them in our carnivore-*ish* diet it's best not to overdo it.

Some proponents of higher-carbohydrate paleo diets have argued that modern hunter-gatherers, like the Hadza or !Kung, consume about half of their calories from tubers.[29] But as many anthropologists have pointed out, these people have been marginalized and forced to change their hunting practices, no longer serving as accurate representations of the generations of indigenous peoples that preceded them.[30] These groups are now forced to live on smaller areas of land and are no longer allowed to hunt the elephants and other large game that their ancestors relied upon for thousands of years.[31] Without being able to live in their traditionally nomadic way, they are forced to use more plant foods to supplement their diets. It is also interesting to note that the height of many indigenous peoples has declined over the last few hundred years, a change that is understood to be related to the marginalization of these groups with resulting changes to their previous way of life.[32,33]

WHAT ABOUT FUNGI?

Mushrooms are another type of food many people ask about on a carnivore-*ish* type diet. Technically, fungi are a separate kingdom from plants, but they do still make many toxins to defend themselves against animal predation. *Agaricus bisporus* is the species commonly known as white button mushrooms, but it also includes portobello and crimini varieties that are common in grocery stores. This species of mushrooms makes a mycotoxin known as agaritine, which is known to be harmful to humans by binding to DNA[34] and causes cancers in animal studies.[35] The good news is that agaritine is mostly denatured by cooking, but do we really want to be putting something like this in our body if it's not necessary? Many mushrooms also contain significant amounts of oxalates, and we have already discussed the documented cases of oxalate toxicity related to over-consumption of chaga.[36]

Rice cultivated with the mold species, *Moascus purpureus,* is known as red yeast rice and contains a mycotoxin moncacolin K, or lovastatin, which inhibits HMG-CoA reductase, just like other statin drugs.[37] From our previous discussions, we know that this is a bad idea if we want to have mitochondria that function well. Overall, mycotoxins are common in fungi, and the bottom line here is that we really don't know how many of these may be affecting us. Studies with mushrooms like lion's mane suggest that there may be some benefit,[38] but I'm not convinced that any species of mushroom is entirely safe as food or provides unique benefits that we cannot derive from living a radical life: exercise, sun, heat, cold, ketosis, fasting, and eating animal foods. It's important to note here that within treatment of mental illness, there is a clear role for the use of fungal-derived molecules like psilocybin in the treatment of depression, anxiety, PTSD, and cancer-related demoralization.[39,40,41,42] I also believe that in many of these psychiatric conditions, underlying brain inflammation should be addressed to achieve the best results.

What to Drink on a Carnivore Diet

Working with clients in my private practice, few things elicit more heart-felt groans of agony than the suggestion that they should eliminate coffee from their diets. Those that are able to make this lifestyle change, however, report more stable energy levels, better sleep, and brighter overall moods.

Coffee is made from the roasted seeds of the *Coffea arabica* and *Coffea canephora* plants. As we've learned previously, the seeds of plants often harbor some of the most dangerous toxins, and coffee beans are no exception to this rule. They contain polyphenols (caffeic acid and chlorogenic acid) that have been found to damage DNA at levels present in a *single cup*.[43] In his paper on plant pesticides, Bruce Ames notes:

> *"Roasted coffee is known to contain 826 volatile chemicals; 21 have been tested chronically and* **16 are rodent carcinogens;** *caffeic acid, a non-volatile rodent carcinogen, is also present. A typical cup of coffee contains at least 10 mg (40 ppm) of rodent carcinogens (mostly caffeic acid, catechol, furfural, hydroquinone and hydrogen peroxide)."*

Dr. Ames isn't the only one to highlight the mutagenic potential of compounds in coffee. Researcher Louise Mennen notes:

> *"Some polyphenols may have carcinogenic or genotoxic effects at high doses or concentrations. Caffeic acid, for example, when present at a 2% level in the diet,* **induced forestomach and kidney tumors in rats and mice. Linear extrapolation of these data indicates appreciable risk at normal dietary levels.***"*[44]

Yes, I know, you hate me right now, and you might have just spit out your morning coffee all over this page. You can always buy a fresh copy and gift this one at a white elephant party. I know your coffee helps you wake up in the morning and poop, but you should be able to do both of those things without stimulants like caffeine, and you will, I promise.

Interventional studies can show improvements with antioxidant status in coffee drinkers, but the story here is very similar to sulforaphane.[45] Coffee polyphenols act as *pro-oxidants* in the human body and trigger the NRF2 pathway, which leads to the formation of increased amounts of glutathione.[46] These increased amounts of glutathione can make it look like oxidative stress parameters improve in the short term. But just like isothiocyanates, the polyphenols in coffee have also been shown to damage DNA and are going to have damaging effects in other parts of the body as well.[47,48]

For most people who drink coffee, caffeine is a valuable part of the package, but this molecule is designed by plants as a defense compound. It's a phytoalexin placed in seeds by the coffee plant to deter animals from eating them. Plants don't want their babies to get eaten! Though it would take a heck of a lot of coffee to kill you (about seventy-five cups), caffeine does have a lethal dose in humans. Drinking a few cups of coffee per day may result in an addiction, however, and can exert negative physiologic effects in humans including raising heart rate, blood pressure, blood glucose, and the subjective experience of acute anxiety.[49] Caffeine addiction has also been linked to chronic depression and anxiety, and withdrawal from this substance can be quite unpleasant.[50,51]

Acrylamide is yet another downside of coffee. It is formed during the roasting of many foods, including nuts, crackers, bread, breakfast cereals, French fries, and potato chips, and is also found in cigarette smoke. Acrylamide is classified as group 2A carcinogen by the the National Cancer Institute and as a potential carcinogen and "extremely hazardous" substance by other United States governmental agencies. After a legal ruling in 2018, 7-Eleven stores in California must now place a *Prop 65* label warning of harmful chemicals in the coffee due to its acrylamide content. Yikes!

Acrylamide has been shown to cause multiple types of cancer in animal models.[52,53] In epidemiology studies in humans, it is associated with renal, endometrial, and ovarian cancers.[54] Mechanistically, acrylamide appears to interfere with hormone signaling, cellular cytoskeleton components, and calcium flux within our cells. There are also concerns that it has deleterious effects on the liver as well as the reproductive, immune, and nervous systems. There's much more research to be done, but do we really want more of this chemical in our bodies?

Unless we're drinking organic coffee, we are also getting a decent dose of man-made pesticides with that cup of joe. Coffee crops are highly sprayed with pesticides like glyphosate and 2-4-D, both of which have been linked to cancer and have been shown to disrupt human biochemistry.[55,56,57-59] After coffee has been harvested, the beans are often stored during processing for long periods of time, during which they can become moldy and contaminated with mycotoxins including ochratoxins A & B, penicillic acid, citrinin, fumonisin, and aflatoxin.[60,61,62] All of these are known to damage DNA in humans and have been linked to both brain and kidney toxicity.[63,64,65,66] Wet processing of coffee beans may decrease levels of mold toxins, but this is rarely done.

Even if we aren't convinced that levels of mycotoxins in coffee are a problem, these compounds have also been found in many other plant foods including grains, wine, beer, dark chocolate, and peanut butter.[67,68,69] Elimination of these plant foods and coffee will unquestionably reduce our exposure to this array of badness.

Polyphenolic compounds in green tea have also been shown to damage DNA and have been linked to liver damage and disordered thyroid hormone synthesis.[48,70,71] As we saw in Chapter Four and Chapter Five, there's no evidence that we need plant compounds to achieve robust levels of glutathione or optimal antioxidant status. From fruit and vegetable depletion studies, we've also seen that when all polyphenols and isothiocyanates are removed, markers of oxidative stress and inflammation do not increase.[72] Risking damage to our DNA for what are likely empty promises of hormetic benefit doesn't sound like a good deal to me.

So when it comes to beverages on a carnivore diet, what should we drink? Pardon me if this sounds pedestrian, but how about good old water? This is what our ancestors have been drinking for the last 4 million years, with perhaps a bit of blood mixed in there as well. When we return to this simple approach, *good quality* water becomes a fundamentally thirst-quenching and enjoyable experience. Notice my emphasis on good quality here. It is worthwhile to consider drinking higher quality water than the fluoride, chlorine, and pharmaceutical-enriched liquid that comes straight out of our faucets.[73] My personal preference is spring water from a source that is regularly tested for contaminants. In the Appendix are resources for finding a spring near you. In the unfortunate situation that there's not a spring nearby, a water filtration system for your house or at least in the kitchen is a good investment. Sparkling mineral water is also an option, and many of these have higher amounts of dissolved good minerals (calcium and magnesium) than tap water. I'd be remiss if I didn't mention that I'm particularly fond of Gerolsteiner and Pellegrino.

WHAT ABOUT ALCOHOL?

I hope that no one reading this is under the impression that alcohol is good for them. This substance is known to be toxic to the liver, and although we can metabolize small quantities of it, any amount puts stress on our body. In Chapter Five, we debunked the myth that resveratrol has a valuable role in our diet, and after the previous discussion of mycotoxins, we've further seen that the notion that wine is beneficial for us is largely a misconception. Finally, much like coffee, conventionally grown grapes are heavily sprayed with pesticides, and many wines have added sulfites. No wonder so many of us suffer from raging headaches after drinking the red stuff. Distilled spirits like vodka or whiskey might contain less of the contaminants that can negatively affect some people. They would probably be the "cleanest" version of alcohol to drink if we choose to indulge in moderation from time to time, but beer and wine are off the team.

WHEN TO EAT ON A CARNIVORE DIET

Eat when you are hungry and consider an eating window most days. I do think the time-restricted eating principle of having a confined eating window, with a longer period of fasting, is a valuable addition to your lifestyle with a carnivore diet.

Very often, people end up eating fewer times throughout the day on this type of diet because they aren't as hungry. After one and a half years of eating a nose-to-tail carnivore diet, I don't even know how I ever ate three or more times a day. Twice per day has become the norm for me and many other people. I practice time-restricted eating on most days, consuming two large meals within a seven-hour eating window between 9 a.m. and 4 p.m. I find that I am so satiated after my first meal that I do not need to snack throughout the day and then eat another moderate-sized meal at 4pm, fasting from then until the next morning.

I prefer to keep my eating window earlier in the day to allow for a large amount of time between my last meal and sleep. Moving the eating window earlier in the day (also known as eTRF) has been shown to result in improvement in many markers, as noted by these authors:

> *"In the morning before breakfast, eTRF increased ketones, cholesterol, and the expression of the stress response and aging gene Sirtuin1 and the autophagy gene LC3A (all p < 0.04), while in the evening, it tended to increase brain-derived neurotropic factor (BNDF; p = 0.10) and also increased the expression of mTOR (p = 0.007)... eTRF also altered the diurnal patterns in cortisol and the expression of several circadian clock genes (p < 0.05).* **eTRF improves 24-hour glucose levels, alters lipid metabolism and circadian clock gene expression, and may also increase autophagy and have anti-aging effects in humans.**"[4]

Impressive findings, right? Kind of makes us think about whether eating dinner is really a good thing after all. Many self-quantifiers have similarly noted improved sleep metrics when finishing their last meal of the day at least three to four hours before going to bed.

For some people, eating once per day, known as OMAD (one meal a day), works well. I have found it difficult to get enough calories with this sort of eating style, but for those with smaller calorie needs on a daily basis who want to maximize the fasting window, this might be a good option.

If a Tier 1 carnivore diet sounds like a good fit, we might start with the low-toxicity plants and add in moderate-toxicity foods to see how these are tolerated. This should be done intentionally and with attention to possible reactions. High-toxicity plants should be avoided in the diet completely. I've provided a carnivore-*ish* diet pyramid that may be helpful in visualizing the foods commonly eaten on this type of a diet.

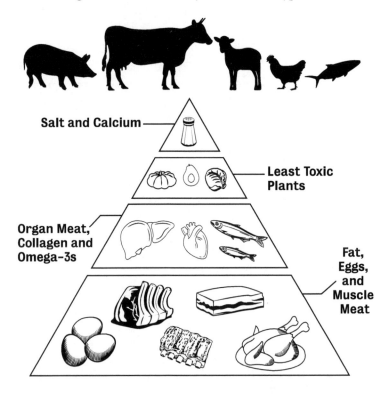

Approximately 85% animal foods, possibly 15% plant foods

Below is a sample of a typical day on a Tier 1 carnivore diet. All of these typical days will vary based on our goals, body composition, and metabolic rate.

What a typical day of Tier 1 Carnivore looks like:

Breakfast:
- 3 eggs with 1 Tbsp of ghee (clarified butter)
- 3 slices of bacon
- 1/2 avocado with salt

Lunch:
- 10 oz grass-fed ribeye steak with salt (other options in clude 10 oz ground beef, 10 oz chick roast, or 10 oz sirloin)
- Cucumber slices, romaine lettuce with olive oil/ vinegar dressing
- 1/2 cup raspberries

Dinner:
- 8 oz lamb chops (other options include 8 oz skirt steak, 8 oz tri-tip, 8 oz sirloin, 8 oz chuck roast, or any other cut)
- Olives
- 1/2 avocado
- 1/2 cup blueberries

TIER 2: THE MEAT AND WATER CARNIVORE DIET

This is the most basic and simplest version of a carnivore diet. It's for people who want to experiment with a whole foods, animal-based diet for short amounts of time within the framework of an elimination diet. In my opinion, this type of carnivore eating is not ideal for the long term, but it can serve as a simple introduction.

On a Tier 2 carnivore diet, "*eat meat, drink water*" is the classic adage. It's a pretty simple formula, and as an elimination diet, it can be a very powerful tool. Though there are a few examples of people doing well long term on a diet such as this, not everyone appears to thrive when eating this way. My main concern beyond short-term use is the possibility of nutrient deficiencies. Although our body's requirements for some things change in the absence of carbohydrates, the RDA's probably still serve as a reasonable guide for most nutrients. While muscle meat is rich in many vitamins and minerals like B_3, B_6, B_{12}, potassium, zinc, iron, and selenium, it lacks in a number of things that humans need to function optimally.

While I do think a Tier 2 carnivore diet can be very helpful for some people, adding a few foods like eggs and occasional seafood will help fill in many of the potential nutrient gaps. Evolutionarily, I also don't believe that we would have eaten only the muscle meat of animals. There are numerous examples from anthropological literature to suggest that indigenous groups consistently prized organ meats.[5]

What a typical day of Tier 2 Carnivore looks like:

Breakfast:

- 10 oz grass fed ribeye steak with salt

Lunch:

- 8 oz lamb burgers with salt, 4 strips of bacon

Dinner:

- 12 oz grass fed NY steak with salt

TIER 3: THE FRESHMAN CARNIVORE DIET

Sometimes we join the freshman team before we make it to junior varsity, and that's totally okay! The freshman carnivore diet adds a few things to the Tier 2 meat and water plan. This is where most folks start out, and then usually progress to Tiers 4 and Tier 5 as they get more interested in eating organ meats. A Tier 3 carnivore diet includes meat, eggs, seafood, and dairy if tolerated. Eggs alone enrich a carnivore diet by adding good amounts of vitamin A, choline, vitamin K2, DHA, and folate, but there still might be some nutritional holes on a Tier 3 carnivore diet. I think most will feel and perform better with a few organ meats in their diet, but a Tier 3 freshman carnivore diet is much more sustainable than a Tier 2 diet of only meat and water.

WHAT ABOUT SEAFOOD ON A CARNIVORE DIET?

Seafood is another valuable part of a carnivore diet. Low-mercury fish like wild salmon and sardines will be good sources of EPA and DHA as well as the iodine needed to make thyroid hormones. Shellfish are also incredibly nutrient-rich with oysters being superheroes when it comes to zinc and omega-3, and mussels are loaded with manganese.

When thinking about seafood, it's also important to remember that humans have sadly polluted oceans and lakes, and in general both freshwater and saltwater seafood may carry a higher toxic burden than freely grazing land animals. Though I do think seafood and some freshwater fish can have a role in a carnivore diet, it's very important to know the heavy metal content of these foods if we choose to consume them. Larger fish like tuna, halibut, king mackerel, swordfish, and shark contain very high levels of mercury and other heavy metals and should be avoided completely. Wild salmon will be much lower in this regard and may be eaten once or twice a week, if desired.

Shellfish can have higher levels of cadmium and other heavy metals as well. Eating mussels, oysters, clams, shrimp, crab, lobster, or scallops once or twice a week is a great addition to a carnivore diet, but if we're making seafood the majority of our animal foods, we should definitely monitor blood levels for heavy metals.

WHAT ABOUT CHICKEN, TURKEY, AND OTHER BIRDS?

Though all of these are totally fine to include on a carnivore diet for variety, most people find that ruminant animals like beef, buffalo, lamb, and venison are more satisfying and enjoyable. From a nutritional perspective, ruminant muscle meat and organs are generally better sources of the vitamins and minerals we need. Dark chicken meat is a good source of vitamin K2, however, and chicken skin is very rich in collagen. Chicken feet, bones, necks, and backs can also be used to make a rich bone broth.

WHAT ABOUT PORK?

Pigs are monogastric animals with one stomach like humans, rather than the multiple stomachs found within the ruminant digestive system. Unless you know a local farmer, it can be very hard to find pigs that are fed high-quality food. Most are given a diet of low-quality grains like corn, soy, and millet. Their menus are much like the diet of a conventionally raised cow in a feedlot. Later in this book, I'll discuss the importance of eating grass-fed meat and the potential for mold toxins in grains fed to animals. The primary point to remember is that what an animal eats affects the quality of its meat and organs. Do we really want to be eating animals fed with grains contaminated with pesticides and mold toxins? We should also keep this in mind when considering the sources of chicken, turkey, and eggs we are consuming. I believe this is a strong argument to eat organic fowl and pork if we choose to include these foods in our diet.

What a typical day of Tier 3 Carnivore looks like:

Breakfast:
- 3 eggs cooked in tallow (rendered cow fat) or ghee
- 4 oz NY strip steak

Lunch:
- 6 oz wild king salmon with butter or ghee
- 3 oz goat milk yogurt

Dinner:
- 6 oz shrimp
- 8 oz grass-fed ribeye steak with salt

TIER 4: THE JUNIOR VARSITY CARNIVORE DIET

This tier is for those courageous souls interested in the carnivore diet who are organ-curious. If we truly hope to turn these corporeal vessels we inhabit into the most finely tuned machines possible, we need to provide them with all of the nutrients they need to get the biochemical engines humming along at the highest RPM possible. The ancestral precedent for eating animals nose-to-tail is backed by contemporary knowledge of the indispensable nutritional value of organ meats. At this level of a carnivore diet, it's also time to think about incorporating tendons and connective tissue into our diet for a bit more glycine to complement methionine-rich muscle meats.

LIVER MAGIC

For those looking to dip a toe into the waters of including organ meats in their diet, liver and heart are a great place to start. By adding these, we'll significantly level up on nutrient adequacy and ascend a notch on the kick-butt meter.

Heart is similar to muscle meat in nutritional content but has a bit more CoQ10. It's got a slightly different flavor and is tender if cooked properly. Beware of overcooked heart though; it can get a bit chewy.

A very important thing to know about liver is that it's **not** the body's filter or full of toxins! It is true that the liver contains the majority of the enzymatic systems involved in detoxification, and through the phase 1 and phase 2 pathways compounds are prepared for excretion in the bile or urine. The liver doesn't store toxins; it chemically transforms them. This is how we get rid of the nasty chemicals and compounds hanging around in our bodies, like sulforaphane, curcumin, resveratrol, flavonoids, and heavy metals.

So the liver isn't a filter. Is it really that uniquely nutritious? You betcha! What nutrients am I talking about here? Liver is particularly rich in many minerals and B vitamins that complement those found in muscle meat.

PER 100 g	Blueberries	Kale	Ribeye	Beef Liver	Fish Roe	Egg Yolk
Vitamin A Retinol	0	0	5 mcg	4968 mcg	90 mcg	191 mcg
Thiamin (B1)	trace	0.1 mg	0.1 mg	0.2 mg	0.3 mg	0.2 mg
Riboflavin (B2)	trace	0.3 mg	0.2 mg	2.8 mg	0.7 mg	0.5 mg
Niacin (B3)	0.4 mg	1.2 mg	3.6 mg	13.2 mcg	1.8 mg	0.02 mg
Vitamin B6	0.05 mg	0.1 mg	0.4 mg	1.1 mg	0.2 mg	0.4 mg
Biotin (B7)	0.5 mg	0	trace	42 mcg	100 mcg	55 mcg
Folate (B9)	6 mcg	62 mcg	3 mcg	290 mcg	80 mcg	146 mcg
Vitamin B12	0 mcg	0 mcg	3 mcg	59.3 mcg	10 mcg	2 mcg
Vitamin C*	9.7 mg	93 mg	3.5 mg	25 mg	16 mg	0
Vitamin D	0	0	4 IU	49 IU	484 IU	218 IU
Vitamin E (mg)	0.6 mg	0.7 mg	0.1 mg	0.4 mg	7 mg	2.6 mg
Vitamin K2	0	0	15 mcg	263 mcg	1 mcg	34 mcg
Calcium	6 mg	254 mg	6 mg	5 mg	22 mg	129 mg
Choline	6 mg	0.4 mg	57 mg	333 mg	335 mg	820 mg
Copper	0.05 mg	0.15 mg	0.1 mg	9.8 mg	0.1 mg	0.1 mg
Iron	0.3 mg	1.6 mg	2.6 mg	4.9 mg	0.6 mg	2.7 mg
Magnesium	6 mg	33 mg	24 mg	18 mg	20 mg	5 mg
Phosphorous	12 mg	55 mg	210 mg	387 mg	402 mg	390 mg
Potassium	77 mg	348 mg	357 mg	313 mg	221 mg	109 mg
Selenium	0.1 mcg	0.9 mcg	24 mcg	40 mcg	40 mcg	56 mcg
Zinc	0.2 mg	0.4 mg	7.8 mg	4 mg	1 mg	2.3 mg

Looking at this previous graphic comparing the nutritional content of animal and plant foods, we can compare muscle meat to liver and quickly notice that the latter is a much richer source of many nutrients, including biotin, folate, riboflavin, vitamin C, choline, vitamin A, vitamin K2, and copper.

On the mineral side, liver is one of the best sources of copper, which is needed for enzymes like super oxide dismutase (SOD). SOD serves a critical role in the redox management system in our bodies by converting the superoxide radical (O_2-) into molecular oxygen (O_2) or hydrogen peroxide (H_2O_2). Copper deficiency can result in accumulation of O_2^-, which leads to disastrous consequences in terms of excess oxidative stress. Deficiency of this mineral is rare, but it can occur if we consume too much zinc without some copper to balance it out. The most common reason for this is excess zinc supplementation, but it is also possible through diet if we get a lot of zinc in muscle meat without liver or other copper-rich foods. Clinical copper deficiency manifests with neurological symptoms that mimic B_{12} deficiency, including difficulty with balance and walking.

Liver is also rich in choline, which is important for the cell membranes throughout our body. We've also discussed the vital importance of vitamin K2 for proper calcium partitioning and cardiac health—and liver is a valuable source of this nutrient as well. From the Rotterdam Study, we saw that those who had the most K2 in their diet showed a clear trend toward less cardiovascular disease, while wimpy K1 from plants did little to help these folks.[76]

The critical roles played by riboflavin and folate in the function of the MTHFR enzyme have already been discussed. These B vitamins are found in robust amounts in organ meats like liver and kidney, but levels are much lower in muscle meat. If we don't include organs in our diet, we can become deficient in these nutrients, leading to rising homocysteine levels and possible issues with methylation reactions within detoxification, neurotransmitter synthesis, and hundreds of other biochemical processes in the body. We've discussed vitamin C at length previously, but it's interesting to note that liver and other organ meats are much richer sources of this nutrient than muscle meat as well.

Biotin, or vitamin B7, is often forgotten about, but it's quite important for healthy hair, skin, and nails. In fact, biotin was originally named "vitamin H," derived from the German phrase "haar und haut," which translates to hair and skin. While we are discussing biotin, it's important to note that while raw egg yolks can be a delicious addition to a steak or tartare, eating raw egg white is a bad idea. In raw egg whites is a compound called **avidin** that can bind biotin and cause a deficiency of this nutrient. The RDA for biotin is 30 micrograms per day, which is present in a few ounces of liver or kidney, but we'd have to consume 21 ounces of steak to get this amount.

Simply put, liver is a nutritional powerhouse that helps complement muscle meat, and by including moderate amounts of it in our diet, we are sure to benefit profoundly.

IS IT POSSIBLE TO EAT TOO MUCH LIVER?

We've probably all heard the lore regarding arctic explorers who were poisoned by excess vitamin A from eating polar bear livers.[77] Although we know that vitamin A is a valuable nutrient, the question of how much we should consume often comes up. There are case reports of toxicity connected to excess vitamin A consumption, but the vast majority of these are related to supplements rather than consumption of vitamin A in liver. Due to studies correlating higher levels of vitamin A intake with birth defects, pregnant women are cautioned against excess consumption, but this research does not differentiate food versus supplemental sources.[78] In experiments with pigs, metabolism of vitamin A from supplements appears to be different than from food.[79] The former continues to elevate blood levels with escalating doses, but this pattern is not observed when pigs were fed liver directly.

While liver from ruminants is a very nutrient-rich food, and much lower in vitamin A than polar bear liver (approximately 180 IU per gram vs. 20,000 IU per gram), it's probably best not to consume excessive amounts of it until this vitamin A research is further fleshed out. For most people, 8–16 ounces of liver per week will be totally safe in terms of vitamin A, and it will provide robust doses of all the other valuable nutrients present in this organ. Current recommendations for pregnant women are to not exceed 10,000 IU (international units) of vitamin A per day, an amount found in about 2 ounces of liver. Liver from non-ruminant animals, like chickens, is a good source of nutrients as well but is not as rich as beef or lamb.

WHY METHIONINE/GLYCINE BALANCE MATTERS

If we've made it to the junior varsity team, it's probably time to think about incorporating connective tissue into our diet to optimize the balance of methionine and glycine. These are two amino acids that participate in a balanced dance within our body. Methionine is an essential sulfur-containing amino acid and a source of methyl groups for many biochemical reactions. Recall that within the folate cycle, MTHFR makes L-Methylfolate, which donates a methyl group to homocysteine, forming the methionine, which is then made into S-adenosylmethionine (SAMe), a molecule with roles as a methyl donor in hundreds of reactions.

Our body controls the flow of methyl groups very carefully, and excess methyl groups in the form of methionine can be buffered by glycine, forming sarcosine, which is then either recycled or excreted. Excess methionine can cause us to waste glycine, potentially leading to low levels of this amino acid. In contrast to methionine, which we must obtain from diet, we can make a small amount of glycine per day, but studies suggest that our manufacturing capacity falls significantly short of our needs and that we really must have a robust supply from our diet for optimal health.[80] Glycine serves many roles in the body, including the formation of both collagen and glutathione, as well as serving as a neu-rotransmitter in the brain.[81]

Some in the health space have stated that high-methionine diets may shorten our lifespan, referring to trials done in rats in the 1990s.[82] What they neglect to mention is that in subsequent studies, when rats were fed diets with similar amounts of methionine along with a balanced amount of glycine, all of the negative effects of the high-methionine diet vanished.[83] It wasn't that a high-methionine diet was harmful, but rather that this type of diet created an insufficiency in glycine, which led to negative health effects. Other studies in animal models have shown that methionine restriction can prolong life,[84] but the story here is the same. It's not about limiting methionine, it's about balancing this amino acid with glycine. When this is done, similar longevity effects are also observed.[85]

The easiest way to get a robust amount of glycine in our diet is to eat tendons and connective tissue like our ancestors did when they ate the whole animal. Though many of us may not be used to it, this means eating the chewy bits of steak or bone broth made from collagenous tissues, like beef knuckles, chicken backs, necks, and feet or tendons. Hydrolyzed collagen supplements can also fill this need in our diet, but we should be sure to select the highest quality source possible for this from grass-finished beef.

The takeaway here is that muscle meat is rich in methionine and connective tissue rich in glycine. Though we don't always see it in the grocery store, animals are about half muscle and half connective tissue. We should probably eat a reasonable amount of each in whatever form is easiest on a daily basis if we want to mimic the way we've been eating animals throughout our evolution and ensure optimal performance of our biochemical engines.

What a typical day of Tier 4 Carnivore looks like:

Breakfast:
- 3 eggs cooked in ghee
- 6 oz tenderloin steak
- 2 oz liver

Lunch
- 8 oysters
- 8 oz bone broth
- 3 oz king salmon

Dinner:
- 8 oz grass-fed NY steak, being sure to eat the "chewy bits"
- 6 oz steamed mussels

TIER 5: THE VARSITY CARNIVORE DIET

This is it! You've made it to the top of the carnivore ladder. Not that I think any of the other tiers are bad diets, but Tier 5 is what I would consider to be the closest thing to an ideal version of the carnivore diet. It's how I eat every day, because I want to perform as optimally as possible. If you want the super sporty Tesla version of the carnivore diet, look no further. A Tier 5 carnivore diet builds on the foundation we've already put in place with the previous tiers, including grass-fed muscle meat, connective tissue, liver, seafood, and eggs. It also adds in more organ meats and considers fat/protein ratios based on performance goals.

One type of seafood I didn't mention in our previous discussion of a Tier 3 or Tier 4 carnivore diet is fish eggs (roe). This is a food that has been treasured by indigenous groups for thousands of years. As you'll see when referring back to the "superfoods" graphic, salmon roe is rich in many nutrients, including DHA, vitamin C, vitamin E, vitamin D, and selenium. It is also lower in many of the heavy metal contaminants found in the meat of fish. In addition, smaller quantities are eaten, which allows us to derive many of the benefits of fish in a more compact package. DHA in salmon roe is also in the phospholipid form, which has been shown to be more bioavailable and better incorporated into our neural tissue than other forms of this omega-3 fatty acid.[86] On a Tier 5 carnivore diet (or any of the tiers), it's worth thinking about incorporating this food from time to time for its unique nutrient composition.

OTHER ORGANS

Though liver is an amazing organ, it's not the only one our ancestors ate, and it should probably be rotated with other organs in our diet. If we're ready to be in the starting lineup on a Tier 5 carnivore diet, kidney is one of the next organ meats we should consider. It's not something we are accustomed to eating in Western cultures, but this organ has been prized by many indigenous groups and is a nutrient powerhouse. Viljalmur Stefansson observed that kidneys were given to Inuit children "somewhat as if they were candy."[87] They don't exactly taste like a Snickers bar, but kidneys have as much riboflavin, K2, folate, and vitamin C as liver. For those looking to get more riboflavin in the diet, which we could all benefit from, kidney is a great option. As an added bonus, for those with histamine-sensitivity issues, kidney contains the enzyme diamine oxidase. Our body uses this enzyme to break these compounds down, and many have found improvement in their symptoms when they include this organ in their diet.

Exploration of organ meats beyond kidneys is definitely for the adventurous. Those who choose to consume them have generally found they feel better overall and have more energy when including a larger variety of these foods in their diet. In a given week, I might eat brain, spleen, pancreas, thymus, and "oysters" (testicles) in addition to my staples of liver and kidney. Did you just make an "ewwww" face? That's totally okay! These aren't required, but they're an option if you are interested. In the forthcoming *The Carnivore Code Cookbook,* there will be many recipe ideas that include different organs for you to add to your diet. If you just can't include organ meats, try using desiccated organ supplements as an intermediate step.

How Much Organ Meat Should We Be Eating?

Previously, we discussed that 8–16 ounces of liver per week is a good amount to include, but what about these other organs? If liver is the lead guitarist, then kidney plays the drums, and who doesn't like a good beat? It's a fantastic addition to our carnivore diet in doses of 8 ounces or so per week. We might think of the other organs like heart, pancreas, spleen, brain, and "oysters" as the backup singers and include them throughout the week in smaller portions. Who's the lead singer of this band? Well, it's really a duet sort of arrangement with muscle meat and fat belting out the sultry vocals. Based on our goals, let's talk more about each of these as we discuss the importance of a carefully considered fat/protein ratio.

How Much Protein and How Much Fat

As we saw in Chapter One, humans are fat-hunters. There is a very large body of anthropological literature to support the notion that indigenous groups and our ancestors sought out this nutrient above all others.[31] As noted by anthropologist David Rockwell:

"The Cree considered fat the most important part of any animal. One reason they valued bears above other animals was because of their body fat."[88]

In addition to the Cree, anthropologists who studied the Inuit (Alaska), and many other Native American tribes, along with Australian Aborigines noted the preferences toward fat as well. At the beginning of our journey together, we discussed that because of the way our human metabolism works, we can really only obtain about 40 percent of our calories from protein before it starts to put stress on our biochemistry. We don't use amino acids directly for fuel—we convert them to glucose through gluconeogenesis when the need arises. Protein is best thought of as a building block, while fat and carbohydrates fuel the metabolic engine. Once we've obtained enough protein to grow and repair the structural components of our body, more of this macronutrient doesn't seem to be helpful, and too much might tax our system in the excretion process of excess nitrogen groups from amino acids.[89]

There appears to be a "sweet spot" for protein intake that provides us with the right amount of building blocks for structural growth and repair but doesn't overly tax our metabolism and biochemistry. This amount will be a bit different for every individual based on each person's level of muscle mass, the type of activities they engage in, and their athletic goals.

A protein intake of 1 gram per pound of body weight per day will place most of us in this sweet spot and be more than enough to maintain muscle mass without taxing our biochemistry. I am five feet, ten inches and weigh about 165 pounds, so for me, this translates to around 170 grams of protein per day. Children, the elderly, or those who are looking to gain muscle might need a bit more, perhaps 1–1.2 grams per pound of body weight, but beyond this amount, there is probably no benefit to more protein.

A pound of muscle meat is 454 grams and contains about 100 grams of protein. The rest of the meat is water weight. Many people are confused by this fact, but think about how much lighter meat is when we make beef jerky. None of the protein has gone away in that process, but the water has been removed. So for me, a "sweet spot" of around 170 grams of protein per day generally means about 28 ounces of meat and organs per day. With the balance of methionine and glycine in mind, I favor cuts of meat that are rich in connective tissue, and I include bone broths made from tendons and other collagenous tissues as well.

From a macronutrient perspective, once we appreciate how much protein to aim for, the rest of our calories will come from fat and carbohydrates. The debate regarding how much of each of these to use in our diet for optimal health rages on, but I believe that the vast majority of us will perform best using fat as our primary fuel. Certainly, this appears to be the case for those with frank diabetes or who have evidence of insulin resistance and metabolic dysfunction.

The benefits of a ketogenic, fat-based metabolism are many. There is evidence that such diets can reverse insulin resistance and diabetes, lower blood pressure, increase mitochondrial biogenesis, turn on longevity genes, and reduce oxidative stress and DNA damage.[90,91,92-95] There is further evidence that these diets can decrease appetite, lead to profound weight loss, improve mood, and be protective for our brain.[96,97,98,99] From a cardiovascular risk standpoint, a ketogenic diet has also been shown to decrease triglycerides and metabolic dyslipidemia while increasing HDL.[100,101] On the other hand, low-fat diets generally increase triglycerides, lower HDL, and raise levels of insulin.[102]

That's an impressive list of benefits for ketogenic diets, isn't it? The real question might just be, why would we *not* want to run on fat most of the time? Some athletes competing at a very high level may benefit from occasional, moderate amounts of carbohydrates, but for the vast majority of us, a predominantly ketogenic metabolism is clearly an upgrade from one based on carbohydrates.

If we choose fat over carbohydrates for our fuel source on a carnivore diet, how much of this should we be eating? Again, this will be a different from person to person, but once we design a dietary framework that gets us the "goldilocks" amount of protein from meat and organs, the rest our calories will come from fat. I generally recommend a 1:1 ratio of fat to protein by grams for most people, but some will eat even more fat than this. For me, this usually translates into about 170 grams of fat per day. I obtain this amount mostly from grass-fed fat trimmings, suet, and egg yolks. With these macros I am easily able to maintain my muscle mass and not gain extra adipose tissue.

Many of us have been wrongly led to believe that eating lots of fat will cause weight gain, but this just isn't true. It's completely possible to lose weight eating fat in a 1:1 ratio with protein on any of the types of carnivore diets I have described. The secret to this is in how *satiating* fat is as a macronutrient. Once we start incorporating more good fat sources in our diet, we may be surprised at how full we feel throughout the day. In this situation, it's incredibly freeing to no longer be controlled by our appetite all of the time as so many are on carbohydrate-heavy diets.

We're not used to thinking of animal fat as a nutrient source, but it's a uniquely valuable food we have sought preferentially throughout our existence that should not be neglected or undervalued. Just like organ meats have a unique nutritional profile, animal fat does as well. I believe that it should be intentionally included on a well-constructed, nose-to-tail carnivore diet. What?! Fat has nutrients? You bet it does! Animal fat is a great source of fat-soluble vitamins like E and K2. Grass-fed animal fat is also a source of the omega-3 fatty acids—EPA, DHA, and DPA.

If we are eating grass-fed meat, there will be some fat with cuts like ribeye and NY strip, but it's not a ton. Most of the fat is now trimmed off our meat by butchers, so we have to specifically ask for trimmings or for the fat around the kidneys, which is known as **suet**. Grain-fed meat is fattier than grass-fed meat, but I have concerns about the accumulation of more toxins like estrogen-mimicking compounds, pesticides, and dioxins. In the Appendix, you'll find resources for where to find the high-quality, grass-fed fat you'll need to fuel your body in the best way possible.

BONES ARE ORGAN MEAT TOO!

Another thing to consider on a Tier 5 carnivore diet as a great source of fat is bone marrow. Countless accounts of indigenous people, past and present, describe the way in which this food has been relished for generations. Bone marrow also provides a good source of calcium, a mineral we haven't talked about much thus far, but which is very important. Just like other minerals, including sodium, potassium, and magnesium, we can't make calcium and must obtain it from our diet. Some people fear that eating calcium-rich foods will increase their risk of arterial calcification, but when our diet contains robust amounts of vitamin K2, this won't be the case. Aside from dairy, which we'll discuss below, sources of calcium on a carnivore diet include bone broth, bone marrow, bone meal and egg shells. Say what? Who the heck eats these things? Our ancestors certainly have, and many indigenous groups do today as well!

If we choose to use bone meal powder for calcium, we must be careful to select one that is low in heavy metals. Sadly, due to human pollution of the earth, bone meal may be contaminated with concentrated environmental toxins, so we must be careful to choose our source from cattle who are drinking clean water. I have listed my preferred sources of bone meal and dosing in the Appendix, and I'll note here that they are obtained from young, grass-fed animals in New Zealand that meet the *Prop 65* standards for lead and other heavy metals.

Egg shells are another good source of calcium on a carnivore diet, but the notion of eating them is sure to raise a few eyebrows. Again, quality is important here, but when sourced from organic chickens, ducks, or turkeys, they are a valuable addition to any carnivore diet. Clinical studies in women with osteoporosis have demonstrated that egg shells reduce pain and arrest bone loss.[103] Further research has also shown that egg-shell calcium is highly bioavailable and that egg shells contain other valuable trace minerals for bone health, including strontium, along with growth factors like **TGF-beta** and **calcitonin**.[104] Fortunately, heavy metals do not concentrate in egg shells and numerous analyses have shown them to be free from these contaminants.[105] Egg shells should be boiled prior to consumption to avoid any possible contamination with *Salmonella* or *Campylobacter* that may be on the outside of the shell.

In order to maximize the amount of calcium contained within it, bone broth can be cooked in an acidic solution (usually with vinegar) for twelve to twenty-four hours. Research into the mineral content of this ancestral elixir has demonstrated that when prepared in this way, the extraction of both calcium and magnesium are increased about sixteen-fold.[106]

If there are any concerns regarding the adequacy of calcium intake, checking the level of parathyroid hormone (PTH) and serum ionized and total calcium levels can be helpful. If serum total calcium is on the upper end of normal, and PTH is in the bottom third of the reference range, it's a good indicator that we are getting enough of this mineral in our diet. For our body to have healthy calcium homeostasis, we also need to obtain adequate levels of vitamins D and K2, which are best obtained from moderate amounts of real sunlight and organ meats.

What About Dairy?

Throughout our evolution, I don't believe that we would have had much exposure to dairy from other animals. Although some modern indigenous groups like the Maasai warriors include dairy in their diet, animal husbandry is a very recent adaptation within human societies and began only about 10,000 years ago.

Most of us don't appear to be well-adapted to dairy from ruminant animals due to a number of proteins contained within it that can activate our immune system. The most common of these is beta-casomorphin, a breakdown product of casein. The name of this molecule looks like "morphine," and it acts in a similar way in the human body. It activates opioid signaling pathways and can *disturb normal satiety signals*, leading to increased hunger and weight gain in many individuals.[107,108] Think about it—do you ever really feel full when you're eating cheese? In my own experiences, I know that I can eat a large amount of dairy foods without experiencing the same satiety signals I get from animal meat and fat, often leading to overeating.

The opiate-like qualities of dairy also make it slightly addicting, likely an evolutionary adaptation that encourages babies to drink a lot of milk so they get as many calories and nutrients as possible. As adults we no longer need to gain weight rapidly and can get all the nutrients we need from solid foods. Milk also contains both sugar (lactose) and fat, a satiety-disrupting combination of macronutrients that occurs very uncommonly in the natural world. There are sources of complex carbohydrates and sugars in plant foods and sources of fat in both plant and animal foods, but milk is one of the only places where these two occur together. The combination of fat and carbohydrates short-circuits our normal appetite-control mechanisms, a fact that junk food manufacturers picked up on decades ago. As we've previously discussed, candy bars, ice cream, and many of the other foods that are difficult for us to stop eating are all composed of sugar and fat. These foods are hijacking our brains and triggering our ancestral programming in negative ways.

In addition to activating the opiate-signaling cascade, casein can also trigger the immune system. It has two variants, A1 and A2, which break down into unique forms of beta-casomorphin. A1 casein is found in the milk of most cows in the United States, and the A2 variant occurs in the milk of other ruminants like buffalo, goat, and sheep. The A1 variant becomes beta-casomorphin 7, a molecule that has been linked to the development of Type I diabetes, celiac disease, Hashimoto's thyroiditis, ulcerative colitis, cardiovascular disease, and other autoimmune illnesses.[109,110,111] Elevated levels of this molecule have also been found in patients with schizophrenia, who improve with subsequent dialysis or casein-free diets.[112]

Derivatives of A1 casein may be damaging to our gut and kindle inappropriate immune responses in susceptible individuals. I don't think A1 dairy should be a part of any diet aimed at achieving improved health. Though some individuals might be able to tolerate A2 dairy from an immunological standpoint, these alternate beta-casomorphin variants will still activate opioid signaling pathways and can affect satiety in negative ways.

I've personally found that all types of dairy trigger my eczema, and exclusion of dairy in the clients I work with consistently allows for increased satiety, less inflammation, and easier weight loss. If we have an autoimmune issue or are interested in losing weight, I'd recommend leaving dairy out for at least the first sixty to ninety days of a carnivore diet. This includes milk, yogurt, butter, and ghee from all animals.

BORON—THE OFTEN OVERLOOKED BUT CRUCIAL MINERAL

One last mineral to think about as we seek to refine our carnivore diet to the highest degree possible is *boron*. Our knowledge of this mineral's role in the human body continues to expand, but there's still much to learn here. What we do know is that boron appears to play key roles in bone mineralization and hormone synthesis.[113] Interventional studies with this mineral in both men and women have shown improved levels of testosterone and other hormones, as well as improved outcomes in people with kidney stones and arthritis.[114,115,116] People in areas of the world with lower boron intake (1 milligram per day) have also been observed to have much higher rates of arthritis than those where dietary levels are higher (3–10 milligrams per day).

Regardless of the dietary strategy we choose to use, this mineral is an important one to include in our diet, and we should make sure we are getting it in adequate doses. On a carnivore diet, the best sources of boron are bone meal and A2 dairy, if tolerated.

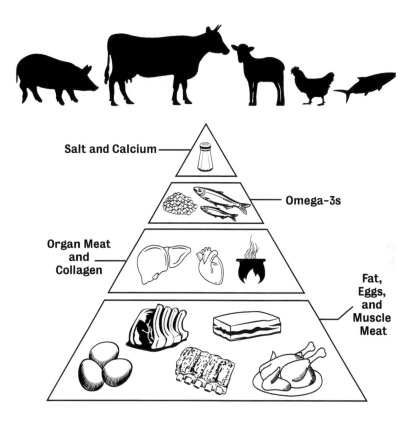

What a typical day of Tier 5 Carnivore looks like for me:

Breakfast:

Upon awakening, I consume about 3 grams of Redmond Real salt with a large glass of spring water. I then meditate and do a light morning workout before jumping into the day. I've found two meals a day works best for me.

10:00 a.m. Lunch:
- 6 egg yolks
- 90 g beef suet/trimmings
- 2 oz liver
- 2 oz kidney
- 14 oz ribeye steak with Redmond Real salt

3:30 p.m. Dinner:

- 3 raw oysters
- 80 g beef suet/trimmings
- 10 oz NY steak
- 2 oz thymus
- 2 oz pancreas
- 2 oz bone marrow
- 8 oz bone broth and 1/2 tsp bone meal

At this point you are probably saying, "Paul, you are crazy!" I've been called worse things! But, to provide you with an alternative of the Tier 5 carnivore diet, I will offer you a "non-Paul" version below:

What a typical day of Tier 5 Carnivore looks like for someone else:

Breakfast:

- 3 eggs cooked in tallow
- 2 oz beef liver
- 1 oz kidney
- 10 oz NY steak with salt
- 14 oz raw goat milk

Lunch:

- 60 g beef suet/trimmings
- 4 oz scallops cooked in tallow
- 2 oz bone marrow and 1/2 tsp bone meal

Dinner:

- 70 g beef suet/trimmings
- 10 oz ribeye steak
- 6 jumbo shrimp
- 8 oz bone broth

We've covered a lot so far about the different ways to eat a carnivore diet. Tier 5 is basically how I eat day in and day out. As I've noted earlier, this type of a carnivore diet may not be for everyone at all times, and don't think that everyone needs to eat just like me in order to derive the benefits of a carnivore diet. Traveling makes eating high-quality animal meats, organs, and fat difficult from time to time. It's totally okay to use Tier 1–4 diets in our life when they are the most appropriate for the current situation or if they work best for us. As I've emphasized previously, any dietary intervention that increases high-quality animal foods and cuts out the most toxic types of plant foods is going to improve our overall quality of life. Let's move on from the types of foods eaten on a carnivore diet to a discussion of some of the other details surrounding how to incorporate such a way of eating into our life and get one step closer to fully crushing it.

How to Live a Radical Life

I began this book with the assertion that the food we eat is the single biggest lever in health and disease. So far we've seen all of the ways in which food can either harm us or be deeply nourishing. From our discussions of the fallacy of xenohormesis and the importance of using environmental hormetics, we've also seen that optimal health is about more than just what we put in our body, it's also about how radically we live our life.

Some would have us believe that this radical life is hard to find, requiring tons of supplements, fancy gadgets, or complex dietary protocols, but our evolutionary history argues otherwise. If it were really that difficult, our ancestors would have perished swiftly, and the human race would not have become the dominant species on the planet. The equation for living a radical life is simple: eating animals nose-to-tail provides all of the nutrients we need to thrive with no associated toxins. We must also be outside in the sun—playing, hunting, and exploring—and sleeping in the dark at night, free from the incessant, low-level stress we all face in Western society. A bit of heat, cold, and some intense exercise are other important parts of this equation, as is spending time with family and community while giving and receiving love as we pursue something we are passionate about in our lives. As we saw with our examination of the Blue Zones, these are the aspects that create a rich and long life by complementing our intentional food choices. When we rediscover these long-forgotten principles of ancestral wisdom and incorporate them into our lives, we will reclaim our vibrant health and thrive as the incredibly capable beings we were meant to be.

The formula is simple: MEAT. PLAY. LOVE.

Clean Carnivore Reset (CCR)

Our immune system has a memory, and it's a darn good one! When we remove the plant foods from our diet that have been damaging the lining of our gut and causing inflammation, it's going to take a bit of time for things to heal and for the immune system to calm down. The half-life of the main type of antibody (IgG) used in our body is twenty-one days.[117] This means that when our immune cells react to an invader or a foreign molecule from food, it's going to take ninety days, or nearly five half-lives, for the antibodies produced during this process to vanish from our circulation. Ninety days! This is why it's so difficult to understand which foods may be triggering our immune system and what can be so powerful about elimination diets. More often than not, it's the process of removing things from our diet, rather than adding whatever the newest "superfood" is, that results in the greatest healing.

Trust me: your fibromyalgia, lupus, Hashimoto's, or eczema is not a turmeric deficiency. It's your immune system being over stimulated because of the foods you are eating that are damaging the gastrointestinal epithelium and causing leaky gut. We're not used to thinking this way, but even if we remove 95 percent of the foods making the immune system angry, those few remaining triggers can cause symptoms to persist and can make it very difficult to tell what the real culprits are. We can think of the decision to improve our health by eliminating plant foods as an experiment. But in order to get the most accurate data, this experiment must be done as carefully as possible. To truly appreciate how plant foods are affecting us, we'll need to avoid them for a full three months as intentionally as we can.

I'm not saying that we need to go from a life of eating plants to never eating another plant in our lives. It's overwhelming for most of us to think about any dietary change as a permanent decision for our entire life, but it's much more approachable to consider it as a ninety-day experiment. There are many within the growing carnivore community who feel the best they ever have without any plants in their diet and don't plan to eat them again in the future, but this doesn't have to be the norm for everyone. Within the context of a **Clean Carnivore Reset**, the carnivore diet can also serve as "the ultimate elimination diet." It can help us get back to a place of radically improved health, from which we can add less toxic plant foods back into our diet with careful attention to possible recurrence of symptoms. I don't love the word "cleanse" because of all of its mainstream connotations and associated images of worthless supplements and silly smoothies, but if we can create a cleanse that consists of real food without the fancy gimmicks, that's something I can get behind. In this light, we might consider the **Clean Carnivore Reset** a type of "steak cleanse." And who doesn't love the sound of that?

CASE STUDIES AND TESTIMONIALS WITH A CARNIVORE DIET

Now that we've learned all about the reasons to avoids plants, the incredible nutritive value of animal foods, and the nuts and bolts of how to eat a carnivore diet, I'd like to share a bit of the published literature on case studies of this way of eating, as well as some personal stories from real people who have adopted the carnivore diet.

Crohn's disease is an autoimmune condition of inflammation in the walls of the gastrointestinal tract so severe that it often erodes completely through the bowel wall. The case of a fourteen-year-old boy diagnosed with Crohn's disease who was unresponsive to traditional therapies and treated with a carnivore diet illustrates the power of such a dietary intervention.[118] He originally suffered with abdominal pain, gastrointestinal bleeding, and anemia and was diagnosed after upper and lower endoscopies were performed. When administration of multiple types of immunosuppressive agents failed to improve his condition, he was placed on a nose-to-tail carnivore diet and experienced immediate impressive results. Within two weeks of this dietary change, his symptoms had improved so significantly that he was able to completely stop his medications. By the fourth week, his anemia had corrected, and his blood levels of inflammatory markers improved significantly. Ultrasound imaging of his intestines over the next six months showed gradual improvements, and after eight months was completely normal, no longer displaying thickening of the terminal ileum. During this time period, his height and weight gradually increased, and intestinal permeability normalized. Impressive stuff!

Ketogenic diets are also well known to reverse insulin resistance and to treat Type II diabetes.[119,120] They have demonstrated superior outcomes relative to reduced-calorie diets in head-to-head trials for this condition.[121] With this in mind, it's not surprising that a carnivore diet, which is ketogenic in nature, has also been reported in the medical literature demonstrating efficacy in treating patients with Type II diabetes.[122]

Rather than arising from insulin resistance, Type I diabetes results from an autoimmune destruction of the pancreatic beta cells. This often occurs in childhood and abolishes the pancreas' ability to regulate blood sugar, requiring those with Type I diabetes to use supplemental insulin throughout their lives. In yet another impressive display of its might, a carnivore diet used shortly after diagnosis of Type I diabetes has been shown to reverse this autoimmune process, allowing the pancreas to continue to secrete insulin on its own.[123,124] Two cases of reversal of Type I diabetes (T1DM) are noted below:

*"Herein, we present a case of a 19-year-old male with newly diagnosed T1DM. The patient was first put on an insulin regime. Twenty days later, he shifted towards the [carnivore diet] and was able to discontinue insulin. Strict adherence to the diet resulted in normal glucose levels and a more than three-fold elevation of C-peptide level indicating restored insulin production. Currently, the patient has been on the [carnivore diet] for 6.5 months. He is free of complaints, and no side effects emerged. **We conclude that the [carnivore diet] was effective and safe in the management of this case of newly diagnosed T1DM."***

*"A nine year- old child with T1DM who initially was on an insulin regime with high carbohydrate diet was then put on the [carnivore diet]. Following dietary shift, glucose levels normalized and he was able to discontinue insulin. No hypoglycemic episodes occurred on the diet and several other benefits were achieved including improved physical fitness, reduction of upper respiratory tract infections and eczema. Currently, he is on the diet for 19 months. **Adopting the [carnivore diet] ensured normoglycemia without the use of external insulin. The diet was sustainable on the long-term. Neither complications nor side effects emerged on the diet."***

Results such as these are unprecedented with mainstream treatments of Type I diabetes, likely because the prevailing paradigm of autoimmune disease does not consider the possibility of food triggers. Clearly, if dietary protocols like the carnivore diet are begun promptly after diagnosis, it is possible to reverse autoimmune illnesses by removing the root cause of the condition and preserve the function of the tissues being damaged in these processes.

A carnivore diet has also proven effective in the treatment of brain cancer, cervical cancer, rectal cancer, Gilbert's syndrome, hypertension, obesity, and childhood absence seizures.[122,125,126-129] As with the ketogenic diet, many more formal studies are needed before the carnivore diet becomes widely accepted in the medical community as a possible therapeutic intervention. The numerous published case reports and the stories of thousands of people who have already benefited from this way of eating strongly suggests its restorative potential and safety.

When it comes to understanding which foods are damaging our guts and triggering our immune systems, elimination is an extremely powerful tool. This is one reason the carnivore diet is so powerful. By eliminating all potential plant food triggers, the carnivore diet is one of the most effective interventions available in the treatment of autoimmune and inflammatory illness, and I strongly believe that over the next few years, more and more clinicians will begin to realize this and incorporate it into their practice for the benefit of thousands of patients.

* * *

JUDY'S STORY: I've always sought to be thin. I thought the best way to achieve that was being vegetarian with the occasional fish. I ate a low-fat, high-fiber diet with spinach salads, daily, for twelve years.

While I was thin and my metabolic markers were "perfect," behind closed doors, I struggled with a crippling eating disorder that was accompanied by bouts of depression and anxiety. When I look back now, I know the lack of fat and meat in my meals always had me craving for more. I kept myself full with bottomless cups of green tea, coffee, and fibrous vegetables. Stomach distention was the only way I knew how to feel full. Full, yes, but never satisfied.

All things came to a crash after I had my first son. When he was six months old, I ended up with mastitis and I had to take antibiotics. The burden of exclusively pumping while barely nourishing my body and lack of sleep finally took a toll. I had a breakdown and, frankly, I don't remember two weeks of my life.

The doctors never were able to explain what happened, but they diagnosed me with severe postpartum depression and I was put on Zyprexa, an anti-psychotic that does not allow you to breastfeed. I stopped breastfeeding while I "lost my mind." In the hospital, each day I was retold the story of why my son wasn't there and how I had stopped nursing. Each time, I would cry and ask for my son. I was told it was heartbreaking to watch. While I write this, it still hurts my heart.

It's like I was in the movie *Groundhog Day* or *50 first dates*, but this was my life.

I never talk about this part of my journey because it's the darkest time of my life. I enrolled in an outpatient eating disorder facility to "cure" myself of my bad eating habits. I was forced to sit with therapists and dietitians while they monitored my meals. No food was off limits, and they encouraged a high-carbohydrate diet with sugary desserts.

Everything in moderation was the cure for eating disorders. Maybe that's why eating disorder relapse rates are often times more than 50 percent.

I was told by my psychiatrist that I was always mildly depressed and that I'd have to take medication for the rest of my life. The imbalance was just a part of me. While I was pregnant with my second child, I created a will and medical directive. I made these just in case I never "woke up" from another breakdown. Thankfully, that day never came.

Once I had my second child, I was determined to be healthier. I found the carnivore diet by way of the ketogenic community, and I've never looked back. I am now almost two years carnivore and I have yet to take anti-depressants or anti-psychotics again.

Once I started eating meat, I was healed. As I write this, I am still nursing my three-year-old son. My eating disorder behaviors are gone. Sure, there are days I can overeat, but the *urge* is no longer there. Cravings are bad mental habits, but the physical urges are gone. I believe so much of what happened was due to my low-fat vegetarian diet. My body needed binges to satisfy the need for fat and, all along, I just thought I had no self-control.

If we sift through nutritional misinformation, we can start to heal. So much of what we struggle with now is not because something is inherently wrong with us. It's because we are nourishing our bodies with the wrong things—things like plant-based, carb-centric, low-fat diets.

Meat has allowed me to have a second chance at life, and I am—from the bottom of my heart—grateful.

Paul's note: Judy Cho can be found @nutritionwithjudy on Instagram and other social media platforms and is the illustrator who helped me create many of the graphics for this book. I'm so glad she could share her own story within these pages and am grateful for all of her help with this project.

* * *

ALYSE'S STORY: My illusion of veganism being the superhuman diet was completely shattered within twenty-four hours.

Well—here goes nothing, I thought to myself as I took my first bite of animal food in four and a half years. In this moment, I had to completely surrender and release all vegan ideologies that I had so deeply woven my entire identity and livelihood around. As a "vegan influencer" with a collective social media following of nearly 1 million people around the world, you can only imagine how surreal this moment felt.

After years of dabbling in all of the plant-based diets under the sun—raw vegan, high-carb low-fat, high-fat low-carb, whole foods, junk food, raw vegan keto, the list goes on—I began reflecting on the state of my health (or lack thereof).

It wasn't until I saw some of my closest friends transitioning their diet and experiencing immense relief and healing that I had even considered the possibility of veganism playing a role in my health deteriorating. I was struggling with digestion, brain fog, memory loss, fatigue, and lack of sex drive, which were all deeply affecting the quality of my day-to-day life.

Once I allowed myself to question the diet, it was as if a veil was slowly being lifted from in front of my eyes. I realized that the only time I was entirely free of digestive discomfort during the extent of my vegan journey was when I was barely consuming enough calories—hence, my digestive system didn't really need to work very hard. My brain fog and fatigue were steadily increasing. My ability to concentrate and communicate clearly was practically non-existent. And as someone who loves learning and creating, I genuinely felt like I started to lose my identity, not being able to carry out the things that were so life-giving to me.

I was at the end of my rope, willing to try anything to feel healthy again. So when my friend proposed thirty days of carnivore—I actually considered it. What felt like a complete 180-degree change somehow seemed very intriguing, dare I say, appealing. After much thought and consideration, I decided to give it seven days.

My first non-vegan meal in almost five years was 8 ounces of smoked salmon. I don't think I will EVER forget the way I felt waking up the next morning. My mind felt more clear and focused than it had been in years. And for me, that was enough. My illusion of veganism being the superhuman diet was completely shattered overnight. I was humbled to say the least.

I have been eating mostly carnivore ever since—eating mainly beef, salmon, and eggs, and I cannot imagine where I would be right now if I had not surrendered to that seven-day experiment. For the first time in so long, I feel like myself again. When I stick to eating mainly carnivore, my digestion is flawless, mental clarity on point, healthy sex drive is present, muscle recovery (plus growth!) is better than ever, and energy is extremely stable.

Every single day, I express thanks to the animals for nourishing my mind and body, as well as for the doctors and public figures who advocate for this style of eating. If it wasn't for the constant inspiration from others, I know this path would feel a bit more lonely. But thankfully, we're all in this together!

Paul's note: Alyse Parker can be found on YouTube, where she has over 700,000 subscribers, and on other social media outlets @alyseparkerr.

* * *

DAVE'S STORY: My name is Dave, I'm a thirty-three-year-old guy from the other side of the world: Melbourne, Australia.

I just want to start by saying thank you, thank you, and thank you!

I absolutely love your content and simply can't express how grateful I am for you making it available to not just me but the broader community. It has quite literally altered the course of my life.

In [a] relatively short time, I've experienced huge changes, both physically and, most interestingly, mentally. The following is a non-exhaustive list of some of the changes I have experienced so far: greatly improved sleep, improved skin and teeth health, flawless digestion, increased energy, shredded body fat, very noticeable increase in lean muscle, complete alleviation of gastric reflux, complete alleviation of GOUT (anything with corn syrup among other things triggers me to have gout), mental clarity like I have never experienced, and most importantly of all—this way of eating appears to have completely abolished my long term anxiety/panic attacks.

The physical improvements are fantastic, no doubt, though I've always been somewhat lean and energetic; it's the mental benefits that I'm most grateful for. For the past sixteen to eighteen years or so, I have had anxiety of varying degrees. The past two years were undoubtedly the worst as I developed serve panic/anxiety attacks a few weeks after having an anaphylactic response to an anti-inflammatory medication (naproxen). I work in a corporate environment as an analyst at a top tier law firm, and as I'm sure you can imagine, thats not an ideal environment to be suffering with an anxiety-related condition. It was affecting my life in a profound way.

And now . . . It's GONE . . . I don't know what else to say. It's just gone. I have a confidence now that I don't think I have ever possessed. I'm in awe and, frankly, amazed. I genuinely thought anxiety was part of me and that I would continue to suffer with it for the remainder of my life. I initially noticed an improvement within the first two to three weeks of going 100 percent carnivore. And now, it's honestly like someone flicked a switch and simply turned it all off.

* * *

BEN'S STORY: Being diagnosed at the age of thirteen with a neurological disease called chronic inflammatory demyelinating polyneuropathy (CIDP) wasn't part of my dream of becoming an Army Ranger, Jedi, and professional athlete that played in the NBA, MLB, and NHL (move over Bo Jackson).

The deterioration of the protective covering of my nerves put a damper on most things, including my reflexes and having enough strength to cut my own food. After being failed by modern medicine and doctors, I decided to give all that conventional knowledge a break for a while. I have always had a very "suck it up" type of a mindset and just figured I would go about my life and pretend that the chronic pain and brain fog wasn't an issue. The nerve damage and my brain not communicating well with my peripheral nervous system wasn't going to have long-term effects, right?

Fast forward a few years and all of a sudden, a few outliers in the medical field were starting to get my attention. I started learning about inflammation and how my risk of cardiovascular disease, diabetes, cancer, and so many other ailments was escalated because of my chronic state of inflammation. I was still sticking to my guns when it came to the whole "avoiding conventional doctors promise" I made to myself, so I decided to do my own research. I learned that the standard American diet was causing the majority of the issues I had. I decided to change my diet, and the psychological warfare being conducted against meat was starting to make a little sense to me for some reason. I decided to buy a juicer and see how long I could go on only freshly juiced fruits and veggies. I went about three weeks at first and felt amazing. I then tried a raw vegan diet but slowly started feeling horrible again. I don't remember how long that lasted, probably because my brain wasn't functioning properly due to lack of nutrition from the real game changer . . . animal fat.

I bounced back and forth from a standard American diet and paleo-*ish* for years until finally committing to a strict paleo way of eating. After about a year of paleo I decided to try keto. My cognitive function was night and day when I was in ketosis, and I really felt a lot of inflammation leaving my body. I love vegetables, so I would experiment with seeing how high I could get my carb and fiber count and still stay in ketosis. I soon realized that the more fiber I ate, the worse I felt.

This wasn't my answer, but I wanted to try something else before I caved and scheduled an appointment with a neurologist. I was having CIDP flare ups that only seemed to get worse. I fortunately discovered another one of those outliers in the medical field that really seemed to care about actually healing people and exploring the cause and effect of our health. Watching videos and podcasts of Dr. Paul Saladino really answered a lot of questions and concerns I had about eating only meat. I decided to give carnivore a try, and to be honest, I wanted it to fail.

I have always loved fruits and vegetables and couldn't imagine life without all the social norms of food that my life revolved around. After ten days of beef, salt, and water, I doubled the amount of pull ups I could do and was finally able to wake up and walk down the stairs like a grown up instead of using both feet on each stair like a toddler (because of the pain I was in). I felt better after ten days of carnivore than I had in twenty-five years. My inflammation was mostly gone, brain fog was gone, and my mood was better than it's been in a long time. I am very confident that a nose-to-tail carnivore diet has put my CIDP in remission, and I encourage everyone to give it a try. Even if you don't think you have anything wrong with you, it will allow you to establish a baseline and slowly add back foods to see how your body reacts. I found that I was sensitive to foods that I had no clue I was. Often times, you don't know how bad you're feeling until you feel amazing!

WRAPPING UP

I'm so grateful to all of these people for sharing their stories with me and allowing me to share them with you as a part of this book, which has truly been a labor of love.

My goal in writing *The Carnivore Code* is not to convince everyone in the world to never eat plants again. It's to help us all understand that plants can be quite toxic, and that by eliminating all or most of them in favor of more nutrient-rich animal foods, we will upgrade ourselves in so many ways. But this will only happen if we are willing to commit ourselves to a certain amount of time following the diet as carefully as possible. If the idea of removing plants from your diet long term is overwhelming, just think about it as a forty-five- or ninety-day experiment and do the clean carnivore reset. I am confident that at the end of this time period, you will be amazed by the positive changes that have occurred.

The road to health and optimal life is not an easy one, however, and there are bound to be some challenges. In the next chapter, we'll discuss pitfalls we might run into when adopting a carnivore diet and answer many of the common questions people have as they embark on this heroic journey.

CHAPTER THIRTEEN

COMMON PITFALLS WHEN STARTING A CARNIVORE DIET

Do you remember that video game *Pitfall!* where you had to swing on vines over booby-trap laden pits? Okay, so maybe you're not a child of the '80s like me, but when I said this journey would be an adventure, I didn't lie! Just as this journey has already led us through some turbulent waters, our individual exploration of a new dietary landscape will have its challenges as well. But never fear, I've got your back. I want you to be successful on your quest, wherever it may lead you.

In this chapter, I'll break down many of the common pitfalls people experience when transitioning to a carnivore diet. I want to help make your experiences with this way of life as easy as possible. I'd like to emphasize that there are always some adjustments that need to be made when eating in a new way, and they do not always represent problematic reactions to the diet. For many people, bumps in the road like these are unpleasant and often lead to a discontinuation of the carnivore diet—or any diet, for that matter—but I'd urge you to push through the first two-to-three-week adjustment phase. There are great treasures awaiting you, including mental clarity, improved mood, weight loss, improved gut health and inflammation, and increased libido! In the Appendix, you'll also find many frequently asked questions to further troubleshoot any issues that may arise.

Disaster Pants

Not surprisingly, the most commonly encountered issues when transitioning to a carnivore diet are gastrointestinal. As we've spoken about throughout this book, the gut is ground zero when it comes to interactions between the food we eat and our immune system. We also know that the composition of the gastrointestinal microbiome is strongly influenced by the foods we consume. When we eat carbohydrates and plant fiber, we preferentially feed populations of bacteria that thrive on these. When our diet is mainly protein, animal fiber, and fat, the gut microbiome adjusts accordingly, and populations of bacteria that prefer these sources of energy expand as the carbohydrate-loving organisms recede.

But the gut is not always a peaceful place where everyone lives in harmony. It's a bit more like Medieval Europe, with multiple groups constantly vying for power and influence over the land. In order for one household to flourish, it must go to war against competing families—and the spoils belong to the victorious. This is exactly how things work amongst different species of bacteria in the gastrointestinal tract. If we feed the "carnivore microbiome," we are essentially giving these families of microbes resources while starving the other organisms who get pushed out, dying off in the process.

Shifts in bacterial populations also happen when we take probiotics or antibiotics, and many people are familiar with the gastrointestinal distress that can occur with either of these interventions. Simply put, when we do something in our life that shifts levels of different bacterial species in our gut, there's going to be fighting amongst the tribes with resulting casualties, and that's not always pleasant for us. In the case of antibiotics, this is usually going to be a bad thing. With a dietary change or probiotics, however, the shift in the microbiome can be for the better, with the most benevolent households coming to power over the medieval lands within us.

One of the most common pitfalls explorers of the carnivore lifestyle encounter is what we might call "disaster pants," aka loose stool or diarrhea. It's certainly no fun, but it usually only lasts for a few days. In some people with underlying gut issues and lots of nasty microbes previously ruling the roost, loose stool can last up to a few weeks. Let's be clear here: this doesn't mean our body isn't built for a carnivore diet. It most likely means our gut had some issues before we started this way of eating and it's going to take a bit more time to heal. Diarrhea at the beginning of a transition to a carnivore diet is often the result of shifting populations of bacteria within the gut as the carbohydrate-loving bacteria die off. It can also be the result of increased bile acid excretion by the gallbladder and biliary tree, which are needed to emulsify the fat content of the diet. Normally, bile acids are reabsorbed in the small intestine, but with these increased amounts of bile, the small intestine may need some time to adapt. As a result, non-absorbed bile acids, which end up in the colon, can often cause diarrhea.

Loose stool isn't a reason to stop eating a carnivore diet, and there are a few things we can do to help calm things down as we transition over to this new way of eating. The first of these is to take supplemental calcium. The extra calcium can help bind the excess bile acids being produced and prevent their cathartic effect in the large intestine. Good calcium sources include bone meal, crushed egg shells, or a calcium supplement. If the latter option is selected, I would strongly recommend avoiding pills with binders like hydroxymethylcellulose, titanium dioxide, or sulfur dioxide. When working with my clients, we use supplements only rarely, and those we select are always free from any binders which could damage the gut or trigger immune reactions.

To further assist with the symptoms of loose bowels, some people find it beneficial to add digestive enzymes, which might include lipase or a desiccated pancreas organ supplement. Depending on the composition of the gut microbiome, probiotics can also be of benefit, but they should be carefully selected, and the strain chosen is very important. If loose stool persists for more than a few weeks, I'd recommend working with a physician to take a look at what's going on in the gut with formal stool testing. I've noted some stool testing options as well as information regarding digestive enzymes, probiotics, and other supplements in the Appendix.

Some would claim that the "carnivore microbiome" isn't a healthy one, and that we must have plant fiber for "healthy" bacteria to thrive in our gut. But as we saw in Chapter Ten, these claims are based on nothing more than conjecture, and the clinical results of those eating a carnivore diet would argue strongly against these unfounded notions. A nose-to-tail carnivore diet provides ample amounts of animal fiber the microbes in our gut can use to make short chain fatty acids, and a carnivore diet has proven to be effective at reducing leaky gut when studied with PEG 400 testing.[1] A "healthy" microbiome is the microbiome that we have when our gut is healthy, and we are free from gastrointestinal symptoms and systemic inflammation.

CONSTIPATION

On the opposite end of the spectrum from disaster pants is traffic-jam city, also known as constipation. This is a less common occurrence on a carnivore diet, but nonetheless, it deserves careful consideration. It's important to note that when transitioning from a plant-fiber-heavy diet to one that is composed of mostly animal foods, it's completely normal to observe changes in stool quality, frequency, and volume. Specifically, those beginning a carnivore diet usually experience decreased frequency and volume of stool with significant improvement in quality and resolution of gas, bloating, and pain symptoms. But what are "normal" or "healthy" bowel habits at baseline? Though most gastroenterologists diagnose constipation only when someone hasn't had a bowel movement in three days or has had less than three bowel movements per week, I believe this criteria is too lenient. If all is well within our gut, and we aren't fasting or eating greatly reduced quantities of food, we should be having a bowel movement every day. If this hasn't been our pattern leading up to a carnivore diet, there is likely a pre-existing issue that may need some fixing. There are many things that can lead to constipation, including small intestinal bacterial overgrowth (SIBO), dysbiosis, and sluggish gut motility. All of these conditions can be potentially improved by eliminating plant foods, but in some cases, additional intervention may be necessary.

There are thousands of people eating a fully carnivorous diet who have easy-to-pass bowel movements on a daily basis. It is clear that we don't need plant fiber to go *number two*, but some do report constipation when they begin an animal-based diet. Often, these are people who had constipation prior to starting a carnivore diet, who then observe an increase in the amount of time between stools when they transition to more animal foods. Though I don't think having a bowel movement every three to four days is normal, this change is likely due to the decreased amount of stool produced when eating an animal-based diet. It is an exceedingly rare occurrence for me to hear of someone who had completely normal bowel habits to suddenly develop constipation when they started a carnivore diet. In the rare case that this does happen, we may need to consider the protein/fat ratio and include more fat in the diet. We could also try probiotics like *Lactobacillus GG* or *Lactobacillus reuteri* that have been shown to have efficacy in cases of constipation.[2]

The takeaway here is that temporary gastrointestinal issues may arise when starting a carnivore diet, and loose stool is much more common than constipation. But the vast majority of people find incredible improvements from gas, bloating, and other previously painful symptoms.

On a personal note, I'll add that I didn't have any issues with gut symptoms prior to the carnivore diet, but I did experience loose stool that lasted for about two weeks when I started eating this way. Since that time, I've been totally regular every morning like clockwork. How many other doctors are radical enough to tell you all about their own bowel habits? In the case of plant-based advocates this is probably a good thing, though. Trust me when I say that you don't want to know about what goes on in those bathrooms, and you wouldn't want to use one immediately after one of these poor, gaseous folks were in there.

THE KETO "FLU"

Many people who join the carnivore club are already practicing a ketogenic way of eating. For these people, the transition to a diet without plant-based carbohydrates is usually pretty smooth. For those who are not eating a ketogenic diet, this adjustment may be a bit of a speed bump on the road to awesome. When we are eating carbohydrates, our body uses them for energy rather than using the "fat burning mode" that produces ketones. By choosing to run on fat rather than carbohydrates, we must switch our metabolic machinery accordingly, an adjustment that takes the body a bit of time to do. During the first three to four days of the transition period, we may feel tired, irritable, and achy— symptoms sometimes referred to as the "keto flu." There's no infection here, however, it's our body gearing up the metabolic machinery to burn fat for fuel.

One of the major changes that occurs when we transition to a ketogenic metabolism is a sharp decline in insulin levels. In the long term this can be a very good thing, as it usually correlates with significantly improved insulin sensitivity, but in the short term, it can take our body a few weeks to get used to. One of the many roles insulin serves in the body is signaling our kidneys to conserve sodium. When levels of this hormone drop during the ketogenic transition, the result is acutely increased losses of this mineral. Though sodium has been vilified for years by the mainstream establishment, it is critical to our survival and serves many vital roles in the human body. Its balance is tightly regulated within our physiology, and when levels are low, we waste other important minerals like magnesium and potassium in our urine. If we don't provide enough sodium to meet the increasing needs at the beginning of ketosis, our body may become depleted of not only sodium, but magnesium and potassium as well. Many of the symptoms of the "keto flu" are likely due to electrolyte imbalance and can be ameliorated with increased attention to intake of sodium, magnesium, and potassium during this transitional period. This process isn't always easy, but our body is building a whole new metabolic engine that burns clean fuel, so it's worth it!

FATIGUE

Though a bit of fatigue may be part of the keto-adaptation period in the very beginning of the transition to a carnivore diet, this shouldn't last more than a week or so. Beyond this, low energy levels on a carnivore diet are often related to less than ideal fat/protein ratios, inadequate salt consumption, or an inadvertent calorie deficit. Remember our previous discussions on the nature of protein as a building block and fat or carbohydrate as fuel. When I hear from someone that they feel like they've "lost a gear" on a carnivore diet, more often than not they are using protein for the majority of their calories and not consuming enough fat. Though eating steak for every meal is probably the easiest way to do a carnivore diet, for most people, this isn't going to provide enough fat. In extreme cases of lean meat consumption, the result may be a condition that is referred to as "rabbit starvation" that results in excess ammonia production. We definitely do not want to construct a carnivore diet out of just lean chicken breast, lean hamburger, or lean steak. This is a recipe for failure.

Some in the health sphere recommend increasing protein and limiting fat in order to lose weight on ketogenic and carnivore diets, but I don't think this should be taken to extremes. Just like there's a sweet spot for protein of around 1 gram per pound of body weight per day, it appears there's a sweet spot for how much fat we should be consuming for overall optimal health. If we choose to limit fat too much and over consume protein, we may lose weight in the short term but will quickly develop imbalances that hamper attainment of long-term goals and full vitality. As we discussed in the previous chapter, I've generally found that a ratio of 1:1 for fat to protein by grams works well for most people in the absence of carbohydrates. Performance and hormonal balance suffers when fat is limited too much.

Losing weight is about creating a caloric deficit, and the easiest way to do this is to eat satiety-promoting foods. Of these, good quality animal fats are king.[3] In the Western world, we aren't used to eating trimmings, bone marrow, and suet, or thinking of these foods as valuable, but they are hidden gold. Grass-fed fat contains a number of valuable micronutrients, including vitamin K2, omega-3 fatty acids (EPA, DHA, DPA), vitamin E and conjugated linoleic acid (CLA). It's also just darn delicious.

Another reason for fatigue when transitioning to a carnivore diet may be inadequate sodium consumption. How much salt should we be eating per day? Depending on body size, most people find 6–10 grams (1.5–2 teaspoons) of salt daily to be ideal, though some prefer even more. If you are currently on a low-sodium diet, please consult your physician before increasing your intake. By salting my food to taste at each of my two meals per day, and beginning the day with a few grams of salt mixed with water, I've found that I consume about 10–12 grams of salt per day with noted improvements in energy and athletic performance. If we're not sure how much salt we are consuming, it may be helpful at first to measure out 8–10 grams at the beginning of each day to see how it feels eating this amount throughout the day. I'd recommend using these numbers as a ballpark figure to see how you feel. If 8 grams is too much or too little, it's okay to adjust this number up or down. Just remember, salt is a key part of the overall equation of electrolyte balance.

In rare cases, fatigue can also be related to not consuming enough calories. If weight loss is our goal, a caloric deficit will be a common feature of our diet, but for those with a focus on performance—hoping to maintain or even gain weight—not getting enough calories can throw a wrench into things. Inadequate calorie consumption can also be related to too much protein relative to fat. As we've talked about before, our body has a threshold for how much protein it wants. If we try to go above this level, protein-rich foods just won't be appetizing to us. On the other hand, fat will always be welcomed by our body if we need more calories. The trick for most of us is figuring out where to get it from because we're not used to eating animal fat as food. Grass-fed trimmings, suet, and bone marrow will be what we need here.

INSOMNIA

There are multiple reports of improvements in obstructive sleep apnea with a carnivore diet, likely related to weight loss and resolution in posterior pharyngeal lymphadenopathy. That's a mouthful, I know! I'm referring to swelling of the lymphatic (immune) tissues in the back of the throat that can occlude the airway at night, causing obstruction and breathing impairment. Cases of rapid improvement in sleep apnea on the carnivore diet are likely related to this decreased swelling of the posterior throat, suggesting that a dietary food-trigger was previously causing immune activation in these lymphatic tissues. Not only are plants potentially activating the immune system in the gut, they can also be triggering immune tissues throughout the body, including the airway.

Though most people have improvement in sleep, occasionally, people do report insomnia on a carnivore diet. In these cases, I again think about too much protein, too little salt, and disordered methylation related to not enough organ meats. We need a number of nutrients for the methylation cycle to work properly. The two most likely to be deficient are riboflavin and folate. Muscle meat just won't have enough of these for most people, but adding liver and kidney to the diet will improve things significantly. To get a sense of how well our methylation cycle is working, we can check blood levels of homocysteine. Anything over 8 μmol per liter suggests a need for more folate and riboflavin from organ meats. If we don't want to eat organ meats, desiccated organ supplements will be a good adjunct to the diet.

In the health space, some have incorrectly suggested that carbohydrates are necessary for tryptophan to enter the brain as a precursor for melatonin. Tryptophan circulates in the body bound to albumin and competes with other amino acids (tyrosine, threonine, methionine, valine, isoleucine, leucine, histidine and phenylalanine) for entry into the brain through the blood-brain barrier. Rising levels of insulin with the ingestion of carbohydrates can cause levels of the other amino acids to decline as they are taken up into the muscle, leading to an effective increase in tryptophan concentration and subsequent uptake into the brain.[4,5]

The movement of tryptophan into the brain is not carbohydrate-dependent, but rather, concentration-dependent, and if levels of this amino acid are low relative to these other amino acids, suboptimal levels might cross the blood-brain barrier—leading to inadequate melatonin production and sleep disturbance. On the other hand, regardless of carbohydrate intake, if relative levels of tryptophan are high, as they are when consuming a protein-rich carnivore diet, this amino acid can easily cross into the brain to make melatonin, and there's no danger of inadequate production of this hormone.

Furthermore, absolute levels of insulin do not provide information about true levels of insulin signaling. We can have lots of insulin around while in a state of insulin resistance and have very little signaling at the cellular level. Conversely, in situations like a ketogenic diet, the overall amount of insulin is low, but signaling is robust due to a high degree of insulin sensitivity in tissue like the brain. Even without carbohydrates on a ketogenic carnivore diet, there's enough insulin signaling and tryptophan to create the concentration gradient needed to get this amino acid into the brain for melatonin production.

Muscle Cramps

Early on in the adaptation period, some people do experience muscle cramping with ketogenic and carnivore diets. This is likely due to electrolyte deficiencies of sodium, magnesium, and potassium, with sodium being the most common deficiency and the most important to correct first. As we previously discussed, during the first few days or weeks of a ketogenic diet, there is excess wasting of sodium and the other minerals due to declining levels of insulin signaling. Eventually, the body adjusts to this, but in this early phase, it's super important to pay attention to intake of this mineral. If we are getting 6–10 grams of a mineral-rich salt and are still experiencing muscle cramps, it might be worth considering magnesium supplementation. We should also look at our diet and be sure that we are getting ample amounts of calcium and boron, as we discussed previously. It might also be helpful to do some lab testing and look at the levels of these minerals in our red blood cells (RBCs). Serum levels of magnesium and potassium aren't an accurate gauge of muscle stores of these minerals, but RBC levels give a better picture.

Though none of this book should be misconstrued as medical advice, I'll make a few general recommendations regarding electrolyte dosing and sources with the caveat that if our kidney function is not normal, adding extra amounts of magnesium or potassium in supplemental form can be dangerous.

For magnesium supplementation, I would recommend starting with 400–600 milligrams per day, from magnesium glycinate powder—free of the binders common in most supplements. Remember that in order to get 400–600 milligrams of magnesium from magnesium glycinate, you will be ingesting about 3 grams of the powder, most of which will be the glycine part of this molecule.

Even moderate doses of magnesium can cause loose stools, but the glycinate salt of this mineral appears to be the least likely to do this. Citrate, oxide, malate, or other forms of magnesium are almost certain to cause loose stools if we exceed doses of more than 200 milligrams at once. If muscle levels of magnesium are low, many people will need to supplement with this mineral for weeks to months to replace these. There is no convincing evidence that topical forms of magnesium are well absorbed or raise total body levels, so I wouldn't use this form as the only way of supplementing.[6]

I do not recommend oral supplementation of potassium, and have not found this to be helpful or necessary. Meat is naturally a good source of this mineral, and if we are getting enough sodium, we will conserve this potassium well. Supplementation with potassium can also be dangerous in those with suboptimal kidney function and should not be done without physician supervision. Eating a carnivore diet with the recommended amounts of protein provides us with plenty of potassium, and I do not believe that additional intake of potassium is beneficial or required in the setting of an animal-based diet.

Other minerals to think about if muscle cramps occur are calcium and boron. In Chapter Twelve, we talked about sources for both of these on a carnivore diet, and I mentioned that my preferences are high-quality bone broth, bone marrow, bone meal powder, egg shells, or dairy if tolerated.

If muscle cramping persists after addressing sodium, magnesium, boron, and calcium, I would recommend working with a physician to look at the levels of a wider array of micronutrients. White spots on the fingernails are one of the clinical signs I often see that indicate a nutrient deficiency. This is a non-specific finding, however, and can be related to a lack of many different nutrients, including zinc, calcium, selenium, manganese, copper, or other minerals. Consequently, it is necessary to apply more specific nutrient-testing to zero-in on what's missing.

Though supplementation with electrolytes is often useful during the transition phase to a carnivore diet, it's usually not necessary long term if we are getting enough salt in our diet and eating a variety of animal foods found on Tier 4 and Tier 5.

HISTAMINE INTOLERANCE

Fresh animal foods do not contain significant amounts of histamine, but aged or processed meats, cheeses, hydrolyzed collagen, bone broth and shellfish can definitely act as triggers for those with histamine sensitivity. The roots of histamine intolerance aren't fully understood, but this condition is likely connected with leaky gut and the inability of the liver to properly break down histamine-containing compounds in food.[7] Genetic polymorphisms in diamine oxidase (DAO), one of the main enzymes in our body that breaks down histamine, can also lead to intolerance of these compounds. Eating only fresh, non-processed animal foods is the most effective intervention for preventing symptoms related to histamine sensitivity, but DAO supplementation may also be helpful for some people. Kidney is also quite rich in DAO, and many have found improvement in their histamine intolerance by including this organ in their diet or by taking a desiccated kidney supplement.

Most of the clients I work with who have histamine intolerance see gradual improvement in symptoms over time with the carnivore diet. This is most likely connected with gut healing after removing damaging plant foods.

TROUBLE DIGESTING FAT OR RED MEAT

Many of us beginning a carnivore diet may have pre-existing nutrient deficiencies, especially if we are coming from a heavily plant-based diet and aren't used to eating animal foods. In these situations, trouble digesting red meat or fat is often seen as an indication that these foods "don't agree with us," and aren't good for our body. Nothing could be further from the truth. As we've seen along our journey, humans have evolved eating animals. These foods are "written" into our book of life as the best sources of the nutrients we need to function optimally. If we're not digesting animal meat or fat well, it's likely because of a nutrient deficiency that we've acquired by *not eating these foods* rather than an indication of an intolerance towards them.

To digest meat, we need a strongly acidic environment within our stomach. In order to generate all of this acid, cells there must have enough zinc and other nutrients commonly found in meat.[8] Zinc supplementation has been shown to improve gastroesophageal reflux by increasing acid production and leading to better functioning of the gastroesophageal sphincter.[9] Guess how many good sources of zinc there are in the plant kingdom? Zero. What's a good source of zinc in the animal world? Red meat! Remember our discussion from Chapter Eight about the huge decrease in zinc absorption from oysters when they were eaten with phytic acid containing foods like beans and tortillas? It should come as no surprise that if we don't eat red meat, or if we commonly eat foods high in phytic acid and oxalates, we have a reasonable chance of becoming deficient in zinc and other nutrients needed to digest this ancestrally valuable food. If we get stomach discomfort from eating beef or lamb, we might try smaller portions. Also, checking our zinc levels is probably a good idea. Ultimately, however, the answer is usually to keep eating these foods in order to obtain the nutrients within them and not to continue avoiding them.

From time to time, I also hear that people have trouble digesting fat. This could be a related to low stomach acid as well, but it's more likely due to inadequate bile or pancreatic enzyme production. Bile is produced in the liver, concentrated in the gallbladder, and released in response to meals containing protein and fat. After food has been partially digested by acid within the stomach, it passes into the duodenum, where it mixes with bile, making the mixture less acidic. Bile salts emulsify the fat within this partially digested food, allowing it to become water-soluble and creating a greater surface area for pancreatic enzymes to act upon. If we don't produce enough bile, fat in the food we eat will pass through our gastrointestinal tract and be excreted in a condition known as malabsorption. The result will be a pale-colored stool rather than a stool with a normal brown hue.

If a person has trouble digesting fat and has pale stool, it may be the result of inadequate bile production. This condition is usually due to a choline deficiency, which has been shown to impair proper transport of bile acids into the bile from the liver.[10] As we've learned previously, appreciable quantities of this nutrient are only found in animal foods. The pattern is the same here: difficulty in digesting fat isn't usually due to the fat itself, it's often due to a deficiency in a nutrient that we can only obtain in adequate quantities by eating a diet rich in animal foods. If you have trouble tolerating the amount of animal fat that I recommend on a carnivore diet, you can back off temporarily while making a strong effort to significantly increase your intake of choline-rich foods like egg yolks and liver. You might also consider a desiccated gallbladder supplement during this time as well. After a few weeks, you should be able to begin increasing intake of fat gradually without gastrointestinal discomfort.

Though less common than choline deficiency, insufficient production of pancreatic enzymes is another possibility in cases of difficulty digesting fat at the beginning of a carnivore diet. In this case, supplementation with digestive enzymes may be helpful during the first few weeks of such a diet as the body adjusts.

WHY GALLBLADDER STONES FORM AND HOW TO AVOID THEM

Bile is composed of bilirubin, bile salts (also known as bile acids), and cholesterol. Bile acids are synthesized in the liver from cholesterol and then transported into the bile ducts, which flow into the gallbladder in a choline-dependent manner. If we don't make enough bile salts, or the bile salts made in the liver can't be transported into the bile, the cholesterol concentration in bile can become too high, leading to the formation of the most common type of gallstones.[11,12] The accumulation of cholesterol-rich gallstones is known as cholelithiasis, a condition found in approximately 15 percent of the US population, though the actual incidence is probably even higher.

If one of these stones becomes lodged in the neck of the gallbladder, bacteria from within the gut can migrate into the stagnant space within it and cause an infection, resulting in acute cholecystitis. When asymptomatic gallstones are detected, the gallbladder will often be removed prophylactically, or the exogenous bile acids ursodiol and chenodiol may be used as pharmaceuticals that help dissolve the cholesterol stones.[13] Ultimately, however, the formation of these gallstones is a disease of inadequate production of bile salts that could be corrected by increasing our intake of choline.[14]

Since this book has been full of bold statements, I'll make another one: cholelithiasis due to cholesterol gallstones is completely preventable if we eat a diet rich in choline. If we have gallstones and still have our gallbladder, or if we want to prevent gallstones, we should be sure to get a robust amount of choline in our diet—egg yolks and liver for the win! Don't give up your gallbladder unnecessarily!

In summary, if we are having trouble digesting fat, it's okay to decrease the amount we are eating in order to give our body time to get nutrients from our animal-based diet that will be needed for this process. If there's a history of gallbladder stones, focusing on choline intake will be crucial, and supplementation with ox bile or desiccated gallbladder may be helpful in the short term. In cases of insufficient pancreatic enzyme production, adding these in supplemental form may help until our body gradually adapts.

LACK OF VARIETY

Usually, when I describe the carnivore diet to people, they respond with a joyful disbelief: "You mean I can eat steak, eggs, scallops, salmon, and oysters all the time and get healthier?" Occasionally, however, those who hear about this way of eating fear a lack of variety and impending food boredom, but this isn't usually what happens in real life once most take the plunge.

Allow me to offer a personal story that illustrates this well. Many years ago, I set off with a friend on one of the most grand adventures of my life: a through-hike of the Pacific Crest Trail. We traveled north through the mountains of California, Oregon, and Washington, and hiked 2,700 miles from the border of Mexico all the way into Canada. When I was packing food for the trip, I was sure things like peanut butter, oatmeal, and other plant foods I relished at the time would never get boring, so I included them as daily rations for the entire trip. For the first few weeks of hiking, I was able to stomach them, but I quickly grew sick of the peanut butter and oatmeal, and by mile 1,000, I threw them out at every resupply or tried to trade that stuff for something better with other hikers. The fascinating thing was that even though I was also eating beef jerky every day, I never got tired of it. In fact, it quickly became the most prized food in my backpack.

During this three-and-a-half month epic adventure, I learned that even the plant foods I thought were the most enjoyable quickly got boring, but animal foods never did. This surprised me at the time, but it now makes total sense. Animal foods are what our body really craves. They provide ultimate nutrition without the toxins found in plants. If we eat the same plant food day after day, the specific toxins contained within it build up in our system, and we steadily develop aversions. Remember, plant foods are survival foods—they aren't meant to be eaten regularly. Once you begin a carnivore diet, I think you'll be surprised at the way you look forward to every meal. Animal foods never seem to get old, boring, or repetitive *because they are what we are programmed to eat,* and they are incredibly nutrient-rich!

Concerns with lack of variety may also indicate that we are using food as entertainment. Yes, food is meant to be enjoyed, and many colorful plant foods provide beautiful displays of artistic expression, but if our goal is health, we may need to seek artistic outlets elsewhere and focus on understanding which foods allow us to achieve the best quality of life possible.

If the idea of eating only animal foods sounds unattainable, I'll ask the following questions: What do we really want? What is our highest quality of life and what are we willing to do to achieve this? Our current environment of constantly available food with unlimited variety requires more discipline than ever before and can easily sabotage our efforts to improve our lifestyle. If we are truly committed to regaining or maintaining optimal health, disciplined food choices are how we achieve this— plain and simple. Thankfully, animal foods are delicious.

CARNIVORE DIET WITH AN APOE4 POLYMORPHISM

Though this isn't really a pitfall encountered with a carnivore diet, questions regarding this polymorphism and FTO are quite common and important to address at this point in the book.

Discussions surrounding APOE4 can quickly become complex, but I think it's safe to say that most of what we have heard about saturated fat being bad with APOE4 is grossly oversimplified. APOE is one of the apolipoproteins that travel on the surface of lipoproteins and serve as markers on these particles. Within the brain, APOE is produced by cells called astrocytes and is the principle carrier of cholesterol, transporting this valuable cargo to neurons. Adequate cholesterol is essential for proper membrane function and fluidity, but cholesterol in the blood doesn't cross the blood-brain barrier, so the brain must make its own. APOE is the *bridge* by which this cholesterol is transported to neurons, and in people with the APOE4 gene variant, this transfer appears to happen more slowly under conditions of insuline resistance. Population studies in the West suggest that individuals carrying one or two copies of the APOE4 variant, rather than APOE3 or APOE2, have a significantly increased risk of developing Alzheimer's disease. This occurrence leads many to believe that this genotype has an ominous prognosis, but the story is more complex than this.[15,16]

Not all individuals with the APOE4 polymorphism develop dementia. In many non-westernized populations with higher exposure to infectious disease and parasites, such as the Bolivian Tsimane and Nigerian Yoruba, this genetic alteration appears to be *protective* with regard to cognitive decline and inflammation.[17,18,19] Evolutionary studies also reveal that APOE4 is the oldest variant. It was the form present in all of our ancestors up until 200,000 years ago when APOE3 appeared, followed by APOE2 120,000 years later.[20,21] This means that for the vast majority of our evolution, APOE4 was the *only* variant of this allele, likely serving a protective role against infection. Do we really believe that all of our ancestors—with the APOE4 allele and eating lots of animal foods—invariably developed significant neurocognitive issues? Sounds like another evolutionary incongruity to me. There must be another piece of this equation today affecting our risk of dementia. Care to take a stab at what it might be?

If you said insulin resistance, you are right. A connection between Alzheimer's disease and insulin resistance is well established, and this type of dementia has been termed "Type III diabetes" because of the associated deficits in insulin signaling.[22] Though the APOE4 variant likely protected us from infectious disease for the last 4 million years, it appears to make us a bit more susceptible to insulin resistance in the brain when we eat foods that aren't consistent with our evolutionary past.[23,24,25] But as we've seen from the Tsimane and Yoruba, *APOE4 does not appear to be harmful in insulin-sensitive populations.* Why is there such a strong association between this genetic variant and Alzheimer's disease in Westerners? When 88 percent of the population demonstrates metabolic dysfunction and insulin resistance, of course APOE4 looks bad![26]

Takeaway: Eating a carnivore diet allows us to join the elite ranks of those with exquisite insulin sensitivity, and having an APOE4 polymorphism won't be harmful in this situation. In fact, when used in individuals with APOE4 variants and cognitive impairment, high-saturated-fat ketogenic diets lead to *improvements* in markers of insulin resistance as well as brain functions that include memory, executive function, and abstract thinking.[27]

THE CARNIVORE DIET WITH AN FTO MUTATION

FTO polymorphisms are another common genetic variant I get asked about with regard to higher saturated fat diets like carnivore. Again, the short answer here is that these are not an issue either, but let's elaborate on a few details.

As its name suggests, polymorphisms in FTO, or the **fat mass and obesity-associated gene**, correlate with an increased predisposition to obesity. In a large population study of 38,759 Europeans, carriers of one copy of the risk allele (rs9939609 T->A) weighed 2.6 pounds more than those with no copies, while individuals homozygous for this variation weighed 6.6 pounds more and had a 1.67 times increased rate of obesity.[28]

Discussions of polymorphisms quickly turn into alphabet soup, but I'll try to simplify things here. The "rs9939609" refers to a specific spot in the genetic sequence of the FTO gene in which some people have the nucleotide base *adenine* (A) in place of *thymine* (T). This is called a "polymorphism," and when only one gene copy possesses such a change, an individual is said to be heterozygous. Homozygosity refers to the situation in which both gene copies are polymorphic at a particular position in the sequence.

Having an FTO polymorphism does not inescapably result in obesity. It is estimated that 74 percent of Caucasians carry at least one copy of this gene variant, including myself, but most of us aren't obese.[98] Much of the concern surrounding FTO in the setting of an animal-based diet comes from one epidemiology study that showed an *association* between the rs9939609 genotype and obesity in individuals with metabolic syndrome, and it was stronger in those who consumed more saturated fat.[30] Immediately we can see the problems here. Attempting to apply an observational epidemiology study of a population with insulin resistance to those of us who reside within the metabolically healthy portion of the population is misguided and myopic. Throughout our journey, we've seen repeatedly that the state of insulin resistance changes everything. Studies done on populations experiencing this are simply not applicable to those who are insulin sensitive. We've also seen the way in which unhealthy user bias can confound studies. Another glaring question with this study is: just what other sorts of junk foods were these individuals eating with their saturated fat?

The FTO gene doesn't exist just to make us gain weight. It serves important roles in the human body involving demethylation of RNA, but much like APOE4, when we move away from an ancestral lifestyle, those with polymorphisms may be more predisposed to the development of negative consequences.

Takeaway: Having a polymorphism in the FTO gene is extremely common and is not a reason to avoid saturated fat on a carnivore diet. The key is to realize that the populations studied are often insulin resistant, severely limiting the applicability of their findings to metabolically healthy individuals. We must not be misled by this bad science and the unfounded hype surrounding the dangers of saturated fat!

WRAPPING UP

I hope that this chapter and the previous one will serve as a comprehensive guide as we begin our own journey with a carnivore diet. I've tried to address as many of the common pitfalls and questions as I could. In the Appendix, there is a list of many frequently asked questions that go beyond this chapter, but we are always learning and there will surely be more to explore in the future. Because of my own experiences, and those of my clients and the carnivore community, I believe more than ever that this is the way that we are fundamentally designed to eat. The research I have done in writing this book has also strengthened my conviction that a nose-to-tail carnivore diet is written into our book of life and is what we find in the user manual that we have searched for so diligently. By eating animals, we have access to the most nutrient-rich foods this planet can provide. By choosing to make them the focus of our diet, while shunning plant foods and the toxins contained within them, we mirror the way our ancestors ate and will reclaim the profound health that is our birthright.

In the final chapter of this book, we'll consider the ethical and environmental impact of consuming animal foods in today's changing world. We will find that, rather than being a part of the problem, ruminants may be one of the only hopes we have of reversing global climate change. The final adventures await.

CHAPTER FOURTEEN

THE END OF THE ROAD
AND BEGINNING A NEW WAY OF LIFE

I am greatly honored that you have chosen to walk this road with me, and that we have arrived at the end of our journey together. It is my greatest hope that I have provided you with information that will be useful and enriching to your own life. I deeply believe that remembering our ancestral design and eating a nose-to-tail carnivore or carnivore-ish diet will bring us radical health and a profoundly increased quality of life. As we approach the end of our road together, I have just one request of you: If you've found value in what I've shared, do not remain quiet. The world needs to know what we have learned. The amount of mis-information present within our culture is overwhelming, and it is ever increasing. Some of this is driven by well-intentioned physicians and others of influence who haven't yet realized that their paradigm is incorrect. For these people, I hope that this book and its message will be a clarion call toward a careful examination of their beliefs. It is also a very heart-breaking reality that much of the incorrect information we encounter arises from corporate interests who have much to gain.

THE ENVIRONMENTAL IMPACTS OF EATING MEAT

If you have any doubts of these motives, remember the recent history of industry involvement in the demonization of animal fats. Take a look at the list of businesses who supported the absurd EAT-Lancet guidelines, which recommended that we consume only 14 grams of meat per day under the guise of helping the environment. A full list of these companies can be found in the Appendix, but included are the likes of Bayer, Monsanto, Kelloggs, Pepsi, Cargill, Nestle, and Syngenta. See a pattern here? Much like businesses benefited enormously from fostering the general public's belief that animal fats were bad and vegetable oils were healthy, these agribusiness enterprises stand to make billions of dollars convincing us that plant-based foods are the healthier option and the responsible environmental choice. So far in this book, we've talked at length about why the claims that animal food is unhealthy and plant food is our salvation are pure hogwash, but now I'd like to spend a bit of time examining the environmental impact of eating animal foods. Spoiler alert: in the United States, these companies produce over ten times the amount of greenhouse gases as cows, and regenerative ruminant agriculture can actually *reduce* the amount of carbon dioxide in the atmosphere!

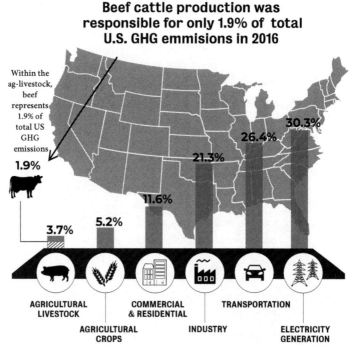

Beef cattle production was responsible for only 1.9% of total U.S. GHG emmisions in 2016

Within the ag-livestock, beef represents 1.9% of total US GHG emissions

1.9%

3.7%   5.2%   11.6%   21.3%   26.4%   30.3%

AGRICULTURAL LIVESTOCK — AGRICULTURAL CROPS — COMMERCIAL & RESIDENTIAL — INDUSTRY — TRANSPORTATION — ELECTRICITY GENERATION

U.S. Environmental Protection Agency, EPA 430-R-16-002 (2016, April) Inventory of U.S. Greenhouse Gas Emissions and Sinks: 1990-2014: Retrieved from https://www.epa.gov/sites/production/-files/2016-04/documents/us-ghg-inventory-2016-main-text.pdf

Let's just cut right to the chase here and ask the most important question: How much do cows actually contribute to the overall greenhouse gas emissions within the United States? The answer is a very small amount. If we look at the figure above, which is based directly on data from the EPA's 2016 report, it quickly becomes apparent exactly how small this contribution is. According to this data, beef as a whole represented only 1.9 percent of the total greenhouse gas emissions in 2016. **1.9 percent!** That's half as much as plant agriculture; ten times less than industry or transportation; and more than fifteen times less than electricity generation, the largest producer of greenhouse gases. Why is it then that all we ever hear from politicians and those who claim to campaign for the environment is talk about methane from ruminants?

Follow the dollar signs, my friends. In addition to being a complete ecological catastrophe, the elimination of animal agriculture in the United States would decrease emissions here by a paltry 2.6 percent, and .36 percent globally.[1,2] Yet this now seems to be the main focus of so many discussions, without any mention of the other 98 percent of contributions. Might this have something to do with the fact that so many big businesses stand to lose hundreds of billions of dollars if the spotlight were turned upon them and they were held accountable for their devastating impact on our environment?

Based on their small contribution to greenhouse gas production and the integral place within grassland ecosystems, the elimination of ruminants is clearly not the answer to our climate woes.

The other part of this equation often overlooked is that methane emissions from livestock is part of the carbon cycle and does not increase the total amount of carbon in the atmosphere. In contrast, the carbon dioxide produced by industry, transportation, and electricity generation represents newly created carbon and adds to the overall amount of this element in the atmosphere. This is a nuanced distinction; let's explore it further by elaborating on how greenhouse gases affect our environment, the natural carbon cycle, and where ruminants (animals like cows, buffalo, sheep, and deer with upper digestive tracts specialized for fermentation of plant matter) fit in.

There are numerous greenhouse gases, including water vapor, carbon dioxide (CO_2), methane (CH_4), nitrous oxide, and ozone, that concentrate in the earth's atmosphere. They all absorb infrared radiation from the sun and warm the surface of the planet. These gases have always been here, and without them the surface of our earth would be a frigid zero degrees Fahrenheit.[3] Since the industrial revolution kicked off in the mid-eighteenth century, the atmospheric concentration of carbon dioxide has increased from 280ppm to 415ppm in 2019.[4] As a result, scientists are concerned that if levels continue to rise, global warming could progress to dangerous levels. Check out what is known as the Keeling Curve if you are interested in seeing how levels of CO_2 in the atmosphere have spiked in the last seventy years.

As part of the carbon cycle, methane produced by ruminants goes into the atmosphere and is broken down into carbon dioxide after a period of about ten years. This atmospheric carbon dioxide is then used by plants during their cellular respiration to make carbohydrates. Cows then eat these plants and digest the carbohydrates, releasing methane back into the environment as the cycle continues. Notice that within this process, the methane produced by cows does not represent new carbon in the atmosphere but rather serves as a portion of the carbon cycle that is necessary for life on earth. The carbons contained within the methane molecules emitted from cows were once part of the carbon dioxide normally present in the atmosphere. This is in stark contrast to the carbon dioxide released from the burning of fossil fuels, which breaks down long-chain carbon-containing molecules from within the earth and releases *new* carbon dioxide into the environment, increasing the overall amount in the atmosphere. It is this new carbon that's raising the amount of carbon dioxide to 415ppm, not the methane from cows, which participates in the carbon cycle and has always been present in the atmosphere. The real problem here is our use of fossil fuels, a crutch that seems inescapable in the present moment—but supports the argument that in the near future, we must move toward other forms of renewable energy sources rather than continuing our dependence on the use of oil and gas. Gas and oil companies aren't going to like that, and neither are the supporters of the EAT-Lancet guidelines, all of whom stand to lose a lot of money with less use of fossil fuel.

Methane from ruminants is also only a fraction of the methane released into the atmosphere on a daily basis. As a whole, methane represents 8 percent of the greenhouse gases in our atmosphere, and the *majority* of this comes from coal mining, natural gas usage, the breakdown of trash in landfills, and natural sources like wetlands and termites. Often, we will hear those who deride animal agriculture stating that methane is the most dangerous greenhouse gas because of its strong ability to contribute to global warming, but these folks never admit that their trash and electrical usage contributes significantly to this as well. Nor do they acknowledge the equal contribution of natural wetlands and insect ecosystems, which are clearly vital for the overall health of the planet. The simple fact here is that methane from ruminants is not the problem. It's always been a part of our planet's atmosphere and pales in comparison to the other sources of greenhouse gases.

In place of ruminants, many suggest that we eat fake meat made from sawdust, bamboo, and oxidized seed oils. They state that such choices are better for the environment, ignoring the fact that these industrially produced burgers contribute more to greenhouse gas emissions than well-raised ruminants. Furthermore, the mono-crop agriculture that is used to grow most plant foods today damages the soil and reduces organic matter by exposing deeper layers of earth to oxidation in the process of tilling.[5] Once these layers are damaged, they are much more susceptible to erosion and runoff when rains arrive. This further depletes the land of the nutrients necessary for healthy plants to grow and destroys natural ecosystems. Sadly, both the EAT-Lancet guidelines and these fake meat products seem to be more about lining the pockets of multi-national corporations than reversing the dangerous changes happening within our environment today. They are certainly not aimed at improving our health.

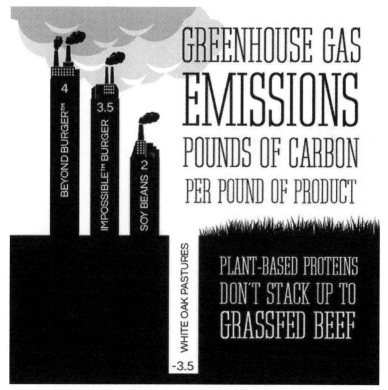

From White Oak Pastures based on *Life Cycle Analysis* done by Quantis.
Available here: https://blog.whiteoakpastures.com/hubfs/WOP-LCA-Quantis-2019.pdf

There is hope, however. Attention is beginning to shift toward solar, wind, and hydroelectric power, and we are learning more about the ability of regenerative agriculture practices to sequester carbon in the soil.

When soil is healthy, plants are able to draw greater amounts of carbon dioxide from the environment into the soil and their root systems. Conversely, traditional farming and mono-crop agriculture deplete the soil of nutrients, decreasing its ability to sequester carbon dioxide and destroying delicate ecosystems. Proper grazing of ruminant animals serves to *enrich* the soil with organic matter and, therefore, increases its carbon-carrying capacity.[6,7] Regenerative agriculture practices promote these evolutionarily appropriate grazing styles, and placing cattle farmed in this manner on depleted grasslands has been shown to revitalize these ecosystems. Analyses of farms like White Oak Pastures in Georgia has demonstrated that regenerative agriculture practices result in a carbon *negative* ecosystem.[8] On farms like this one and others employing similar grazing practices, more carbon is sequestered into the soil than is released into the atmosphere. The result is a net *decrease* in greenhouse gas emissions as grass-fed cattle are raised on the land. Doesn't that just turn the tables and cast things in a new light? **Rather than decreasing the amount of beef raised on this planet, increasing the farming of grass-fed regeneratively raised cattle might just be our best hope to become healthier humans and to preserve the environment around us.**

Soil Organic Matter

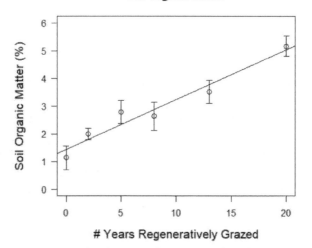

 # Years Regeneratively Grazed

From White Oak Pastures based on soil analyses performed there.

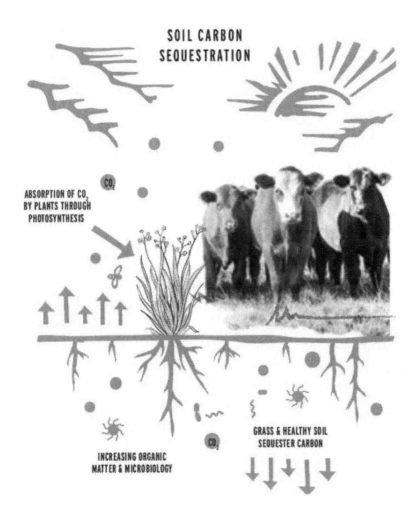

SOIL CARBON SEQUESTRATION

ABSORPTION OF CO_2 BY PLANTS THROUGH PHOTOSYNTHESIS

CO_2

INCREASING ORGANIC MATTER & MICROBIOLOGY

CO_2

GRASS & HEALTHY SOIL SEQUESTER CARBON

We must not be misled by the assertions of those who seek to demonize ruminants with misleading messages that are based on incorrect information. If we truly hope to be good stewards of this planet, we must become the healthiest and most resourceful people that we can be by eating animal foods that nourish our bodies and brains. We can then use our collective creativity to address the real sources of climate change in industry and develop viable long-term strategies to arrest and reverse the damages that have already been done.

SUMMING IT ALL UP

Throughout this book, there have been a number of themes that have arisen repeatedly worth reflecting on as we come to the end of our journey together. Perhaps the most striking of these is the profoundly negative way in which insulin resistance influences our physiology and is the underlying "bad guy" in so many diseases. We know that insulin resistance is to blame for illnesses like diabetes, hypertension, and PCOS, and in Chapter Eleven we saw that it also makes our LDL and arterial walls more sticky and is likely the real villain in the process of atherosclerosis. It would be evolutionarily inconsistent for a part of our biology, like LDL, to be both good and bad for us at the same time. When we are healthy, we have nothing to fear from this lipoprotein that serves so many vital and protective roles in our physiology.

In our discussions of Alzheimer's dementia, insulin resistance was again implicated as a major driver of the development of this debilitating cognitive impairment. We found that those possessing the APOE4 polymorphism are more susceptible due to apparent worsening of insulin signaling when they diverge from an ancestral diet. Individuals with the FTO polymorphism also appear more prone to weight gain and obesity in the setting of insulin resistance. Those of us who carry these genetic variants but are insulin sensitive, however, avoid any such issues. The good news with insulin resistance is that it's easy to avoid by eating a nose-to-tail carnivore diet, maintaining a healthy weight, and eliminating foods that damage our gut and cause inflammation. As insulin sensitive individuals, we are part of an elite tribe, my friends.

Another theme along our journey has been the fundamental limitations of epidemiology, which is too often confounded by healthy and unhealthy user biases. This type of observational science can easily be distorted to support specific claims that don't hold up in controlled, interventional studies. When looking at epidemiology studies, it's also critical to remember that 88 percent of the U.S. population is metabolically unhealthy, and correlations must be interpreted within this context. With most of those around us possessing some degree of insulin resistance, we must be careful with interpretations of research. We must always be vigilant to view it through this lens and compare it to interventional studies and studies done in populations where metabolic dysfunction is not present. As we've seen throughout our journey, this type of scientific evidence tells a much different story.

Viewing health and medicine through an ancestral lens, so many of the points used to challenge a carnivore diet make little sense. Why would a food such as meat, which we've been eating for more than 4 million years and which allowed our brains to grow rapidly, be bad for us? Why would plants be good for us when they have developed chemical defenses to discourage predation, and why would they contain magical health-promoting compounds? There are no magical plant compounds that we need to become the best versions of ourselves, and anyone who claims otherwise is likely trying to sell you something. On the contrary, using animal foods for the majority of our nutrition is absolutely the best way to optimize our health, performance, and longevity.

FINAL THOUGHTS

Discussions of the environmental impact of our food choices remind us of our inextricable connection with the land and the soil of the earth. Our ancestors knew this and acted accordingly, generally being careful not to over-hunt or destroy the ecosystems they depended upon for nourishment and livelihood. Though we now live in a modern world, too often separated from these fundamentally human practices, it's instructive to recall this ethos. That's what this book is really all about. One of my favorite proverbs reminds us of this.

> *"When the blood in your veins returns to the sea, and the earth in your bones returns to the ground, perhaps then you will remember that this land does not belong to you, but it is you who belong to this land."*
>
> *-Anonymous*

Eating a nose-to-tail carnivore diet is about more than knowing which foods humans should eat to be optimally healthy. At its core, this movement is about remembering the ways our ancestors lived that are written in our own *book of life*. For millions of years, we have been eating animals as our primary food. This has allowed us to grow into the intelligent, problem-solving beings we are today. At the same time, we've also been moving in natural landscapes. We've been feeling the sun on our skin and the dirt under our feet. We've been sipping from natural bodies of water, and we've been building tribes of people that we truly care about. If we really want to flourish and become the prodigious beings we are designed to be, we must remember more than just how our ancestors ate—we must remember the way they *lived*.

The carnivore diet is about adopting a lifestyle in which we make efforts to do what we were designed for as often as possible. It's about walking in the woods with bare feet and taking the time to play. It's about moving and jumping outdoors—in the sunlight, in the snow, and in cold lakes and rivers. It's about celebrating the communities around us that give our life meaning. This book began with a foreword from Mark Sisson, one of the people who has done such a good job of reminding us of the joys that come from returning to our primal lifestyle roots.

As we come to the end of our journey together, let us not forget that one day, we will all leave this earth. Perhaps nothing is more important than living the short number of days that we have here with as much joy and vigor as possible. It is my deepest hope that this book will dispel the untruths that too often cloud our vision and confuse our efforts to live dazzling lives, and that it will provide us with the tools necessary to reclaim the radical health that is our ancestral birth right. Our ancestors have shown us the way. We have only to listen to what they teach us in order to become the beautiful, powerful, and vibrant humans we were designed to be.

Stay radical!

FREQUENTLY ASKED QUESTIONS

When I started writing this book, I knew that I would never be able to address every single possible question that arose from it—that's what my next books are for. In an effort to be as comprehensive as possible, however, I am including this section to address many commonly asked questions. As has been the case throughout this book, I've made an effort to include as many references as possible to allow readers in search of more information to "go further down the rabbit holes" on their own.

IS GRASS-FED MEAT BETTER THAN GRAIN-FED MEAT?

Absolutely.

Grass-fed meat is better than grain-fed meat in so many ways. From the environmental perspective, the nutritional perspective, and the toxin perspective, cows raised and finished on grass are superior sources of food for humans.

In the final chapter of this book, we talked about the environmental implications of eating meat and discussed the fact that ruminant agriculture contributes a very small amount to the overall greenhouse gas emissions. Of this contribution, fully grass-fed ruminant agriculture is clearly superior to traditional grain-finishing methods and produces less green house gases. In addition to feeding animals with grass throughout their lifecycle, many farms are now beginning to use the work of Alan Savory to implement regenerative agriculture practices. This type of farming seeks to mimic the grazing practices of wild animals. Farms such as White Oak Pastures in Georgia and Belcampo in Northern California have been using these methods and have proven to be net-carbon negative, sequestering more green house gases into the soil than are produced during livestock cultivation.

Grass-fed meat is also a more nutritious food source. Studies of grass-fed meat have demonstrated higher levels of vitamin C, vitamin E, and glutathione when compared to traditional grain-fed meat.[1] They also provide a more favorable fatty acid profile with increased levels of EPA, DHA, DPA, and CLA.[2] Intuitively, this makes sense—cows and buffalo fed the foods they've evolved eating are going to be much healthier than those confined to a feedlot that are fed inferior food. Sounds a bit like humans, doesn't it? If we eat what we've evolved to eat, we'll be the best version of ourselves, but if we rely on fallback foods, our health is sure to gradually decline. I don't know about you, but eating the healthiest cows sounds like a good investment to me.

The most striking differences in the quality of grass-fed versus grain-fed meat are found when we *compare the toxin loads between these two.* Grain fed to cows is sprayed with pesticides and often highly contaminated with mold. Cows fed these grains are exposed to higher levels of glyphosate, 2-4-D, atrazine, and mycotoxins, all of which can bioaccumulate and end up in the meat and fat of these animals. Grain-fed cattle are also likely to have a higher exposure to persistent organic pollutants like dioxins from pentachlorophenol-treated wood used for the water tanks in feedlots.[3] These animals are also routinely fed other manufacturing byproducts, including candy, cookie crumbs, and potato waste, while housed in feedlots.[4] In Chapter Twelve, we discussed issues surrounding the pesticides glyphosate and 2-4-D, both of which are potentially quite harmful for humans. Atrazine is a fat-soluble herbicide with known endocrine-disrupting properties as an estrogen mimetic, and it is commonly sprayed on corn fed to cattle.[5] Strikingly, when male frogs are exposed to moderate doses of atrazine early in development, this compound turns them into females due to its estrogenic activity.[6] Ummm, I like my hormones the way they are, thank you!

The downsides of grain-fed meat don't stop there, however. Remember mycotoxins from our discussion of coffee? One of those was fumonisin, produced by fusarium mold, which is also known to contaminate much of the corn in the United States. What are cows fed in feed lots? Much of their diet will be corn and other moldy, pesticide-laden grains. Fumonisin and related mycotoxins are also endocrine disruptors with estrogenic effects. They are widely distributed in cereal grains and can be detected in basically all grain-based foods we eat.[7,8] Yikes! If we can avoid these toxins and support more intentional and healthy farming practices in the process, why don't we? Are these really things we want in the meat and organs we are eating? Though grass-fed animal foods are slightly more expensive, they sound like a pretty good investment to me.

Before we move on from the grass-fed versus grain-fed discussion here, it's quite important to point out that the term "pasture-raised" is often used in a misleading manner. It is not the same as a grass-fed, grass-finished animal. I've even seen grocery stores label grain-finished meat as "pasture-raised" without clarifying that these animals were fed grain in feedlots at the end of their life. Don't be fooled by this shady sort of advertising, which is known as "greenwashing"!

WHAT DO I DO WHEN I FALL OFF THE WAGON?

Don't beat yourself up; just start eating as intentionally and cleanly as possible again.

We don't need to do any special cleanse involving expensive supplements if we eat not so great foods. Our body will take care of the detoxification and rebalancing on its own when we provide it with all of the amazing nutrients in animal foods. We might consider fasting for a period of twenty-four to forty-eight hours after a bump in the road, but I have some reservations about recommending something that may be viewed as a "punishment." If we don't view fasting in a negative light, then this might be a good intervention after periods of particularly poor eating, but it's not required.

HOW SHOULD I COOK MY MEAT?

Though meat cooked on a grill or at high temperatures tastes pretty good, there is some evidence that heterocyclic amines and polycyclic aromatic hydrocarbons do induce some degree of oxidative stress, activating the NRF2 pathway in the liver.[9] Our ancestors probably would have eaten meat cooked over an open fire, and we do have biochemical pathways to deal with moderate amounts of these compounds, but if we really want to create the least amount of oxidative stress possible, cooking our meat more gently is probably a good idea most of the time.

Using lower temperature cooking methods, like a pressure cooker, crock pot, steam convection oven, or slow cooking in a pan will lower the formation of HCAs and PAH significantly. If we elect to cook our meat in a pan, I'd recommend against the use of oils as these can become oxidized with heating. The best option for this is to use a high quality stainless-steel pan. Avoid using non-stick coated pans of any kind as the chemical coatings on these can also be toxic for humans.

HOW SHOULD I GET MY FAT?

Make friends with a butcher who can source from grass-fed farms! Getting to know a butcher who can provide high-quality meat, organs, and fat will be hugely helpful in our quest to acquire the best foods on the planet. If our butcher can get us grass-fed trimmings (the fat trimmed off of steaks) or suet, then we should write them a thank you note, bring them flowers, or serenade them, because he or she will quickly become one of our favorite people.

If this isn't a possibility, there are resources for farms that sell grass-fed fat in the Appendix of this book. I prefer actual fat from animals to the liquid-rendered fats like tallow or ghee that are more common today. Un-rendered fat may contain more fat-soluble nutrients and has accompanying connective tissues that provide a source of collagen. It's also easier to digest for many people.

WHAT ABOUT MARIJUANA?

Marijuana contains polyphenols, and just like all of the other polyphenols discussed in Chapter Five, these have also been shown to be potentially harmful to humans by damaging DNA and decreasing levels of testosterone and other androgens. When studied in cell culture at doses obtainable with recreational use, the cannabinoids cannabidiol and cannabidivirin were found to have negative effects:

> *"Our findings show that **low concentrations of cannabidiol and cannabidivirin cause damage of the genetic material in human-derived cells**. Furthermore, earlier studies showed that they cause chromosomal aberrations and micronuclei in bone marrow of mice. Fixation of damage of the DNA in the form of chromosomal damage is generally considered to be essential in the multistep process of malignancy, therefore the currently available data are indicative for potential carcinogenic properties of the cannabinoids."*[10]

I believe marijuana and its related compounds may have utility for some medical applications, but I don't think they are a beneficial addition to the lifestyle of healthy individuals. If marijuana is helpful for our anxiety or sleep, it may serve a temporary adjunctive role, but we should look diligently for the causes of these issues as well. Working with a physician who is savvy enough to help us search for the roots of illnesses and using this book as guide toward changing our diet in positive ways will likely get us to a place where we no longer need marijuana or cannabinoids.

Doesn't protein putrefy in our gut? Isn't it the hardest thing for our body to digest?

Urban legends, anyone?

Contrary to popular belief, meat is much more easily digestible than plant matter. After learning in this book about the many ways plants conspire to prevent us from digesting them, this should come as no surprise. With our acidic stomachs and long small intestines, we are uniquely adapted to absorb the nutrients present in animal foods very efficiently, but the same cannot be said for plant foods. The simple proof of this can be found in our poop! Those eating a carnivore diet quickly notice that the volume of stool decreases significantly, and undigested food is never seen in the toilet after a bowel movement like it might be after eating salad or other plant foods.

The notion that meat putrefies in the colon is just plain wrong as well. Unless there is a major problem with our digestion, undigested proteins from animal foods do *not* make it to the large bowel in any appreciable amounts. Time to put this myth to rest. I dare you to challenge a plant eater to a "who's poop is prettier" contest!

Where did our ancestors get sodium from, and how much were they eating?

This is a fascinating question that ties into discussions of the other electrolytes. During the eight-to-twelve-week period of keto adaptation, our needs for sodium appear to increase significantly as insulin levels drop sharply. Many people find that during this period and beyond, intakes of salt as high as 6–10 grams per day can be very helpful. Large epidemiology studies suggest that those consuming this amount of salt have the lowest cardiovascular death rates and overall mortality,[11] contrary to the fear-mongering talk about salt that we've so often heard.

It seems likely that our ancestors would have sought out salt deposits to obtain this nutrient, as many other animals do. In more recent history, salt has been treasured and used as a form of payment, from which the term "salary" is derived. Wars have been fought over salt, and salt brine was used to pay soldiers in the field during the War of 1812. Tales of a mountain of salt of innumerable value near the Missouri River were given to Congress by President Thomas Jefferson as justification for Lewis and Clark's 1804 expedition to the Louisiana Territory.

We should not fear salt, but instead remember the incredible value this substance has had throughout human history. My preferred source is Redmond Real Salt, which is derived from an underground inland deposit in Utah. It is free from **microplastics** and other contaminants that are common in traditional sea salts.

WHERE DID OUR ANCESTORS GET MAGNESIUM/POTASSIUM FROM?

Most of the magnesium our ancestors consumed was probably from their water. Spring water is much higher in magnesium and other minerals than the municipal tap water available today. The mineral water *Gerolsteiner* contains 100 milligrams of magnesium and 345 milligrams of calcium per liter, and tap water simply pales in comparison.[12] Muscle meat also contains a decent amount of magnesium, with about 100 milligrams per pound. Drinking a few liters of spring water per day and eating as little as 1 pound of muscle meat can easily get us to the RDA for magnesium from highly bio-available sources.

Furthermore, the notion that plants are the best source of magnesium is just plain wrong. It's actually pretty hard to get the 400 milligrams of RDA from plant sources. We'd have to eat 2 pounds of kale in order to achieve this level! I don't even want to think about how much gas and stomach pain I'd have after that. Remember also that the magnesium found in plants is not very bio-available due to the chelating properties of phytic acid and oxalates.

Meat is also a rich source of potassium, with over 1,400 milligrams per pound. There's no RDA for this mineral, and I don't think anyone really knows how much is ideal. Epidemiology studies suggest that intakes of potassium over 2,000 milligrams per day are associated with decreased all-cause mortality, but cardiovascular disease mortality does not improve with higher amounts.[11] With these findings in mind, aiming for 2,000 milligrams per day seems reasonable, but I do not think we need to worry about obtaining massive amounts of potassium. There's no interventional data to suggest that this is beneficial as long as our blood pressure is within normal range. If blood pressure is elevated, the first thing to think about is addressing possible underlying insulin resistance.

Take home: Eating animal foods and drinking water from a good source will provide us with ample amounts of these minerals as long as we are thinking about sodium consumption from an ancestral perspective. Proper maintenance of mineral balance must also consider sources of calcium and boron as discussed in Chapter Twelve.

IS COCONUT OIL OK? WHAT ABOUT OLIVE OIL?

Animal fats are a much richer source of fat-soluble vitamins like K2 than plant fats, and I recommend them over coconut, olive, or avocado oils when transitioning to a carnivore or carnivore-*ish* diet. Furthermore, though we often think of plant oils as only fat, they also contain proteins known as **oleosins**, which can act as *immune triggers* in some people.[13] Oleosins in peanut and sesame oils are known to cause strong allergic reactions in sensitive individuals.[14,15] Oleosins isolated from both coconut and olive oils may do the same.[16,17,18] If our goal is to eliminate the plant foods that may be triggering our immune system, *avoiding all plant oils* is a good idea.

There's a ton of hype around the polyphenols in olive oil, but I'm far from convinced that these provide a unique benefit in humans. Refer back to Chapter Five for a discussion of the not so magical nature of polyphenols. These are plant molecules made by plants, for plants, and they don't play well with our biology, nor is there solid evidence that we need them to be optimal.

Both olive oil and coconut oil also contain salicylates—yet another reason to avoid them.

WHERE DO COCONUTS FALL IN THE PLANT TOXICITY SPECTRUM?

I would place coconuts somewhere in the middle of the spectrum. They appear to be better tolerated than other nuts and seeds but can definitely still cause issues for some people, perhaps because of their salicylate content. We spoke briefly about salicylates in Chapter Five and discussed them as a common plant toxin found in many foods.

A fairly good list of salicylate-containing foods can be found by visiting this web address:

atpscience.com/salicylate-foods-sensitivity-intolerances-and-food-list

If we are really trying to clearly understand which foods might be triggering immune reactions, coconuts are best left out of our diet. They may have a limited role in a carnivore-*ish* diet but should be reintroduced carefully with attention to possible symptoms.

DO I NEED SUPPLEMENTS ON A CARNIVORE DIET.

No.

Everyone comes from a unique position of nutritional adequacy/inadequacy when they begin a new dietary change. If we include a variety of organ meats, we can meet all of our nutritional needs. This assumes adequate nutrient absorption and a reasonably healthy gut, however. There are conditions, such as celiac disease, small bowel overgrowth, and autoimmunity, that affect the stomach and the gastrointestinal tract and which can result in malabsorption and limit our body's ability to assimilate the nutrients in food. If our bowel habits are normal, and we don't have gastrointestinal symptoms, chances are we absorb the nutrients in our food just fine. If we're not sure, a stool test that includes fecal fat and measures gastrointestinal inflammation can determine if malabsorption is a problem.

In cases of pre-existing nutritional deficiency, some supplementation may be useful, but this must be determined with our physician on a case-by-case basis depending on detailed lab testing.

WILL MY LDL/CHOLESTEROL RISE ON A CARNIVORE DIET?

It may.

LDL doesn't rise for everyone who eats this way, but for many people, LDL will rise, and *that's probably a good thing*. If you're still fearful of LDL, you may want to refer to our previous extensive discussion of the many valuable roles this particle has in the body and all of the data suggesting that—in people who aren't insulin resistant—more LDL is probably protective due to its immunological functions.

In Chapter Eleven, we also discussed that LDL probably rises on a carnivore diet due to increased production of cholesterol within the shared synthesis pathway with ketones. I don't think a rising LDL on a ketogenic or carnivore diet is anything to worry about *as long as markers of insulin sensitivity and inflammation are low*. If you're not sure about these, working with a physician who is familiar with ketogenic physiology will be helpful.

Take home: LDL is not the enemy, and there is no evidence that it is enough to initiate atherosclerosis on its own.

What bloodwork should I get before or after beginning a carnivore diet?

I know a lot of people will ask this question so I've placed this information in the Appendix.

What if I don't want to eat organ meats?

A lot of people are in this boat when they begin a carnivore diet. We understand that organ meats may be very nutritious, but we haven't grown up eating them, don't know how to cook them, and find the flavors or textures to be odd. In this situation, desiccated organs from high-quality grass-fed animals are a great option. Because the freeze drying process is very gentle and involves low-temperature dehydration, it preserves the nutrients in organs very well. In the Appendix, I've recommended the best sources for this type of supplement.

A word of caution here: because of the increasing awareness of the effectiveness and convenience of desiccated organs, many companies are beginning to bring very low-quality versions of these to market. I would only recommend organ complex supplements sourced from grass-fed animals within the United States or from New Zealand. Assays show that organ supplements sourced from Argentina and other South American countries are of much lower quality and purity. These should be avoided until supplies from these countries demonstrate improved standards.

The other good news here is that I will be releasing a nose-to-tail carnivore cookbook with my friends Ashley and Sarah Armstrong with 150 amazing recipes, many of which will include organ meats. Keep your eye out for *The Carnivore Code Cookbook*!

Can I do a carnivore diet if I don't have a gallbladder?

Absolutely.

As we discussed above in Chapter Thirteen, bile is made in the liver and transported into the biliary tree where it is stored in the gallbladder. Your liver still makes the same amount of bile after you've had your gallbladder removed, but it is now stored within the bile ducts, which often dilate to accommodate a larger volume post cholecystectomy. Even without a gallbladder, we will release bile from the biliary tree when we eat food. In this situation, a choline-rich diet remains the key to adequate bile salt production, so there's no reason to limit consumption of animal foods.

HOW MUCH SHOULD I BE EATING ON A CARNIVORE DIET?

Let satiety be your guide.

If you are hungry, eat. If you're not, don't. One of the challenges for many individuals as they transition into a carnivore diet is *breaking old habits of snacking or using food as entertainment between meals.* When transitioning from eating this way, many find that their cravings are significantly decreased and are much less tempted to "cheat" on a carnivore diet.

I don't count calories, nor do I think you should need to on a carnivore diet. Most people will remain at a healthy weight on a nose-to-tail carnivore diet or lose weight if they are obese. If you find yourself gaining weight unexpectedly, there's probably something else going on. The cause might be thyroid issues or metabolic dysfunction, and you may want to talk to your physician about this to look for the root cause.

WHAT ABOUT FASTING?

Fasting is great, but it's not required.

If weight loss is your goal, incorporating fasting into your carnivore diet occasionally or on a regular basis will help you achieve your goals sooner. For those of us at a healthy body weight but with autoimmune or inflammatory issues, fasting might also be a useful intervention because it *allows the gut to rest and provides an opportunity for the immune system to calm down.* I would recommend against fasting for those who are trying to gain weight or who are coming from a place of nutritional inadequacy.

Though fasting is touted for its **autophagy** (cellular "housecleaning") benefits, remember that a ketogenic diet leads to many of the same biochemical changes within the body even in the fed state.[19] Time-restricted eating will also result in some autophagy during the daily fasting window,[20] an effect that will be accentuated by low-carbohydrate diets.

It's also important to point out that if you are not keto-adapted (which may take a few weeks on a diet with less than 20 grams of carbohydrates per day), fasting from a carbohydrate-based metabolism is likely going to be pretty miserable. If fasting is something we are interested in, it's best to do at least a week of low-carbohydrate eating prior to beginning such an endeavor.

WHAT ABOUT CHEAT MEALS?

I'm not a fan.

Many diets today allow for cheat meals from time to time, but I don't think these are a good idea. Remember the quality of life equation from the introduction of this book. It's one thing to decide that our highest quality of life may not be eating a carnivore diet from time to time, but it's entirely different to feel as though we are depriving ourselves six days of the week, only to finally be allowed to eat junk food on the seventh day. In a completely backwards framework, this creates an atmosphere of scarcity most of the week and *positions junk food as a reward.*

A carnivore diet is not about limiting what we can eat, it's about understanding that on this type of diet, we are able to eat the most life-giving, nutrient-rich foods on the planet all of the time. It's a diet of abundance for us, as it was for our ancestors who treasured animals foods when they could obtain them. Using cheat meals incorrectly shifts us to a scarcity mindset and positions junk food as abundance. It sabotages our efforts to make a lasting, positive lifestyle change. It's going to be hard to shift from our previous dietary habits and mindset, but making positive choices for our health isn't about depriving ourselves of things we enjoy. It's about understanding which foods foster fundamental health and celebrating these.

From an immunologic standpoint, cheat meals are also a train wreck. Remember that the immune system has a memory, and if we keep reminding it of the triggering foods, it won't be able to fully calm down. The point of the Clean Carnivore Reset is to allow enough time to understand how it feels to be well and then investigate which foods might be triggering us with careful reintroduction. Cheat meals completely undermine this valuable self-experimentation. As we make our transition to a carnivore diet, I'd strongly recommend considering forty-five to ninety days of a Carnivore Reset to see how good you can really feel before muddying the waters with the inclusion of cheat meals.

WHAT ABOUT PERSISTENT ORGANIC POLLUTANTS (POPs) IN ANIMAL FOODS?

These are not something to worry about if we are eating grass-fed meat, fat, and organs.

POP exposure has declined 95 percent since the 1970s, and the main source of our exposure today is probably that camp fire we had on the beach last summer.[21,22] As we spoke about in the discussion of grass-fed versus grain-fed meat, the quality of the food we eat affects our exposure to compounds like dioxins and many other harmful chemicals. The main sources of exposure for animals to dioxins are incinerator waste added to feed (which is no longer allowed) and feeding troughs constructed of pentachlorophenol-treated wood in feedlots.[3] Grass-fed ruminants would not be exposed to these and are much less likely to contain elevated levels of dioxins and other toxins.

The notion that dioxins are found only in animal food is also incorrect. When the levels of dioxins in different foods have been measured across various countries like the Netherlands, Finland, and Greece, many plant products have also been found to have high levels.[23,24,25] Amounts in both plant and animal foods appear to vary considerably between samples.

IS A KETOGENIC DIET HARMFUL TO THE BODY? DOES IT RAISE CORTISOL?

Nope.

As we talked about in the last chapter, ketogenic diets have been shown to decrease oxidative stress at the level of the mitochondria, to reduce blood pressure, and to be neuroprotective in models of traumatic brain injury.[26,27,28,29] Multiple studies have found that after a short period of keto-adaptation, low-carbohydrate diets do not increase the level of cortisol or activate the sympathetic nervous system.[30,31] Conversely, there is evidence from interventional trials that carbohydrates may increase cortisol levels and amplify the body's stress response through the hypothalamic-pituitary-adrenal axis.[32] Well now, that casts things in a different light, doesn't it?

Ketogenic diets have been found to have no adverse consequences when studied for six months in obese individuals.[33] They have also been found to improve fertility in women with PCOS.[34,35] In studies of vascular function, no changes were found in children after two years on a ketogenic diet.[36] Studies of autonomic nervous system function have also shown no change in heart rate variability, a measure of activation of the sympathetic ("fight or flight") nervous system.[37]

Though thyroid labs typically change on a ketogenic diet, claims that this way of eating are harmful to hormonal balance are unfounded. Discussions of thyroid hormones quickly become complex, but I'll break this down briefly. The main lab most physicians look at to get a sense of thyroid function is TSH, or thyroid stimulating hormone, which is released from the anterior pituitary as a signal to the thyroid to produce thyroxine, or T4. This is released into the blood stream and converted into triiodothyronine, or T3, which is the main active form of thyroid hormone. On ketogenic diets, TSH doesn't usually change, but T3 might decline a little, almost always remaining within the reference range. Much like the situation with insulin, it appears that in a ketogenic state, our *tissue sensitivity* to thyroid hormones increases, leading to lower levels. This does not appear to be a pathological change, but a reflection of adjustments in our physiology. The lack of change in TSH with no observed changes in basal metabolic rate indicate no overall decline in thyroid function in this situation.[38,39,40] Furthermore, low-carbohydrate diets have been shown to *improve* autoimmune thyroid conditions and lead to a decrease in multiple types of anti-thyroid antibodies.[41] Your thyroid and other hormones will be just fine on a ketogenic carnivore diet!

Takeaway: Ketogenic diets are very safe, and there's a substantial amount of evidence that they are protective in many ways.

WHAT IF I AM AN ATHLETE AND WANT TO DO THE CARNIVORE DIET?

There are now many elite athletes using slightly modified versions of a carnivore diet and finding great success. These include one-hundred-mile running world record holder Zach Bitter and Kona Iron Man champion Pete Jacobs.

Studies of ketogenic diets in endurance athletes suggest a performance advantage with this way of eating and show that after a six-to-eight-week period of keto adaptation, rates of glycogen storage and replenishment are equivalent with those of carbohydrate-focused athletes.[40,42]

> *"Compared to highly trained ultra-endurance athletes consuming a high-carbohydrate diet, long-term keto-adaptation results in extraordinarily high rates of fat oxidation, **whereas muscle glycogen utilization and repletion patterns during and after a 3-hour run are similar.**"*[43]

These studies also show that keto adapted athletes are much better at using fat for fuel during exertion, which allows them to use more efficient metabolic machinery during extended efforts.

At a basic level, explosive activities like sprinting and lifting weights rely on stores of creatine and glycogen. With a carnivore diet, our creatine stores will be topped off and the above noted studies suggest that after a period of keto adaptation, glycogen stores and replenishment look just like those athletes relying on carbohydrates. It should also be noted that many traditional ketogenic diets used to treat children with epilepsy prescribed large amounts of fat with very limited protein consumption, with ratios of around 4:1 fat to protein by grams. In these extreme cases of both protein and carbohydrate restriction, muscle glycogen stores may become depleted. But with significantly greater amounts of protein and less fat, as recommended in Chapter Twelve, this will not be a problem.

During very long aerobic exertion efforts, like a marathon or beyond, we will need to refuel during races and in training in order to avoid complete depletion of glycogen stores. This is probably best done with "clean" source of carbohydrates, like dextrose or honey, rather than highly processed gels and other supplements. For efforts that aren't long and intense enough to deplete glycogen, carbohydrates are not necessary during workouts and consumption of a carnivore diet after exertion will allow for full replenishment of glycogen stores.

In a twelve-week study comparing a ketogenic diet to a standard high-carbohydrate diet, no difference was found in high-intensity continuous or intermittent exercise, maximal cardiovascular performance, or heart rate variability.[37] This means that even during the period of keto-adaptation, no performance decline was seen with a ketogenic diet during high-intensity interval training or maximal efforts. In this study, there was also no evidence of negative effect on the sympathetic nervous system.

I recently completed one of the hardest workouts of my life, appropriately named "the barbarian," in a completely ketogenic state after eating a purely Tier 5 carnivore diet for the last eighteen months. It consisted of walking a mile up and down hills with 70 pounds on my back, pulling a 120-pound sled over asphalt, and carrying two 70-pound kettlebells with 10 pounds strapped on each ankle. That was a total of 350 pounds of suffering strapped to my body. Needless to say, it was brutal, and I suffered mightily. It took me one hour and fifty-three minutes to complete, but I never felt limited by my cardiovascular fitness or energy levels. I was limited only by the strength of my 170-pound frame that had to carry more than twice its bodyweight over this distance. I traditionally don't train for this type of masochistic endeavor but prefer activities like martial arts and surfing that favor a balance of strength, quickness, and flexibility.

My point here is that I could never have done this without large stores of glycogen in my muscles. It also illustrates that long, intense efforts are absolutely possible without any carbohydrate prior to, during, or afterwards. The jury is still out on whether carbohydrates lead to better strength gains. As we know from previous discussions, we can trigger mTOR with protein in a targeted fashion if we want maximal anabolic signaling. As long as I am getting enough calories and eating lots of fat alongside my "sweet spot" amount of protein, I haven't noticed any decline in my physical performance and feel much better overall from an athletic standpoint than I did eating a moderate amount of carbohydrates on a paleo diet. Whether or not we choose to use carbohydrates will depend on our sport of choice and goals, but I believe that most will not need them once they have allowed time for keto-adaptation. If strength gains are our main goal, eating more frequently throughout the day to trigger mTOR as much as possible would be a reasonable strategy.

WHAT IF MY SYMPTOMS DON'T GET BETTER ON A CARNIVORE DIET?

Check the gut. Turn over other stones.

A carnivore diet removes all plant toxins and the vast majority of foods that are potentially damaging to the gut, but some people continue to experience symptoms even with this powerful lifestyle change. In this case, I recommend working with a physician to take a close look at what's going on in the gastrointestinal tract and consider other possible causes of inflammation, such as exposure to heavy metals or other toxins. A carnivore diet is an incredibly powerful tool, but it might not be enough to get rid of pathogenic organisms in your gut if there is a significant toxic burden. Adjunctive therapies may help you get back to optimal health faster. Very rarely, some people may be sensitive to beef, pork, chicken, or another meat eaten on a carnivore diet, and in such a case, leaving the type of meat to which you are sensitive out and relying on the other types of animal food might be helpful.

DO I NEED PROBIOTICS ON A CARNIVORE DIET?

No.

For most people, the collagenous connective tissues in animal foods will be just fine as "animal fiber" for the production of short-chain fatty acids. In certain cases of pre-existing gastrointestinal issues, like small intestinal bacterial overgrowth, probiotics may be helpful, but they're not needed for most people.

Kombucha and other fermented beverages are not great for our teeth, and promises of improved gut health from these are mostly empty. It's really just expensive, fizzy, acidic sugar water. Spend your money on good mineral water instead.

DO I NEED FERMENTED FOODS FOR A HEALTHY GUT MICRO-BIOME?

Nope.

Fermention appears to have been used by our ancestors to detoxify plant foods. If we are going to eat plants, it might not be a bad idea to ferment them in order to break down harmful compounds like isothiocyanates, but the fermentation process doesn't appear to add any unique value to these foods. The lactobacillus organisms that predominate in fermented cultures are ubiquitous in the environment, and we are exposed to them constantly. If testing of our gut shows that we are lacking in this type of critter, it's likely because of another underlying issue like **dysbiosis** (imbalanced bacterial populations in the gastrointestinal tract) or gut inflammation, and eating fermented plants and other fermented foods is unlikely to solve this problem

The acids formed during the process of fermentation can also be quite damaging to the enamel of our teeth, and many cases of damage have been reported from over consumption of fermented foods.[44] Many of these also have capsicum (hot pepper) spices added, which have been shown to disrupt the integrity of the gut lining.

Kombucha? Let it go. Kim chi? Nah. Sauerkraut? Better than raw cabbage but still just survival food.

IS A CARNIVORE DIET REALLY HEALTHY LONG TERM?

Yes, I believe it is.

A common critique of the carnivore diet is that we don't have studies of people who have eaten this way long term, but in fact, we do! Remember our old buddy Vilhjalmur Stefansson who lived with the Inuit? When he came back from his adventures in the arctic, he spoke about his experiences widely, unable to contain his excitement about what he had learned. The medical establishment was skeptical, however, and did not believe he could have lived on only animal foods for years without developing scurvy or other illnesses. Sound familiar? In order to prove to the doubters that he was telling the truth, Vilhjalmur and a friend agreed to eat a nose-to-tail carnivore diet while living in Bellevue Hospital *for an entire year under the observation of physicians.* They didn't call it a Tier 5 carnivore diet, but it was! It included muscle, liver, kidney, brain, bone marrow, salt, and fat! In 1930, a study was published with the findings of this grand experiment and guess what it showed?

> *"At the end of the year the subjects were mentally alert, physically active, and showed no physical changes in any system of the body...vitamin deficiencies did not occur...kidney function tests revealed no evidence of kidney damage...the clinical studies and laboratory evidence gave no indication that any ill effects had occurred from prolonged use of the exclusive meat diet."*[45]

Pretty cool right? We actually do have a long term, controlled study of a nose-to-tail carnivore diet, and it's ninety years old! Time for another mic drop? I think so!

In case you're wondering about the macronutrient ratios eaten while these two were in Bellevue, they look a whole lot like what I've recommended on a Tier 5 diet: 100–160 grams of protein, with about 170 grams of fat daily. These guys were definitely in ketosis!

IS A KETOGENIC CARNIVORE DIET DIFFERENT FOR WOMEN?

Men and women are different from a hormonal perspective, but we are pretty similar at the biochemical level. Both sexes would also have been exposed to the same environments throughout evolution and eaten the same foods, enjoying the bounty of a successful hunt together. Men and women can approach a carnivore diet similarly. They should both think about how much protein they will need to support lean body mass and obtain the rest of their calories from fat while including as many organ meats as possible.

Many of the trials previously cited that demonstrated the safety and efficacy of a ketogenic diet included both men and women. A number of studies have also been done on female-only cohorts that have demonstrated similar results, as well as the superiority of ketogenic diets over low-fat diets for weight loss in this specific population.[46,47] Ketogenic diets are also well known to reverse polycystic ovarian syndrome and other disorders of insulin resistance in women.[35]

The major pitfall for women appears to be inadvertent calorie restriction due to the satiating effects of these types of diets. If you are looking to lose weight, this is a good thing, but women looking to maintain weight or gain muscle should be careful to ensure adequate calories.

In a caloric deficit, menstrual irregularities may occur, but with attention to this aspect, most women should not experience any irregularities with a ketogenic or carnivore diet.

Takeaway: A carnivore diet is totally awesome for both women and men, and there aren't any special considerations for non-pregnant women when eating in this way. See the next question regarding pregnancy and lactation.

IS A KETOGENIC CARNIVORE DIET OKAY FOR PREGNANCY, BREASTFEEDING, AND CHILDREN?

I believe it is, yes.

There aren't any formal studies to address this question, but throughout evolution, countless healthy pregnancies have occurred in a state of ketosis with diets based mainly on animal foods. If this were not the case, how would northern cultures like the Inuit, Aleut, Mongol, or Sami have continued throughout history?

During early development, ketosis is also very common in humans. Most infants less than one year old spend the majority of their time in ketosis, quickly switching to this fat-based metabolism within a few hours of not eating and demonstrating ketones in the blood.[48] The finding that ketones can be directly converted to cholesterol for cell membranes in the brain and the body demonstrates the central role these molecules play in the rapid neuronal development of infants and children.[49] It again reinforces the indispensable roles these molecule play in human biology. Women with healthy pregnancies have also been shown to often be in ketosis, with levels of ketones that are significantly higher than when in the non-pregnant state.[50] Being in ketosis appears to be totally safe for both mom and baby.

A nose-to-tail carnivore diet will provide all of the nutrients both mother and developing child will need to thrive. The main consideration in pregnancy and lactation will be ensuring that we can get enough calories to fuel both parties. If you want to eat a carnivore diet in these states, make sure to include lots of high-quality fat to provide the energy necessary for your body and the growing fetus or nursing infant.

For children, questions often arise about the possibility of limited growth on a ketogenic or carnivore diet. Studies of children using ketogenic diets to control Type I diabetes have not demonstrated evidence for growth delay,[51] but further research is needed here. Remember from previous discussions of mTOR and IGF-1 that both protein and carbohydrates can provide anabolic signals to the body.

Takeaway: Being in a state of ketosis has been a common occurrence for pregnant mothers, infants, and young children throughout history. A nose-to-tail carnivore diet is rich in and provides all the nutrients we need to be fertile and to nurture healthy children. Getting enough calories to meet the increased requirements of pregnancy and lactation will be key if we choose to eat a carnivore diet during these periods.

IS A CARNIVORE DIET REALLY EXPENSIVE?

It definitely does not have to be!

Quality matters when it comes to food, and I strongly believe that obtaining the highest quality foods is one of the best long-term investments we can make. I also understand that finances may be a limiting factor for some. One of the awesome things about a nose-to-tail carnivore diet is that muscle meat is only part of the equation. Many butchers will give you fat trimmings for free and sell you nutrient-rich organ meats for a fraction of the of the cost of a ribeye. When the majority of your diet comes from these foods, a carnivore diet gets much more affordable. Using ground beef or chuck roast as your source of muscle meat, you could eat a completely grass-fed, nose-to-tail carnivore diet for less than fifteen dollars per day. Still think this is an expensive diet?

HOW DOES DR. PAUL EAT A CARNIVORE DIET?

With a big smile on his face.

I described most of this during the discussion of a Tier 5 carnivore diet. You better believe I am on the varsity team—I just wrote a whole book about it! I make a conscious attempt to source my grass-finished meat, fat, and organs from farms that I know well and trust. White Oak Pastures and Belcampo are amazing examples of farms using regenerative agriculture practices to enrich the land while raising animals in the healthiest way possible. By using these methods, they have been able to become "carbon negative," enriching the quality of the soil and sequestering more greenhouse gases than they produce. Though it is more expensive than conventionally raised meat, I believe that, by "voting with my dollars," this is one of the best investments I can make.

How does Dr. Paul exercise?

I prefer to be outside interacting with the natural world when I work out. This means that the majority of my exercise comes in the form of surfing, backcountry skiing, climbing, and occasionally, running up mountains as fast as I can. There's nothing quite like catching a beautiful wave and feeling the ocean move underneath me or floating through the snow down the side of mountain. Doing these things helps me feel connected to the wilderness and reminds me that—even though I live in the modern world—this is where I've come from.

Though it's not outside, I'll make an exception to train martial arts or with kettlebells with some of my friends in San Diego from time to time as well. I also enjoy bodyweight movements, gymnastics (inspired by the work of Ido Portal), or even a bit of traditional deadlifting.

My goal is to be able to maintain my body as a strong and supple instrument that I can use to experience the world around me for the majority of my life.

APPENDIX

The tools you need to kick the most butt on a nose-to-tail carnivore diet.

REGENERATIVE FARMS:

White Oak Pastures in Georgia: WhiteOakPastures.com
Belcampo in California: Belcampo.com
Force of Nature Meats: ForceOfNatureMeats.com
Joyce Farms: Joyce-Farms.com

FIND A FARMER NEAR YOU TO SOURCE GOOD-QUALITY MEAT:

EatWild.com

BLOODWORK:

<u>Basic Labs To Start With</u>

Complete Blood Count w/Differential
Comprehensive Metabolic Panel
GGT
Serum Magnesium, Phosphorous
hs-CRP
Fasting Insulin
C Peptide
Hemoglobin A1c (though somewhat inaccurate, as discussed
    in the book)
Fructoasamine
Lipid Panel
Calcium, Total and Ionized
PTH

Homocysteine
Iron Panel
Thyroid Panel: Free and total T3/T4, TSH, reverseT3, anti-thyro-
globulin antibody, anti-thyroid peroxidase antibody
Uric Acid
Hormones: FSH/LH, free/total Testosterone, DHEA-S, Estradiol,
Progesterone, Prolactin, SHBG, AM cortisol
Urinalysis

More Advanced Labs

NMR Lipid Panel
Fasting Leptin
IGF-1
F2-Isoprostanes/Creatinine Ratio (urine)
Myeloperoxidase
ADMA/SDMA Ratio
8 OH 2 Deoxy Guanosine
Lipid Peroxides
Glutathione (total and fractionated oxidized/reduced)
24 Salivary Cortisol Curve with Cortisol Awakening Response.
Stool Testing: GI Map
Alpha Diversity Analysis: Onegevity (dietary recommendations are
likely to be inaccurate)
Nutritional Testing: Genova Nutreval
Toxins:
Great Plains GPL TOX (non metals)
Serum Heavy Metals Panel (including lead, mercury, arsenic,
cadmium, and tin)
Urine Heavy Metals

PROBIOTICS:

I generally don't think probiotics are necessary on a carnivore diet, but in
cases of constipation or diarrhea, they may have some utility. If you are
going to take a probiotic, I'd recommend the following strains:

Lactobacillus GG (Culturelle)
Lactobacillus Reuteri DSM 17938 and L. *Reuteri ATCC PTA 6475* (*Bio
Gaia Gastrus*)
S. Boulardii Lyo CNCM I 745 (Florastor)

General "Supplements":

Bone Meal: Bones from a regenerative-fed farm, like White Oak Pastures or Traditional Foods Market Whole Bone Calcium

Collagen: Great Lakes hydrolyzed collagen (1–2 scoops daily)

Supplements That May Be Helpful for Loose Stools:

Lipase
Desiccated Pancreas/Gallbladder
Ox Bile (in cases of bile acid malabsorption, this may worsen loose stools)
Egg Shell Powder

Companies Funding The EAT-Lancet Guidelines:

Baker Mackenzie
BASF
Bayer
BCG
Bohler
Cargill
Cermaq
C.P Group
Danone
Deloitte
DSM
Dupont
Edelman Financial
Evonik
Givaudan
Google
Ikea
IFF
KDD
Kellogg's
Nestle
Olam
Pepsi
Protix
Quantis

Sigma
Sonae
Storaenso
Symrise
Syngenta
Unilever
YARA

WATER:

FindASpring.com

Reverse osmosis filters remove flouride and other contaminants, but filtered water should be remineralized.

REFERENCES

Chapter 1

1. Zink, K. D., & Lieberman, D. E. (2016). Impact of meat and lower palaeolithic food processing techniques on chewing in humans. *Nature, 531*(7595), 500-503. doi:10.1038/nature16990
2. Nowell, A., & Davidson, I. (2011). *Stone tools and the evolution of human cognition.* Boulder, CO: University Press of Colorado.
3. Grine, F. E., Fleagle, J. G., & Leakey, R. E. (2009). *The first humans: Origin and early evolution of the genus Homo.* Berlin, Germany: Springer Science & Business Media.
4. Domínguez-Rodrigo, M. (2002). Hunting and scavenging by early humans: The state of the debate. *Journal of world prehistory, 16*(1), 1-54. doi:10.1023/A:1014507129795
5. Blasco, R., Rosell, J., Arilla, M., Margalida, A., Villalba, D., Gopher, A., & Barkai, R. (2019). Bone marrow storage and delayed consumption at middle pleistocene qesem cave, Israel (420 to 200 ka). *Science Advances, 5*(10), eaav9822. doi:10.1126/sciadv.aav9822
6. Arnold, D. C. (1961). Possible origin of the use of fire by early man. *Nature, 192*(4809), 1318-1318. doi:10.1038/1921318a0
7. Milton, K. (2003). The critical role played by animal source foods in human (Homo) evolution. *The Journal of Nutrition, 133*(11), 3886S-3892S. doi:10.1093/jn/133.11.3886s
8. Balter, V., Braga, J., Télouk, P., & Thackeray, J. F. (2012). Evidence for dietary change but not landscape use in South African early Hominins. *Nature, 489*(7417), 558-560. doi:10.1038/nature11349
9. Cordain, L., Miller, J. B., Eaton, S. B., Mann, N., Holt, S. H., & Speth, J. D. (2000). Plant-animal subsistence ratios and macronutrient energy estimations in worldwide hunter-gatherer diets. *The American Journal of Clinical Nutrition, 71*(3), 682-692. doi:10.1093/ajcn/71.3.682
10. Mann, N. (2007). Meat in the human diet: An anthropological perspective. *Nutrition & Dietetics, 64*(s4 The Role of), S102-S107. doi:10.1111/j.1747-0080.2007.00194.x
11. Stefánsson, V. (2018). The home life of stone age man. In *the fat of the land.* (pp. 48)
12. Speth, J. D. (2010). *The paleoanthropology and archaeology of big-game hunting: Protein, fat, or politics?* Berlin, Germany: Springer Science & Business Media.
13. Ingold, T., & Lee, R. B. (1981). The !kung san: Men, women and work in a foraging society. *Man, 16*(1), 153. doi:10.2307/2801993
14. Rockwell, D. (2003). *Giving voice to bear: North American Indian myths, rituals, and images of the bear.* Roberts Rinehart.
15. Tindale, N. B. 1972. The Pitjandjara. In Bicchieri, M. G. (ed.), Hunters and gatherers today: A socioeconomic study of eleven such cultures in the twentieth century, 217-268. New York: Holt, Rinehart and Winston
16. Speth, J. D., & Spielmann, K. A. (1983). Energy source, protein metabolism, and hunter-gatherer subsistence strategies. *Journal of Anthropological Archaeology, 2*(1), 1-31. doi:10.1016/0278-4165(83)90006-5
17. Bilsborough, S., & Mann, N. (2006). A review of issues of dietary protein intake in humans. *International Journal of Sport Nutrition and Exercise Metabolism, 16*(2), 129-152. doi:10.1123/ijsnem.16.2.129
18. Beasley, D. E., Koltz, A. M., Lambert, J. E., Fierer, N., & Dunn, R. R. (2015). The evolution of stomach acidity and its relevance to the human microbiome. *PLOS ONE, 10*(7), e0134116. doi:10.1371/journal.pone.0134116
19. Fohl, A. L., & Regal, R. E. (2011). Proton pump inhibitor-associated pneumonia: Not a breath of fresh air after all? *World Journal of Gastrointestinal Pharmacology and Therapeutics, 2*(3), 17. doi:10.4292/wjgpt.v2.i3.17
20. Jordakieva, G., Kundi, M., Untersmayr, E., Pali-Schöll, I., Reichardt, B., & Jensen-Jarolim, E. (2019). Country-wide medical records infer increased allergy risk of gastric acid inhibition. *Nature Communications, 10*(1). doi:10.1038/s41467-019-10914-6
21. Aiello, L. C. (1997). Brains and guts in human evolution: The expensive tissue hypothesis. *Brazilian Journal of Genetics, 20*(1), 141-148. doi:10.1590/s0100-84551997000100023
22. Perry, G. H., Kistler, L., Kelaita, M. A., & Sams, A. J. (2015). Insights into hominin phenotypic and dietary evolution from ancient DNA sequence data. *Journal of Human Evolution, 79*, 55-63. doi:10.1016/j.jhevol.2014.10.018
23. Rogers, A. R., Bohlender, R. J., & Huff, C. D. (2017). Early history of Neanderthals and Denisovans. *Proceedings of the National Academy of Sciences, 114*(37), 9859-9863. doi:10.1073/pnas.1706426114
24. Ben-dor, M. (2018). *The causal association between megafaunal extinction and Neandertal extinction in Western Europe – Application of the obligatory dietary fat bioenergetic model* (Unpublished doctoral dissertation). Tel Aviv University, Tel Aviv, Israel.

25. Innis, S. M. (2008). Dietary omega 3 fatty acids and the developing brain. *Brain Research, 1237*, 35-43. doi:10.1016/j.brainres.2008.08.078

26. Coletta, J. M., Bell, S. J., & Roman, A. S. (2010). Omega-3 fatty acids and pregnancy. *Reviews in obstetrics & gynecology, 3*(4), 163–171.

27. Dyall, S. C. (2015). Long-chain omega-3 fatty acids and the brain: a review of the independent and shared effects of EPA, DPA and DHA. *Frontiers in Aging Neuroscience, 7*. doi:10.3389/fnagi.2015.00052

28. Kuhn, J. E. (2016). Throwing, the shoulder, and human evolution. *Am J Orthop (Belle Mead NJ), 45*(3), 110-114. Retrieved from https://www.ncbi.nlm.nih.gov/pubmed/26991561

29. Bramble, D. M., & Lieberman, D. E. (2004). Endurance running and the evolution of Homo. *Nature, 432*(7015), 345-352. doi:10.1038/nature03052

30. Holowka, N. B., & Lieberman, D. E. (2018). Rethinking the evolution of the human foot: insights from experimental research. *The Journal of Experimental Biology, 221*(17), jeb174425. doi:10.1242/jeb.174425

31. Kobayashi, H., & Kohshima, S. (2001). Unique morphology of the human eye and its adaptive meaning: comparative studies on external morphology of the primate eye. *Journal of Human Evolution, 40*(5), 419-435. doi:10.1006/jhev.2001.0468

CHAPTER 2

1. Diamond, J. M. (1987). *The worst mistake in the history of the human race* (pp. 64-66). New York City, NY: Discover Magazine.

2. Gurven, M., & Kaplan, H. (2007). Longevity among hunter- gatherers: A cross-cultural examination. *Population and Development Review, 33*(2), 321-365. doi:10.1111/j.1728-4457.2007.00171.x

3. Araújo, J., Cai, J., & Stevens, J. (2019). Prevalence of optimal metabolic health in american adults: National health and nutrition examination survey 2009–2016. *Metabolic Syndrome and Related Disorders, 17*(1), 46-52. doi:10.1089/met.2018.0105

4. Depression. (2019, December 4). Retrieved from https://www.who.int/news-room/fact-sheets/detail/depression

5. Cordain, L., Eaton, S., Miller, J. B., Mann, N., & Hill, K. (2002). The paradoxical nature of hunter-gatherer diets: meat-based, yet non-atherogenic. *European Journal of Clinical Nutrition, 56*(S1), S42-S52. doi:10.1038/sj.ejcn.1601353

6. Cordain, L., Miller, J. B., Eaton, S. B., Mann, N., Holt, S. H., & Speth, J. D. (2000). Plant-animal subsistence ratios and macronutrient energy estimations in worldwide hunter-gatherer diets. *The American Journal of Clinical Nutrition, 71*(3), 682-692. doi:10.1093/ajcn/71.3.682

7. Pontzer, H., Wood, B. M., & Raichlen, D. A. (2018). Hunter-gatherers as models in public health. *Obesity Reviews, 19*, 24-35. doi:10.1111/obr.12785

8. Kaplan, H., Thompson, R. C., Trumble, B. C., Wann, L. S., Allam, A. H., Beheim, B., … Thomas, G. S. (2017). Coronary atherosclerosis in indigenous South American Tsimane: a cross-sectional cohort study. *The Lancet, 389*(10080), 1730-1739. doi:10.1016/s0140-6736(17)30752-3

9. Goodman, A. and Armelagos, G. (1985) Disease and death at Dr. Dickson's Mounds. Natural History Magazine, 94, 12-18.

10. Latham, K. J. (2013). Human health and the neolithic revolution: an Overview of impacts of the agricultural transition on oral health, epidemiology, and the human body. *Nebraska Anthropologist, 28*, 95-102.

11. Grasgruber, P., Sebera, M., Hrazdíra, E., Cacek, J., & Kalina, T. (2016). Major correlates of male height: A study of 105 countries. *Economics & Human Biology, 21*, 172–195. doi: 10.1016/j.ehb.2016.01.005

12. Perkins, J. M., Subramanian, S., Davey Smith, G., & Özaltin, E. (2016). Adult height, nutrition, and population health. *Nutrition Reviews, 74*(3), 149-165. doi:10.1093/nutrit/nuv105

13. Conference on Paleopathology and Socioeconomic Change at the Origins of Agriculture, Cohen, M. N., Armelagos, G. J., Wenner-Gren Foundation for Anthropological Research., & State University of New York College at Plattsburgh. (1984). *Paleopathology at the origins of agriculture.* New York: Academic Press.

14. Price, W. A., & Price-Pottenger Nutrition Foundation. (2003). *Nutrition and physical degeneration.* (pp. 124-126, 253) La Mesa, CA: Price-Pottenger Nutrition Foundation.

15. Stefansson, V. (1935, November). Adventures in diet (part I). *Harper's Magazine.*

CHAPTER 3

1. Mithöfer, A., & Maffei, M. E. (2017). General mechanisms of plant defense and plant toxins. *Plant Toxins*, 3-24. doi:10.1007/978-94-007-6464-4_21

2. Ames, B. N., Profet, M., & Gold, L. S. (1990). Dietary pesticides (99.99% all natural). *Proceedings of the National Academy of Sciences of the United States of America, 87*(19), 7777–7781. doi:10.1073/pnas.87.19.7777

3. Van Kranendonk, M. J., Deamer, D. W., & Djokic, T. (2017, August). Life on earth came from a hot volcanic pool, not the sea, new evidence suggests. *Scientific*

American, 27(3). Retrieved from https://www.scientificamerican.com/article/
life-on-earth-came-from-a-hot-volcanic-pool-not-the-sea-new-evidence-suggests/

4. Damer, B., & Deamer, D. (2015). Coupled phases and combinatorial selection in fluctuating hydrothermal pools: A scenario to guide experimental approaches to the origin of cellular life. *Life, 5*(1), 872-887. doi:10.3390/life5010872

5. Young, J., Dragsted L.O.*, Haraldsdóttir, J., Daneshvar, B., Kall, M., Loft, S., … Sandström, B. (2002). Green tea extract only affects markers of oxidative status postprandially: lasting antioxidant effect of flavonoid-free diet. *British Journal of Nutrition, 87*(4), 343-355. doi:10.1079/bjnbjn2002523

6. Crane, T. E., Kubota, C., West, J. L., Kroggel, M. A., Wertheim, B. C., & Thomson, C. A. (2011). Increasing the vegetable intake dose is associated with a rise in plasma carotenoids without modifying oxidative stress or inflammation in overweight or obese postmenopausal women. *The Journal of Nutrition, 141*(10), 1827-1833. doi:10.3945/jn.111.139659

7. Møller, P., Vogel, U., Pedersen, A., Dragsted, L. O., Sandström, B., & Loft, S. (2003). No effect of 600 grams fruit and vegetables per day on oxidative dna damage and repair in healthy nonsmokers. *Cancer Epidemiology, Biomarkers & Prevention, 12*, 1016-1022.

8. Peluso, I., Raguzzini, A., Catasta, G., Cammisotto, V., Perrone, A., Tomino, C., … Serafini, M. (2018). Effects of high consumption of vegetables on clinical, immunological, and antioxidant markers in subjects at risk of cardiovascular diseases. *Oxidative Medicine and Cellular Longevity, 2018*, 1-9. doi:10.1155/2018/5417165

9. Bjelakovic, G., Nikolova, D., Gluud, L. L., Simonetti, R. G., & Gluud, C. (2008). Antioxidant supplements for prevention of mortality in healthy participants and patients with various diseases. *Cochrane Database of Systematic Reviews.* doi:10.1002/14651858.cd007176

10. Vivekananthan, D. P., Penn, M. S., Sapp, S. K., Hsu, A., & Topol, E. J. (2003). Use of antioxidant vitamins for the prevention of cardiovascular disease: meta-analysis of randomised trials. *The Lancet, 361*(9374), 2017-2023. doi:10.1016/s0140-6736(03)13637-9

11. Liguori, I., Russo, G., Curcio, F., Bulli, G., Aran, L., Della-Morte, D., … Abete, P. (2018). Oxidative stress, aging, and diseases. *Clinical interventions in aging, 13*, 757–772. doi:10.2147/CIA.S158513

12. Wild Herbivores Cope with Plant Toxins. (n.d.). Retrieved from https://www.webpages.uidaho.edu/range556/appl_behave/projects/toxins-wildlife.htm

13. Mithöfer, A., & Maffei, M. E. (2017). General mechanisms of plant defense and plant toxins. *Plant Toxins*, 3-24. doi:10.1007/978-94-007-6464-4_21

14. Wöll, S., Kim, S. H., Greten, H. J., & Efferth, T. (2013). Animal plant warfare and secondary metabolite evolution. *Natural Products and Bioprospecting, 3*(1), 1-7. doi:10.1007/s13659-013-0004-0

15. Van Ohlen, M., Herfurth, A., & Wittstock, U. (2017). Herbivore adaptations to plant cyanide defenses. *Herbivores.* doi:10.5772/66277

16. Laycock, W. A. (1978). Coevolution of poisonous plants and large herbivores on rangelands. *Journal of Range Management, 31*(5), 335. doi:10.2307/3897355

17. Freeland, W. J., & Janzen, D. H. (1974). Strategies in herbivory by mammals: The role of plant secondary compounds. *The American Naturalist, 108*(961), 269-289. doi:10.1086/282907

18. Pfister, J. (1999). Behavioral strategies for coping with poisonous plants. *Bulletin*, 45.

CHAPTER 4

1. Ishidate, M., Harnois, M., & Sofuni, T. (1988). A comparative analysis of data on the clastogenicity of 951 chemical substances tested in mammalian cell cultures. *Mutation Research/Reviews in Genetic Toxicology, 195*(2), 151-213. doi:10.1016/0165-1110(88)90023-1

2. Randerath, K., Randerath, E., Agrawal, H. P., Gupta, R. C., Schurdak, M. E., & Reddy, M. V. (1985). Postlabeling methods for carcinogen-DNA adduct analysis. *Environmental Health Perspectives, 62*, 57. doi:10.2307/3430093

3. Kassie, F., Parzefall, W., Musk, S., Johnson, I., Lamprecht, G., Sontag, G., & Knasmüller, S. (1996). Genotoxic effects of crude juices from Brassica vegetables and juices and extracts from phytopharmaceutical preparations and spices of cruciferous plants origin in bacterial and mammalian cells. *Chemico-Biological Interactions, 102*(1), 1-16. doi:10.1016/0009-2797(96)03728-3

4. Baasanjav-Gerber, C., Hollnagel, H. M., Brauchmann, J., Iori, R., & Glatt, H. (2010). Detection of genotoxicants in Brassicales using endogenous DNA as a surrogate target and adducts determined by 32P-postlabelling as an experimental end point. *Mutagenesis, 26*(3), 407-413. doi:10.1093/mutage/geq108

5. Latté, K. P., Appel, K., & Lampen, A. (2011). Health benefits and possible risks of broccoli – An overview. *Food and Chemical Toxicology, 49*(12), 3287-3309. doi:10.1016/j.fct.2011.08.019

6. Socała, K., Nieoczym, D., Kowalczuk-Vasilev, E., Wyska, E., & Wlaź, P. (2017). Increased seizure susceptibility and other toxicity symptoms following acute sulforaphane treatment in mice. *Toxicology and Applied Pharmacology, 326*, 43-53. doi:10.1016/j.taap.2017.04.010

7. Smith, T. K., Mithen, R., & Johnson, I. T. (2003). Effects of Brassica vegetable juice on the induction of apoptosis and aberrant crypt foci in rat colonic mucosal crypts in vivo. *Carcinogenesis, 24*(3), 491-495. doi:10.1093/carcin/24.3.491

8. Lynn, A., Collins, A., Fuller, Z., Hillman, K., & Ratcliffe, B. (2006). Cruciferous vegetables and colo-rectal cancer. *Proceedings of the Nutrition Society, 65*(1), 135-144. doi:10.1079/pns2005486

9. Baasanjav-Gerber, C., Hollnagel, H. M., Brauchmann, J., Iori, R., & Glatt, H. (2010). Detection of genotoxicants in Brassicales using endogenous DNA as a surrogate target and adducts determined by 32P-postlabelling as an experimental end point. *Mutagenesis, 26*(3), 407-413. doi:10.1093/mutage/geq108

10. Lynn, A., Fuller, Z., Collins, A. R., & Ratcliffe, B. (2015). Comparison of the effect of raw and blanched-frozen broccoli on DNA damage in colonocytes. *Cell Biochemistry and Function, 33*(5), 266-276. doi:10.1002/cbf.3106

11. Heres-Pulido, M. E., Dueñas-García, I., Castañeda-Partida, L., Santos-Cruz, L. F., Vega-Contreras, V., Rebollar-Vega, R., ... Durán-Díaz, Á. (2010). Genotoxicity studies of organically grown broccoli (Brassica oleracea var. italica) and its interactions with urethane, methyl methanesulfonate and 4-nitroquinoline-1-oxide genotoxicity in the wing spot test of Drosophila melanogaster. *Food and Chemical Toxicology, 48*(1), 120-128. doi:10.1016/j.fct.2009.09.027

12. Basu, A. (2018). DNA damage, mutagenesis and cancer. *International Journal of Molecular Sciences, 19*(4), 970. doi:10.3390/ijms19040970

13. Sharma, R., Sharma, A., Chaudhary, P., Pearce, V., Vatsyayan, R., Singh, S. V., ... Awasthi, Y. C. (2010). Role of lipid peroxidation in cellular responses to d,l-sulforaphane, a promising cancer chemopreventive agent. *Biochemistry, 49*(14), 3191-3202. doi:10.1021/bi100104e

14. Bajaj, J. K., Salwan, P., & Salwan, S. (2016). Various possible toxicants involved in thyroid dysfunction: A review. *Journal of Clinical and Diagnostic Research*. doi:10.7860/jcdr/2016/15195.7092

15. Felker, P., Bunch, R., & Leung, A. M. (2016). Concentrations of thiocyanate and goitrin in human plasma, their precursor concentrations in brassica vegetables, and associated potential risk for hypothyroidism. *Nutrition Reviews, 74*(4), 248-258. doi:10.1093/nutrit/nuv110

16. Eastman, C. J., & Zimmermann, M. B. (2018). The iodine deficiency disorders. *Endotext [Internet]*. Retrieved from www.endotext.org

17. Lamberg, B. (1991). Endemic goitre—iodine deficiency disorders. *Annals of Medicine, 23*(4), 367-372. doi:10.3109/07853899109148075

18. Truong, T., Baron-Dubourdieu, D., Rougier, Y., & Guénel, P. (2010). Role of dietary iodine and cruciferous vegetables in thyroid cancer: a countrywide case–control study in New Caledonia. *Cancer Causes & Control, 21*(8), 1183-1192. doi:10.1007/s10552-010-9545-2

19. Chandra, A. K., & De, N. (2010). Goitrogenic/antithyroidal potential of green tea extract in relation to catechin in rats. *Food and Chemical Toxicology, 48*(8-9), 2304-2311. doi:10.1016/j.fct.2010.05.064

20. Chandra, A. K., & De, N. (2012). Catechin induced modulation in the activities of thyroid hormone synthesizing enzymes leading to hypothyroidism. *Molecular and Cellular Biochemistry, 374*(1-2), 37-48. doi:10.1007/s11010-012-1503-8

21. Patel, Satish & Nag, Mukesh Kumar & Daharwal, S.J. & Rawat Singh, Manju & Singh, Deependra. (2013). Plant toxins: An overview. *Research J. Pharmacology and Pharmacodynamics*. 5. 283-288.

22. National Research Council. 1973. *Toxicants occurring naturally in foods*. Washington, DC: The National Academies Press. https://doi.org/10.17226/21278.

23. Van Ohlen, M., Herfurth, A., & Wittstock, U. (2017). Herbivore adaptations to plant cyanide defenses. *Herbivores*. doi:10.5772/66277

24. Bongiovanni, A. M. (1974). Endemic goitre and cassava. *The Lancet, 304*(7889), 1143. doi:10.1016/s0140-6736(74)90906-4

25. Mlingi, N. L., Bokanga, M., Kavishe, F. P., Gebre-Medhin, M., & Rosling, H. (1996). Milling reduces the goitrogenic potential of cassava. *International Journal of Food Sciences and Nutrition, 47*(6), 445-454. doi:10.3109/09637489609031873

26. Akindahunsi, A. A., Grissom, F. E., Adewusi, S. R., Afolabi, O. A., Torimiro, S. E., & Oke, O. L. (1998). Parameters of thyroid function in the endemic goitre of Akungba and Oke-Agbe villages of Akoko area of southwestern Nigeria. *Afr J Med Med Sci, 27*(3-4), 239-242.

27. Jiang, X., Liu, Y., Ma, L., Ji, R., Qu, Y., Xin, Y., & Lv, G. (2018). Chemopreventive activity of sulforaphane. *Drug design, development and therapy, 12*, 2905–2913. doi:10.2147/DDDT.S100534

28. De Figueiredo, S., Binda, N., Nogueira-Machado, J., Vieira-Filho, S., & Caligiorne, R. (2015). The antioxidant properties of organosulfur compounds (sulforaphane). *Recent Patents on Endocrine, Metabolic & Immune Drug Discovery, 9*(1), 24-39. doi:10.2174/1872214809666150505164138

29. Wong, C. P., Hsu, A., Buchanan, A., Palomera-Sanchez, Z., Beaver, L. M., Houseman, E. A., ... Ho, E. (2014). Effects of sulforaphane and 3,3'-diindolylmethane on genome-wide promoter methylation in normal prostate epithelial cells and prostate cancer cells. *PLoS ONE, 9*(1), e86787. doi:10.1371/journal.pone.0086787

30. Glaser, J., & Holzgrabe, U. (2016). Focus on PAINS: false friends in the quest for selective anti-protozoal lead structures from Nature? *MedChemComm, 7*(2), 214-223. doi:10.1039/c5md00481k

31. Ferreira de Oliveira, J. M., Costa, M., Pedrosa, T., Pinto, P., Remédios, C., Oliveira, H., … Santos, C. (2014). Sulforaphane induces oxidative stress and death by p53-independent mechanism: Implication of impaired glutathione recycling. *PLoS ONE, 9*(3), e92980. doi:10.1371/journal.pone.0092980

32. Zhao, S., Ghosh, A., Lo, C., Chenier, I., Scholey, J. W., Filep, J. G., … Chan, J. S. (2017). NRF2 Deficiency upregulates intrarenal angiotensin-converting enzyme-2 and angiotensin 1-7 receptor expression and attenuates hypertension and nephropathy in diabetic mice. *Endocrinology, 159*(2), 836-852. doi:10.1210/en.2017-00752

33. Simmons, S. O., Fan, C., Yeoman, K., Wakefield, J., & Ramabhadran, R. (2011). NRF2 oxidative stress induced by heavy metals is cell type dependent. *Current Chemical Genomics, 5*, 1-12. doi:10.2174/1875397301105010001

34. Müller, T., & Hengstermann, A. (2012). NRF2: Friend and foe in preventing cigarette smoking-dependent lung disease. *Chemical Research in Toxicology, 25*(9), 1805-1824. doi:10.1021/tx300145n

35. Jadeja, R. N., Upadhyay, K. K., Devkar, R. V., & Khurana, S. (2016). Naturally occurring NRF2 activators: potential in treatment of liver injury. *Oxidative Medicine and Cellular Longevity, 2016*, 1-13. doi:10.1155/2016/3453926

36. Varady, J., Gessner, D. K., Most, E., Eder, K., & Ringseis, R. (2012). Dietary moderately oxidized oil activates the NRF2 signaling pathway in the liver of pigs. *Lipids in Health and Disease, 11*(1), 31. doi:10.1186/1476-511x-11-31

37. Crane, T. E., Kubota, C., West, J. L., Kroggel, M. A., Wertheim, B. C., & Thomson, C. A. (2011). Increasing the vegetable intake dose Is associated with a rise in plasma carotenoids without modifying oxidative stress or inflammation in overweight or obese postmenopausal women. *The Journal of Nutrition, 141*(10), 1827-1833. doi:10.3945/jn.111.139659

38. Møller, P., Vogel, U., Pedersen, A., Dragsted, L. O., Sandström, B., & Loft, S. (2003). No effect of 600 grams fruit and vegetables per day on oxidative dna damage and repair in healthy nonsmokers. *Cancer Epidemiology, Biomarkers & Prevention, 12*, 1016-1022.

39. Peluso, I., Raguzzini, A., Catasta, G., Cammisotto, V., Perrone, A., Tomino, C., … Serafini, M. (2018). Effects of high consumption of vegetables on clinical, immunological, and antioxidant markers in subjects at risk of cardiovascular diseases. *Oxidative Medicine and Cellular Longevity, 2018*, 1-9. doi:10.1155/2018/5417165

40. Young, J., Dragsted L.O.*, Haraldsdóttir, J., Daneshvar, B., Kall, M., Loft, S., … Sandström, B. (2002). Green tea extract only affects markers of oxidative status postprandially: lasting antioxidant effect of flavonoid-free diet. *British Journal of Nutrition, 87*(4), 343-355. doi:10.1079/bjnbjn2002523

41. Kumsta, C., Chang, J. T., Schmalz, J., & Hansen, M. (2017). Hormetic heat stress and HSF-1 induce autophagy to improve survival and proteostasis in C. elegans. *Nature Communications, 8*(1). doi:10.1038/ncomms14337

42. Ohtsuka, Y., Yabunaka, N., Fujisawa, H., Watanabe, I., & Agishi, Y. (1994). Effect of thermal stress on glutathione metabolism in human erythrocytes. *European Journal of Applied Physiology and Occupational Physiology, 68*(1), 87-91. doi:10.1007/bf00599247

43. Siems, W. G., Van Kuijk, F. J., Maass, R., & Brenke, R. (1994). Uric acid and glutathione levels during short-term whole body cold exposure. *Free Radical Biology and Medicine, 16*(3), 299-305. doi:10.1016/0891-5849(94)90030-2

44. Duthie, S. J., Duthie, G. G., Russell, W. R., Kyle, J. A., Macdiarmid, J. I., Rungapamestry, V., … Bestwick, C. S. (2017). Effect of increasing fruit and vegetable intake by dietary intervention on nutritional biomarkers and attitudes to dietary change: a randomised trial. *European Journal of Nutrition, 57*(5), 1855-1872. doi:10.1007/s00394-017-1469-0

45. Palani, K., Harbaum-Piayda, B., Meske, D., Keppler, J. K., Bockelmann, W., Heller, K. J., & Schwarz, K. (2016). Influence of fermentation on glucosinolates and glucobrassicin degradation products in sauerkraut. *Food Chemistry, 190*, 755-762. doi:10.1016/j.foodchem.2015.06.012

46. Albertini, B., Schoubben, A., Guarnaccia, D., Pinelli, F., Della Vecchia, M., Ricci, M., … Blasi, P. (2015). Effect of Fermentation and Drying on Cocoa Polyphenols. *Journal of Agricultural and Food Chemistry, 63*(45), 9948-9953. doi:10.1021/acs.jafc.5b01062

CHAPTER 5

1. Bellavia, A., Larsson, S. C., Bottai, M., Wolk, A., & Orsini, N. (2013). Fruit and vegetable consumption and all-cause mortality: a dose-response analysis. *The American Journal of Clinical Nutrition, 98*(2), 454-459. doi:10.3945/ajcn.112.056119

2. Crane, T. E., Kubota, C., West, J. L., Kroggel, M. A., Wertheim, B. C., & Thomson, C. A. (2011). Increasing the vegetable intake dose is associated with a rise in plasma carotenoids without modifying oxidative stress or inflammation in overweight or obese postmenopausal women. *The Journal of Nutrition, 141*(10), 1827-1833. doi:10.3945/jn.111.139659

3. Møller, P., Vogel, U., Pedersen, A., Dragsted, L. O., Sandström, B., & Loft, S. (2003). No effect of 600 grams fruit and vegetables per day on oxidative dna damage and repair in healthy nonsmokers. *Cancer Epidemiology, Biomarkers & Prevention, 12*, 1016-1022.
4. Peluso, I., Raguzzini, A., Catasta, G., Cammisotto, V., Perrone, A., Tomino, C., ... Serafini, M. (2018). Effects of high consumption of vegetables on clinical, immunological, and antioxidant markers in subjects at risk of cardiovascular diseases. *Oxidative Medicine and Cellular Longevity, 2018*, 1-9. doi:10.1155/2018/5417165
5. Young, J., Dragsted L.O.*, Haraldsdóttir, J., Daneshvar, B., Kall, M., Loft, S., ... Sandström, B. (2002). Green tea extract only affects markers of oxidative status postprandially: lasting antioxidant effect of flavonoid-free diet. *British Journal of Nutrition, 87*(4), 343-355. doi:10.1079/bjnbjn2002523
6. Lee, J. E., McLerran, D. F., Rolland, B., Chen, Y., Grant, E. J., Vedanthan, R., ... Sinha, R. (2013). Meat intake and cause-specific mortality: a pooled analysis of Asian prospective cohort studies. *The American Journal of Clinical Nutrition, 98*(4), 1032-1041. doi:10.3945/ajcn.113.062638
7. Sauvaget, C., Nagano, J., Hayashi, M., & Yamada, M. (2004). Animal protein, animal fat, and cholesterol intakes and risk of cerebral infarction mortality in the adult health study. *Stroke, 35*(7), 1531-1537. doi:10.1161/01.str.0000130426.52064.09
8. Shrank, W. H., Patrick, A. R., & Alan Brookhart, M. (2011). Healthy user and related biases in observational studies of preventive interventions: A primer for physicians. *Journal of General Internal Medicine, 26*(5), 546-550. doi:10.1007/s11606-010-1609-1
9. Appleby, P. N., Key, T. J., Thorogood, M., Burr, M. L., & Mann, J. (2002). Mortality in British vegetarians. *Public Health Nutrition, 5*(1), 29-36. doi:10.1079/phn2001248
10. Burgos-Morón, E., Calderón-Montaño, J. M., Salvador, J., Robles, A., & López-Lázaro M, M. (2010). The dark side of curcumin. *Int J Cancer, 126*(7), 1771-1775. doi: 10.1002/ijc.24967
11. Hewlings, S., & Kalman, D. (2017). Curcumin: A review of its' effects on human health. *Foods, 6*(10), 92. doi:10.3390/foods6100092
12. Fang, J., Lu, J., & Holmgren, A. (2005). Thioredoxin reductase is irreversibly modified by curcumin. *Journal of Biological Chemistry, 280*(26), 25284-25290. doi:10.1074/jbc.m414645200
13. Collins, H. M., Abdelghany, M. K., Messmer, M., Yue, B., Deeves, S. E., Kindle, K. B., ... Heery, D. M. (2013). Differential effects of garcinol and curcumin on histone and p53 modifications in tumour cells. *BMC Cancer, 13*(1). doi:10.1186/1471-2407-13-37
14. Hallman, K., Aleck, K., Dwyer, B., Lloyd, V., Quigley, M., Sitto, N., ... Dinda, S. (2017). The effects of turmeric (curcumin) on tumor suppressor protein (p53) and estrogen receptor (ERα) in breast cancer cells. *Breast Cancer: Targets and Therapy, Volume 9*, 153-161. doi:10.2147/bctt.s125783
15. Singh, J., Dubey, R. K., & Atal, C. K. (1986). Piperine-mediated inhibition of glucuronidation activity in isolated epithelial cells of the guinea-pig small intestine: evidence that piperine lowers the endogenous UDP-glucuronic acid content. *J Pharmacol Exp Ther, 236*(2), 488-493. Retrieved from http://jpet.aspetjournals.org/content/236/2/488.long
16. Bjelakovic, G., Nikolova, D., Gluud, L. L., Simonetti, R. G., & Gluud, C. (2007). Mortality in randomized trials of antioxidant supplements for primary and secondary Prevention. *JAMA, 297*(8), 842. doi:10.1001/jama.297.8.842
17. Vivekananthan, D. P., Penn, M. S., Sapp, S. K., Hsu, A., & Topol, E. J. (2003). Use of antioxidant vitamins for the prevention of cardiovascular disease: meta-analysis of randomised trials. *The Lancet, 361*(9374), 2017-2023. doi:10.1016/s0140-6736(03)13637-9
18. Miksicek, R. J. (1993). Commonly occurring plant flavonoids have estrogenic activity. *Mol Pharmacol, 44*(1), 37-43. Retrieved from https://www.ncbi.nlm.nih.gov/pubmed/8341277
19. Collins-Burow, B. M., Burow, M. E., Duong, B. N., & McLachlan, J. A. (2000). Estrogenic and antiestrogenic activities of flavonoid phytochemicals through estrogen receptor binding-dependent and -independent mechanisms. *Nutrition and Cancer, 38*(2), 229-244. doi:10.1207/s15327914nc382_13
20. Messina, M. (2016). Soy and health update: Evaluation of the clinical and epidemiologic literature. *Nutrients, 8*(12), 754. doi:10.3390/nu8120754
21. Bar-El Dadon, S., & Reifen, R. (2010). Soy as an endocrine disruptor: Cause for caution? *Journal of Pediatric Endocrinology and Metabolism, 23*(9). doi:10.1515/jpem.2010.138
22. Habito, R., Montalto, J., Leslie, E., & Ball, M. (2000). Effects of replacing meat with soybean in the diet on sex hormone concentrations in healthy adult males. *British Journal of Nutrition, 84*(4), 557-563. doi:10.1017/S0007114500001872
23. Dinsdale, E. C., & Ward, W. E. (2010). Early exposure to soy isoflavones and effects on reproductive health: a review of human and animal studies. *Nutrients, 2*(11), 1156-1187. doi:10.3390/nu2111156
24. Chavarro, J. E., Toth, T. L., Sadio, S. M., & Hauser, R. (2008). Soy food and isoflavone intake in relation to semen quality parameters among men from an infertility clinic. *Human Reproduction, 23*(11), 2584-2590. doi:10.1093/humrep/den243
25. Mennen, L. I., Walker, R., Bennetau-Pelissero, C., & Scalbert, A. (2005). Risks and safety of polyphenol consumption. *The American Journal of Clinical Nutrition, 81*(1), 326S-329S. doi:10.1093/ajcn/81.1.326s

26. Chandra, A. K., & De, N. (2012). Catechin induced modulation in the activities of thyroid hormone synthesizing enzymes leading to hypothyroidism. *Molecular and Cellular Biochemistry, 374*(1-2), 37-48. doi:10.1007/s11010-012-1503-8

27. Ferguson, J., Ryan, M., Gibney, E., Brennan, L., Roche, H., & Reilly, M. (2014). Dietary isoflavone intake is associated with evoked responses to inflammatory cardiometabolic stimuli and improved glucose homeostasis in healthy volunteers. *Nutrition, Metabolism and Cardiovascular Diseases, 24*(9), 996-1003. doi:10.1016/j.numecd.2014.03.010

28. Resende, F. A., De Oliveira, A. P., De Camargo, M. S., Vilegas, W., & Varanda, E. A. (2013). Evaluation of estrogenic potential of flavonoids using a recombinant yeast strain and MCF7/BUS cell proliferation assay. *PLoS ONE, 8*(10), e74881. doi:10.1371/journal.pone.0074881

29. Van Duursen, M. B., Sanderson, J. T., Chr. de Jong, P., Kraaij, M., & Van den Berg, M. (2004). Phytochemicals inhibit catechol-o-methyltransferase activity in cytosolic fractions from healthy human mammary tissues: Implications for catechol estrogen-induced DNA damage. *Toxicological Sciences, 81*(2), 316-324. doi:10.1093/toxsci/kfh216

30. Ju, Y. H., Carlson, K. E., Sun, J., Pathak, D., Katzenellenbogen, B. S., Katzenellenbogen, J. A., & Helferich, W. G. (2000). Estrogenic effects of extracts from cabbage, fermented cabbage, and acidified brussels sprouts on growth and gene expression of estrogen-dependent human breast cancer (MCF-7) cells. *Journal of Agricultural and Food Chemistry, 48*(10), 4628-4634. doi:10.1021/jf000164z

31. Socci, V., Tempesta, D., Desideri, G., De Gennaro, L., & Ferrara, M. (2017). Enhancing human cognition with cocoa flavonoids. *Frontiers in Nutrition, 4.* doi:10.3389/fnut.2017.00019

32. Sarwar Gilani, G., Wu Xiao, C., & Cockell, K. A. (2012). Impact of antinutritional factors in food proteins on the digestibility of protein and the bioavailability of amino acids and on protein quality. *British Journal of Nutrition, 108*(S2), S315-S332. doi:10.1017/s0007114512002371

33. Griffiths, D. W. (1986). The inhibition of digestive enzymes by polyphenolic compounds. *Advances in Experimental Medicine and Biology,* 509-516. doi:10.1007/978-1-4757-0022-0_29

34. Song, J., Kwon, O., Chen, S., Daruwala, R., Eck, P., Park, J. B., & Levine, M. (2002). Flavonoid inhibition of sodium-dependent vitamin C transporter 1 (SVCT1) and glucose transporter isoform 2 (GLUT2), intestinal transporters for vitamin C and glucose. *Journal of Biological Chemistry, 277*(18), 15252-15260. doi:10.1074/jbc.m110496200

35. Hussein, L., & Abbas, H. (1986). Nitrogen balance studies among boys fed combinations of faba beans and wheat differing in polyphenolic contents. *AGRIS (International System for Agricultural Science and Technology), 31*(1), 67-81.

36. Van Huijsduijnen, R. A., Alblas, S. W., De Rijk, R. H., & Bol, J. F. (1986). Induction by salicylic acid of pathogenesis-related proteins and resistance to alfalfa mosaic virus infection in various plant species. *Journal of General Virology, 67*(10), 2135-2143. doi:10.1099/0022-1317-67-10-2135

37. Weinshilboum, R. M. (1986). Phenol sulfotransferase in humans: Properties, regulation, and function. *Federation Proceedings, 45*(8), 2223-2228.

38. Lawrence, J. R., Peter, R., Baxter, G. J., Robson, J., Graham, A. B., & Paterson, J. R. (2003). Urinary excretion of salicyluric and salicylic acids by non-vegetarians, vegetarians, and patients taking low dose aspirin. *Journal of Clinical Pathology, 56*(9), 651-653. doi:10.1136/jcp.56.9.651

39. Sommer, D. D., Rotenberg, B. W., Sowerby, L. J., Lee, J. M., Janjua, A., Witterick, I. J., ... Nayan, S. (2016). A novel treatment adjunct for aspirin exacerbated respiratory disease: the low-salicylate diet: A multicenter randomized control crossover trial. *International Forum of Allergy & Rhinology, 6*(4), 385-391. doi:10.1002/alr.21678

40. Kjær, T. N., Ornstrup, M. J., Poulsen, M. M., Stødkilde-Jørgensen, H., Jessen, N., Jørgensen, J. O., ... Pedersen, S. B. (2017). No beneficial effects of resveratrol on the metabolic syndrome: A randomized placebo-controlled clinical trial. *The Journal of Clinical Endocrinology & Metabolism, 102*(5), 1642-1651. doi:10.1210/jc.2016-2160

41. Heebøll, S., Kreuzfeldt, M., Hamilton-Dutoit, S., Kjær Poulsen, M., Stødkilde-Jørgensen, H., Møller, H. J., ... Grønbæk, H. (2016). Placebo-controlled, randomised clinical trial: high-dose resveratrol treatment for non-alcoholic fatty liver disease. *Scandinavian Journal of Gastroenterology, 51*(4), 456-464. doi:10.3109/00365521.2015.1107620

42. Kjaer, T. N., Ornstrup, M. J., Poulsen, M. M., Jørgensen, J. O., Hougaard, D. M., Cohen, A. S., ... Pedersen, S. B. (2015). Resveratrol reduces the levels of circulating androgen precursors but has no effect on, testosterone, dihydrotestosterone, PSA levels or prostate volume. A 4-month randomised trial in middle-aged men. *The Prostate, 75*(12), 1255-1263. doi:10.1002/pros.23006

43. Ahmad, A., Syed, F. A., Singh, S., & Hadi, S. (2005). Prooxidant activity of resveratrol in the presence of copper ions: Mutagenicity in plasmid DNA. *Toxicology Letters, 159*(1), 1-12. doi:10.1016/j.toxlet.2005.04.001

44. Gadacha, W., Ben-Attia, M., Bonnefont-Rousselot, D., Aouani, E., Ghanem-Boughanmi, N., & Touitou, Y. (2009). Resveratrol opposite effects on rat tissue lipoperoxidation: pro-oxidant during day-time and antioxidant at night. *Redox Report, 14*(4), 154-158. doi:10.1179/135100009x466131

CHAPTER 6

1. Wang, Z., Zheng, Y., Zhao, B., Zhang, Y., Liu, Z., Xu, J., … Abliz, Z. (2015). Human metabolic responses to chronic environmental polycyclic aromatic hydrocarbon exposure by a metabolomic approach. *Journal of Proteome Research, 14*(6), 2583-2593. doi:10.1021/acs.jproteome.5b00134

2. Prasad, R., & Shivay, Y. S. (2017). Oxalic acid/oxalates in plants: From self-defense to phytoremediation. *Current Science, 112*(08), 1665. doi:10.18520/cs/v112/i08/1665-1667

3. Korth, K. L., Doege, S. J., Park, S., Goggin, F. L., Wang, Q., Gomez, S. K., … Nakata, P. A. (2006). Medicago truncatula mutants demonstrate the role of plant calcium oxalate crystals as an effective defense against chewing insects. *Plant Physiology, 141*(1), 188-195. doi:10.1104/pp.106.076737

4. Sippy, J. J. (1919). Death from rhubarb leaves due to oxalic acid poisoning. *Journal of the American Medical Association, 73*(8), 627. doi:10.1001/jama.1919.02610340059028

5. James, L. F. (1972). Oxalate toxicosis. *Clinical Toxicology, 5*(2), 231-243. doi:10.3109/15563657208991002

6. Sanz, P., & Reig, R. (1992). Clinical and pathological findings in fatal plant oxalosis. *The American Journal of Forensic Medicine and Pathology, 13*(4), 342-345. doi:10.1097/00000433-199212000-00016

7. Farre, M. (1989). Fatal oxalic acid poisoning from sorrel soup. *The Lancet, 334*(8678-8679), 1524. doi:10.1016/s0140-6736(89)92967-x

8. Makkapati, S., D'Agati, V. D., & Balsam, L. (2018). "Green smoothie cleanse" causing acute oxalate nephropathy. *American Journal of Kidney Diseases, 71*(2), 281-286. doi:10.1053/j.ajkd.2017.08.002

9. Park, H., Eom, M., Won Yang, J., Geun Han, B., Ok Choi, S., & Kim, J. S. (2014). Peanut-induced acute oxalate nephropathy with acute kidney injury. *Kidney Research and Clinical Practice, 33*(2), 109-111. doi:10.1016/j.krcp.2014.03.003

10. Ellis, D., & Lieb, J. (2015). Hyperoxaluria and genitourinary disorders in children ingesting almond milk products. *The Journal of Pediatrics, 167*(5), 1155-1158. doi:10.1016/j.jpeds.2015.08.029

11. Christison, R., & Coindet, C. W. (1823). An experimental inquiry on poisoning by oxalic acid. *Edinburgh medical and surgical journal, 19*(76), 323–337.

12. Beug, M. W. (2019). Oxalates in chaga – a potential health threat. *North American Mycological Association.* Retrieved from https://namyco.org/

13. Tsai, M., Chang, W., Lui, C., Chung, K., Hsu, K., Huang, C., … Chuang, Y. (2005). Status epilepticus induced by star fruit intoxication in patients with chronic renal disease. *Seizure, 14*(7), 521-525. doi:10.1016/j.seizure.2005.08.004

14. Wahl, R., Fuchs, R., & Kallee, E. (1993). Oxalate in the human thyroid gland. *Clinical Chemistry and Laboratory Medicine, 31*(9). doi:10.1515/cclm.1993.31.9.559

15. Frishberg, Y., Feinstein, S., Rinat, C., & Drukker, A. (2000). Hypothyroidism in primary hyperoxaluria type 1. *The Journal of Pediatrics, 136*(2), 255-257. doi:10.1016/s0022-3476(00)70112-0

16. Konstantynowicz, J., Porowski, T., Zoch-Zwierz, W., Wasilewska, J., Kadziela-Olech, H., Kulak, W., … Kaczmarski, M. (2012). A potential pathogenic role of oxalate in autism. *European Journal of Paediatric Neurology, 16*(5), 485-491. doi:10.1016/j.ejpn.2011.08.004

17. Gonzalez, J. E., Caldwell, R. G., & Valaitis, J. (1991). Calcium oxalate crystals in the breast. Pathology and significance. *The American Journal of Surgical Pathology, 15*(6), 586-591. doi: 10.1097/00000478-199106000-00007

18. Castellaro, A. M., Tonda, A., Cejas, H. H., Ferreyra, H., Caputto, B. L., Pucci, O. A., & Gil, G. A. (2015). Oxalate induces breast cancer. *BMC Cancer, 15*(1). doi:10.1186/s12885-015-1747-2

19. Ermer, T., Eckardt, K., Aronson, P. S., & Knauf, F. (2016). Oxalate, inflammasome, and progression of kidney disease. *Current Opinion in Nephrology and Hypertension, 25*(4), 363-371. doi:10.1097/mnh.0000000000000229

20. Mulay, S. R., Kulkarni, O. P., Rupanagudi, K. V., Migliorini, A., Darisipudi, M. N., Vilaysane, A., … Anders, H. (2012). Calcium oxalate crystals induce renal inflammation by NLRP3-mediated IL-1β secretion. *Journal of Clinical Investigation, 123*(1), 236-246. doi:10.1172/jci63679

21. Balcke, P., Zazgornik, J., Sunder-Plassmann, G., Kiss, A., Hauser, A., Gremmel, F., … Schmidt, P. (1989). Transient hyperoxaluria after Ingestion of chocolate as a high risk factor for calcium oxalate calculi. *Nephron, 51*(1), 32-34. doi:10.1159/000185238

22. Holmes, R. P., Goodman, H. O., & Assimos, D. G. (2001). Contribution of dietary oxalate to urinary oxalate excretion. *Kidney International, 59*(1), 270-276. doi:10.1046/j.1523-1755.2001.00488.x

23. Tang, M., Larson-Meyer, D. E., & Liebman, M. (2008). Effect of cinnamon and turmeric on urinary oxalate excretion, plasma lipids, and plasma glucose in healthy subjects. *The American Journal of Clinical Nutrition, 87*(5), 1262-1267. doi:10.1093/ajcn/87.5.1262

24. Gasińska, A., & Gajewska, D. (2007). Tea and coffee as the main sources of oxalate in diets of patients with kidney oxalate stones. *Rocz Panstw Zakl Hig, 58*(1), 61-67.

25. Abratt, V. R., & Reid, S. J. (2010). Oxalate-degrading bacteria of the human gut as probiotics in the management of kidney stone disease. *Advances in Applied Microbiology*, 63-87. doi:10.1016/s0065-2164(10)72003-7

CHAPTER 7

1. Sandlin, D. (2013, September 30). The elvis impersonator, the karate instructor, a fridge full of severed heads, and the plot 2 kill the president. *GQ Magazine.* Retrieved from https://www.gq.com/story/paul-kevin-curtis-elvis-impersonator-ricin-assassinations

2. Sperti, S., Montanaro, L., Mattioli, A., & Stirpe, F. (1973). Inhibition by ricin of protein synthesisin vitro: 60S ribosomal subunit as the target of the toxin (Short Communication). *Biochemical Journal, 136*(3), 813-815. doi:10.1042/bj1360813

3. Hayes, A. W., & Kruger, C. L. (2014). *Hayes' principles and methods of toxicology, sixth edition.* Boca Raton, FL: CRC Press.

4. Rodhouse, J. C., Haugh, C. A., Roberts, D., & Gilbert, R. J. (1990). Red kidney bean poisoning in the UK: An analysis of 50 suspected incidents between 1976 and 1989. *Epidemiology and Infection, 105*(3), 485-491. doi:10.1017/s095026880004810x

5. De Oliveira, J., Pusztai, A., & Grant, G. (1988). Changes in organs and tissues induced by feeding of purified kidney bean (Phaseolus vulgaris) lectins. *Nutrition Research, 8*(8), 943-947. doi:10.1016/s0271-5317(88)80133-7

6. Ceri, H., Banwell, J. G., & Fang, R. (1998). Lectin ingestion: changes in mucin secretion and bacterial adhesion to intestinal tissue. *Lectin Methods and Protocols,* 495-504. doi:10.1385/0-89603-396-1:495

7. Shen, H., Lu, Z., Xu, Z., & Shen, Z. (2017). Diet-induced reconstruction of mucosal microbiota associated with alterations of epithelium lectin expression and regulation in the maintenance of rumen homeostasis. *Scientific Reports, 7*(1). doi:10.1038/s41598-017-03478-2

8. Dicker, A. J., Crichton, M. L., Cassidy, A. J., Brady, G., Hapca, A., Tavendale, R., ... Chalmers, J. D. (2017). Genetic mannose binding lectin deficiency is associated with airway microbiota diversity and reduced exacerbation frequency in COPD. *Thorax, 73*(6), 510-518. doi:10.1136/thoraxjnl-2016-209931

9. Banwell, J. G., Howard, R., Kabir, I., & Costerton, J. W. (1988). Bacterial overgrowth by indigenous microflora in the phytohemagglutinin-fed rat. *Canadian Journal of Microbiology, 34*(8), 1009-1013. doi:10.1139/m88-177

10. Ceri, H., Falkenberg-Anderson, K., Fang, R., Costerton, J. W., Howard, R., & Banwell, J. G. (1988). Bacteria–lectin interactions in phytohemagglutinin-induced bacterial overgrowth of the small intestine. *Canadian Journal of Microbiology, 34*(8), 1003-1008. doi:10.1139/m88-176

11. Shanshan Kong, Yanhui H. Zhang, and Weiqiang Zhang, "Regulation of Intestinal Epithelial Cells Properties and Functions by Amino Acids," *BioMed Research International,* vol. 2018, Article ID 2819154, 10 pages, 2018. https://doi.org/10.1155/2018/2819154.

12. Fasano, A. (2011). Zonulin and its regulation of intestinal barrier function: The biological door to inflammation, autoimmunity, and cancer. *Physiological Reviews, 91*(1), 151-175. doi:10.1152/physrev.00003.2008

13. Fasano, A. (2012). Zonulin, regulation of tight junctions, and autoimmune diseases. *Annals of the New York Academy of Sciences, 1258*(1), 25-33. doi:10.1111/j.1749-6632.2012.06538.x

14. Hansson, G. C. (2012). Role of mucus layers in gut infection and inflammation. *Current Opinion in Microbiology, 15*(1), 57-62. doi:10.1016/j.mib.2011.11.002

15. Pellegrina, C. D., Perbellini, O., Scupoli, M. T., Tomelleri, C., Zanetti, C., Zoccatelli, G., ... Chignola, R. (2009). Effects of wheat germ agglutinin on human gastrointestinal epithelium: Insights from an experimental model of immune/epithelial cell interaction. *Toxicology and Applied Pharmacology, 237*(2), 146-153. doi:10.1016/j.taap.2009.03.012

16. Elli, L., Dolfini, E., & Bardella, M. T. (2003). Gliadin cytotoxicity and in vitro cell cultures. *Toxicology Letters, 146*(1), 1-8. doi:10.1016/j.toxlet.2003.09.004

17. Clemente, M. G., Virgiliis, S. D., Kang, J. S., Macatagney, R., Musu, M. P., Di Pierro, M. R., ... Drago, S. (2003). Early effects of gliadin on enterocyte intracellular signaling involved in intestinal barrier function. *Gut, 52*(2), 218-223. doi:10.1136/gut.52.2.218

18. Rivabene, R., Mancini, E., & De Vincenzi, M. (1999). In vitro cytotoxic effect of wheat gliadin-derived peptides on the Caco-2 intestinal cell line is associated with intracellular oxidative imbalance: implications for coeliac disease. *Biochimica et Biophysica Acta (BBA) - Molecular Basis of Disease, 1453*(1), 152-160. doi:10.1016/s0925-4439(98)00095-7

19. Ryder, S. D., Jacyna, M. R., Levi, A., Rizzi, P. M., & Rhodes, J. M. (1998). Peanut ingestion increases rectal proliferation in individuals with mucosal expression of peanut lectin receptor. *Gastroenterology, 114*(1), 44-49. doi:10.1016/s0016-5085(98)70631-6

20. Wang, Q., Yu, L., Campbell, B. J., Milton, J. D., & Rhodes, J. M. (1998). Identification of intact peanut lectin in peripheral venous blood. *The Lancet, 352*(9143), 1831-1832. doi:10.1016/s0140-6736(05)79894-9

21. Pramod, S. N., Venkatesh, Y. P., & Mahesh, P. A. (2007). Potato lectin activates basophils and mast cells of atopic subjects by its interaction with core chitobiose of cell-bound non-specific immunoglobulin E. *Clinical & Experimental Immunology, 148*(3), 391-401. doi:10.1111/j.1365-2249.2007.03368.x

22. Haas, H., Falcone, F. H., Schramm, G., Haisch, K., Gibbs, B. F., Klaucke, J., ... Schlaak, M. (1999). Dietary lectins can induce in vitro release of IL-4 and IL-13 from human basophils. *European Journal of Immunology, 29*(03), 918-927. doi:10.1002/(sici)1521-4141(199903)29:03<918::aid-immu918>3.3.co;2-k

23. Svensson, E., Horváth-Puhó, E., Thomsen, R. W., Djurhuus, J. C., Pedersen, L., Borghammer, P., & Sørensen, H. T. (2015). Vagotomy and subsequent risk of Parkinson's disease. *Annals of Neurology, 78*(4), 522-529. doi:10.1002/ana.24448

24. Zheng, J., Wang, M., Wei, W., Keller, J. N., Adhikari, B., King, J. F., … Laine, R. A. (2016). Dietary plant lectins appear to be transported from the gut to gain access to and alter dopaminergic neurons of caenorhabditis elegans, a potential etiology of Parkinson's disease. *Frontiers in Nutrition, 3.* doi:10.3389/fnut.2016.00007

25. Goedert, M., Spillantini, M. G., Del Tredici, K., & Braak, H. (2012). 100 years of Lewy pathology. *Nature Reviews Neurology, 9*(1), 13-24. doi:10.1038/nrneurol.2012.242

26. Anselmi, L., Bove, C., Coleman, F. H., Le, K., Subramanian, M. P., Venkiteswaran, K., … Travagli, R. A. (2018). Ingestion of subthreshold doses of environmental toxins induces ascending Parkinsonism in the rat. *npj Parkinson's Disease, 4*(1). doi:10.1038/s41531-018-0066-0

27. Shechter, Y. (1983). Bound lectins that mimic insulin produce persistent insulin-like activities. *Endocrinology, 113*(6), 1921-1926. doi:10.1210/endo-113-6-1921

28. Kamikubo, Y., Dellas, C., Loskutoff, D., Quigley, J., & Ruggeri, Z. (2008). Contribution of leptin receptor N-linked glycans to leptin binding. *Biochemical Journal, 410*(3), 595-604. doi:10.1042/bj20071137

29. Gundry, S. R. (2018). Abstract P238: remission/cure of autoimmune diseases by a lectin limite diet supplemented with probiotics, prebiotics, and polyphenols. *Circulation, 137*(1), 238.

30. Nachbar, M. S., & Oppenheim, J. D. (1980). Lectins in the United States diet: a survey of lectins in commonly consumed foods and a review of the literature. *The American Journal of Clinical Nutrition, 33*(11), 2338-2345. doi:10.1093/ajcn/33.11.2338

31. Freed, D. L. (1999). Do dietary lectins cause disease? *BMJ, 318*(7190), 1023-1024. doi:10.1136/bmj.318.7190.1023

CHAPTER 8

1. Rae, C., Digney, A. L., McEwan, S. R., & Bates, T. C. (2003). Oral creatine monohydrate supplementation improves brain performance: a double–blind, placebo–controlled, cross–over trial. *Proceedings of the Royal Society of London. Series B: Biological Sciences, 270*(1529), 2147-2150. doi:10.1098/rspb.2003.2492

2. Benton, D., & Donohoe, R. (2010). The influence of creatine supplementation on the cognitive functioning of vegetarians and omnivores. *British Journal of Nutrition, 105*(7), 1100-1105. doi:10.1017/s0007114510004733

3. Burke, D. G., Chilibeck, P. D., Parise, G., Candow, D. G., Mahoney, D., & Tarnopolsky, M. (2003). Effect of creatine and weight training on muscle creatine and performance in vegetarians. *Medicine & Science in Sports & Exercise, 35*(11), 1946-1955. doi:10.1249/01.mss.0000093614.17517.79

4. Zeisel, S. H., & Da Costa, K. (2009). Choline: an essential nutrient for public health. *Nutrition Reviews, 67*(11), 615-623. doi:10.1111/j.1753-4887.2009.00246.x

5. Derbyshire, E. (2019). Could we be overlooking a potential choline crisis in the United Kingdom? *BMJ Nutrition, Prevention & Health,* bmjnph-2019-000037. doi:10.1136/bmjnph-2019-000037

6. Yin, J., Nielsen, M., Li, S., & Shi, J. (2019). Ketones improves apolipoprotein E4-related memory deficiency via sirtuin 3. *Aging.* doi: 10.18632/aging.102070

7. Miller, V. J., Villamena, F. A., & Volek, J. S. (2018). Nutritional ketosis and mitohormesis: Potential implications for mitochondrial function and human health. *Journal of Nutrition and Metabolism, 2018,* 1-27. doi:10.1155/2018/5157645

8. Stephens, F. B., Marimuthu, K., Cheng, Y., Patel, N., Constantin, D., Simpson, E. J., & Greenhaff, P. L. (2011). Vegetarians have a reduced skeletal muscle carnitine transport capacity. *American Journal of Clinical Nutrition, 94*(3), 938-944. doi:10.3945/ajcn.111.012047

9. Nasca, C., Bigio, B., Lee, F. S., Young, S. P., Kautz, M. M., Albright, A., … Rasgon, N. (2018). Acetyl-l-carnitine deficiency in patients with major depressive disorder. *Proceedings of the National Academy of Sciences, 115*(34), 8627-8632. doi:10.1073/pnas.1801609115

10. Hagen, T. M., Liu, J., Lykkesfeldt, J., Wehr, C. M., Ingersoll, R. T., Vinarsky, V., … Ames, B. N. (2002). Feeding acetyl-l-carnitine and lipoic acid to old rats significantly improves metabolic function while decreasing oxidative stress. *Proceedings of the National Academy of Sciences, 99*(4), 1870-1875. doi:10.1073/pnas.261708898

11. Wang, S., Han, C., Lee, S., Patkar, A. A., Masand, P. S., & Pae, C. (2014). A review of current evidence for acetyl-l-carnitine in the treatment of depression. *Journal of Psychiatric Research, 53,* 30-37. doi:10.1016/j.jpsychires.2014.02.005

12. Veronese, N., Stubbs, B., Solmi, M., Ajnakina, O., Carvalho, A. F., & Maggi, S. (2018). Acetyl-l-carnitine supplementation and the treatment of depressive symptoms: A systematic review and meta-analysis. *Psychosomatic Medicine, 80*(2), 154-159. doi:10.1097/psy.0000000000000537

13. Harris, R. C., Wise, J. A., Price, K. A., Kim, H. J., Kim, C. K., & Sale, C. (2012). Determinants of muscle carnosine content. *Amino Acids, 43*(1), 5-12. doi:10.1007/s00726-012-1233-y

14. Everaert, I., Mooyaart, A., Baguet, A., Zutinic, A., Baelde, H., Achten, E., ... Derave, W. (2010). Vegetarianism, female gender and increasing age, but not CNDP1 genotype, are associated with reduced muscle carnosine levels in humans. *Amino Acids, 40*(4), 1221-1229. doi:10.1007/s00726-010-0749-2

15. Krajcovicová-Kudláčková, M., Sebeková, K., Schinzel, R., & Klvanová, J. (2002). Advanced glycation end products and nutrition. *Physiol Res, 51*(3), 313-316.

16. Huang, J., Chuang, L., Guh, J., Yang, Y., & Hsu, M. (2008). Effect of taurine on advanced glycation end products-induced hypertrophy in renal tubular epithelial cells. *Toxicology and Applied Pharmacology, 233*(2), 220-226. doi:10.1016/j.taap.2008.09.002

17. Wu, J., & Prentice, H. (2010). Role of taurine in the central nervous system. *Journal of Biomedical Science, 17*(Suppl 1), S1. doi:10.1186/1423-0127-17-s1-s1

18. Laidlaw, S. A., Shultz, T. D., Cecchino, J. T., & Kopple, J. D. (1988). Plasma and urine taurine levels in vegans. *The American Journal of Clinical Nutrition, 47*(4), 660-663. doi:10.1093/ajcn/47.4.660

19. Baines, S., Powers, J., & Brown, W. J. (2007). How does the health and well-being of young Australian vegetarian and semi-vegetarian women compare with non-vegetarians? *Public Health Nutrition, 10*(5), 436-442. doi:10.1017/s1368980007217938

20. Burkert, N. T., Muckenhuber, J., Großschädl, F., Rásky, É., & Freidl, W. (2014). Nutrition and health – the association between eating behavior and vsaarious health parameters: A matched sample study. *PLoS ONE, 9*(2), e88278. doi:10.1371/journal.pone.0088278

21. Matta, J., Czernichow, S., Kesse-Guyot, E., Hoertel, N., Limosin, F., Goldberg, M., ... Lemogne, C. (2018). Depressive symptoms and vegetarian diets: results from the constances cohort. *Nutrients, 10*(11), 1695. doi:10.3390/nu10111695

22. Michalak, J., Zhang, X., & Jacobi, F. (2012). Vegetarian diet and mental disorders: results from a representative community survey. *International Journal of Behavioral Nutrition and Physical Activity, 9*(1), 67. doi:10.1186/1479-5868-9-67

23. Meesters, A. N., Maukonen, M., Partonen, T., Männistö, S., Gordijn, M. C., & Meesters, Y. (2016). Is There a relationship between vegetarianism and seasonal affective disorder? A pilot study. *Neuropsychobiology, 74*(4), 202-206. doi:10.1159/000477247

24. Dowlati, Y., Herrmann, N., Swardfager, W., Liu, H., Sham, L., Reim, E. K., & Lanctôt, K. L. (2010). A meta-analysis of cytokines in major depression. *Biological Psychiatry, 67*(5), 446-457. doi:10.1016/j.biopsych.2009.09.033

25. Lindqvist, D., Janelidze, S., Hagell, P., Erhardt, S., Samuelsson, M., Minthon, L., ... Brundin, L. (2009). Interleukin-6 is elevated in the cerebrospinal fluid of suicide attempters and related to symptom severity. *Biological Psychiatry, 66*(3), 287-292. doi:10.1016/j.biopsych.2009.01.030

26. Rosenblat, J. D., Brietzke, E., Mansur, R. B., Maruschak, N. A., Lee, Y., & McIntyre, R. S. (2015). Inflammation as a neurobiological substrate of cognitive impairment in bipolar disorder: Evidence, pathophysiology and treatment implications. *Journal of Affective Disorders, 188*, 149-159. doi:10.1016/j.jad.2015.08.058

27. Lönnerdal, B. (2000). Dietary factors influencing zinc absorption. *The Journal of Nutrition, 130*(5), 1378S-1383S. doi:10.1093/jn/130.5.137

28. Solomons, N. W, Jacob, R. A, Pineda, O., & Viteri, F. (1979). Studies on the bioavailability of zinc in man. II. Absorption of zinc from organic and inorganic sources. *Journal of laboratory and clinical medicine, 94*, 335-343.

29. Bohn, T., Davidsson, L., Walczyk, T., & Hurrell, R. F. (2004). Fractional magnesium absorption is significantly lower in human subjects from a meal served with an oxalate-rich vegetable, spinach, as compared with a meal served with kale, a vegetable with a low oxalate content. *British Journal of Nutrition, 91*(4), 601-606. doi:10.1079/bjn20031081

30. Amalraj, A., & Pius, A. (2014). Bioavailability of calcium and its absorption inhibitors in raw and cooked green leafy vegetables commonly consumed in India – An in vitro study. *Food Chemistry, 170*, 430-436. doi:10.1016/j.foodchem.2014.08.031

31. Hunt, J. R. (2003). Bioavailability of iron, zinc, and other trace minerals from vegetarian diets. *The American Journal of Clinical Nutrition, 78*(3), 633S-639S. doi:10.1093/ajcn/78.3.633s

32. De Bortoli, M. C., & Cozzolino, S. M. (2008). Zinc and Selenium Nutritional Status in Vegetarians. *Biological Trace Element Research, 127*(3), 228-233. doi:10.1007/s12011-008-8245-1

33. Craig, W. J. (2009). Health effects of vegan diets. *The American Journal of Clinical Nutrition, 89*(5), 1627S-1633S. doi:10.3945/ajcn.2009.26736n

34. Gibson, R. S., Heath, A. M., & Szymlek-Gay, E. A. (2014). Is iron and zinc nutrition a concern for vegetarian infants and young children in industrialized countries? *The American Journal of Clinical Nutrition, 100*(suppl_1), 459S-468S. doi:10.3945/ajcn.113.071241

35. Kadrabová, J., Madarič, A., Kováčiková, Z., & Ginter, E. (1995). Selenium status, plasma zinc, copper, and magnesium in vegetarians. *Biological Trace Element Research, 50*(1), 13-24. doi:10.1007/bf02789145

36. Fields, H., Ruddy, B., Wallace, M. R., Shah, A., Millstine, D., & Marks, L. (2016). How to monitor and advise vegans to ensure adequate nutrient intake. *The Journal of the American Osteopathic Association, 116*(2), 96. doi:10.7556/jaoa.2016.022

37. Krajčovičová-Kudláčková, M., Bučková, K., Klimeš, I., & Šeboková, E. (2003). Iodine deficiency in vegetarians and vegans. *Annals of Nutrition and Metabolism, 47*(5), 183-185. doi:10.1159/000070483

38. Kristensen, N. B., Madsen, M. L., Hansen, T. H., Allin, K. H., Hoppe, C., Fagt, S., … Pedersen, O. (2015). Intake of macro- and micronutrients in Danish vegans. *Nutrition Journal, 14*(1). doi:10.1186/s12937-015-0103-3

39. Pawlak, R., Berger, J., & Hines, I. (2016). Iron Status of Vegetarian Adults: A Review of Literature. *American Journal of Lifestyle Medicine, 12*(6), 486-498. doi:10.1177/1559827616682933

40. Young, I., Parker, H., Rangan, A., Prvan, T., Cook, R., Donges, C., … O'Connor, H. (2018). Association between haem and non-haem iron intake and serum ferritin in healthy young women. *Nutrients, 10*(1), 81. doi:10.3390/nu10010081

41. Hooda, J., Shah, A., & Zhang, L. (2014). Heme, an essential nutrient from dietary proteins, critically impacts diverse physiological and pathological processes. *Nutrients, 6*(3), 1080-1102. doi:10.3390/nu6031080

42. Lynch, S. R., Beard, J. L., Dassenko, S. A., & Cook, J. D. (1984). Iron absorption from legumes in humans. *The American Journal of Clinical Nutrition, 40*(1), 42-47. doi:10.1093/ajcn/40.1.42

43. Krajčovičová-Kudláčková, M., Blažíček, P., Kopčová, J., Béderová, A., & Babinská, K. (2000). Homocysteine levels in vegetarians versus omnivores. *Annals of Nutrition and Metabolism, 44*(3), 135-138. doi:10.1159/000012827

44. Gröber, U., Kisters, K., & Schmidt, J. (2013). Neuroenhancement with vitamin B12—underestimated neurological significance. *Nutrients, 5*(12), 5031-5045. doi:10.3390/nu5125031

45. Moore, E., Mander, A., Ames, D., Carne, R., Sanders, K., & Watters, D. (2012). Cognitive impairment and vitamin B12: a review. *International Psychogeriatrics, 24*(4), 541-556. doi:10.1017/s1041610211002511

46. Vogiatzoglou, A., Refsum, H., Johnston, C., Smith, S. M., Bradley, K. M., De Jager, C., … Smith, A. D. (2008). Vitamin B12 status and rate of brain volume loss in community-dwelling elderly. *Neurology, 71*(11), 826-832. doi:10.1212/01.wnl.0000325581.26991.f2

47. Gregory, J. F. (1989). Bioavailability of vitamin B-6 from plant foods. *The American Journal of Clinical Nutrition, 49*(4), 717-717. doi:10.1093/ajcn/49.4.717

48. McNulty, H., Dowey, L. R., Strain, J., Dunne, A., Ward, M., Molloy, A. M., … Scott, J. M. (2006). Riboflavin lowers homocysteine in individuals homozygous for the MTHFR 677C→T polymorphism. *Circulation, 113*(1), 74-80. doi:10.1161/circulationaha.105.580332

49. Lietz, G., Oxley, A., Boesch-Saadatmandi, C., & Kobayashi, D. (2012). Importance of β,β-carotene 15,15'-monooxygenase 1 (BCMO1) and β,β-carotene 9',10'-dioxygenase 2 (BCDO2) in nutrition and health. *Molecular Nutrition & Food Research, 56*(2), 241-250. doi:10.1002/mnfr.201100387

50. Tang, G. (2010). Bioconversion of dietary provitamin A carotenoids to vitamin A in humans. *The American Journal of Clinical Nutrition, 91*(5), 1468S-1473S. doi:10.3945/ajcn.2010.28674g

51. Groenen-van Dooren, M. M., Soute, B. A., Jie, K. G., Thijssen, H. H., & Vermeer, C. (1993). The relative effects of phylloquinone and menaquinone-4 on the blood coagulation factor synthesis in vitamin K-deficient rats. *Biochemical Pharmacology, 46*(3), 433-437. doi:10.1016/0006-2952(93)90519-3

52. Geleijnse, J. M., Vermeer, C., Grobbee, D. E., Schurgers, L. J., Knapen, M. H., Van der Meer, I. M., … Witteman, J. C. (2004). Dietary intake of menaquinone is associated with a reduced risk of coronary heart disease: The rotterdam study. *The Journal of Nutrition, 134*(11), 3100-3105. doi:10.1093/jn/134.11.3100

53. Gast, G., De Roos, N., Sluijs, I., Bots, M., Beulens, J., Geleijnse, J., … Van der Schouw, Y. (2009). A high menaquinone intake reduces the incidence of coronary heart disease. *Nutrition, Metabolism and Cardiovascular Diseases, 19*(7), 504-510. doi:10.1016/j.numecd.2008.10.004

54. Guesnet, P., & Alessandri, J. (2011). Docosahexaenoic acid (DHA) and the developing central nervous system (CNS) – Implications for dietary recommendations. *Biochimie, 93*(1), 7-12. doi:10.1016/j.biochi.2010.05.005

55. Esmaeili, V., Shahverdi, A. H., Moghadasian, M. H., & Alizadeh, A. R. (2015). Dietary fatty acids affect semen quality: a review. *Andrology, 3*(3), 450-461. doi:10.1111/andr.12024

56. Swanson, D., Block, R., & Mousa, S. A. (2012). Omega-3 fatty acids EPA and DHA: Health benefits throughout Life. *Advances in Nutrition, 3*(1), 1-7. doi:10.3945/an.111.000893

57. Aksoy, Y., Aksoy, H., Altınkaynak, K., Aydın, H. R., & Özkan, A. (2006). Sperm fatty acid composition in subfertile men. *Prostaglandins, Leukotrienes and Essential Fatty Acids, 75*(2), 75-79. doi:10.1016/j.plefa.2006.06.002

58. Dyall, S. C. (2015). Long-chain omega-3 fatty acids and the brain: a review of the independent and shared effects of EPA, DPA and DHA. *Frontiers in Aging Neuroscience, 7*. doi:10.3389/fnagi.2015.00052

59. Kiliaan, A., & Königs, A. (2016). Critical appraisal of omega-3 fatty acids in attention-deficit/hyperactivity disorder treatment. *Neuropsychiatric Disease and Treatment, Volume 12*, 1869-1882. doi:10.2147/ndt.s68652

60. Davis, B. C., & Kris-Etherton, P. M. (2003). Achieving optimal essential fatty acid status in vegetarians: current knowledge and practical implications. *The American Journal of Clinical Nutrition, 78*(3), 640S-646S. doi:10.1093/ajcn/78.3.640s

61. Forsythe, L., Wallace, J., & Livingstone, M. (2008). Obesity and inflammation: The effects of weight loss. *Nutrition Research Reviews, 21*(2), 117-133. doi:10.1017/S0954422408138732

62. Giraldo, M., Buodo, G., & Sarlo, M. (2019). Food processing and emotion regulation in vegetarians and omnivores: An event-related potential investigation. *Appetite, 141*, 104334. doi:10.1016/j.appet.2019.104334

CHAPTER 9

1. Bielefeldt, K., Levinthal, D. J., & Nusrat, S. (2015). Effective constipation treatment changes more than bowel frequency: A systematic review and meta-analysis. *Journal of Neurogastroenterology and Motility, 22*(1), 31-45. doi:10.5056/jnm15171

2. Yang, J. (2012). Effect of dietary fiber on constipation: A meta analysis. *World Journal of Gastroenterology, 18*(48), 7378. doi:10.3748/wjg.v18.i48.7378

3. Sullivan, P. B., Alder, N., Shrestha, B., Turton, L., & Lambert, B. (2011). Effectiveness of using a behavioural intervention to improve dietary fibre intakes in children with constipation. *Journal of Human Nutrition and Dietetics, 25*(1), 33-42. doi:10.1111/j.1365-277x.2011.01179.x

4. Ho, K. (2012). Stopping or reducing dietary fiber intake reduces constipation and its associated symptoms. *World Journal of Gastroenterology, 18*(33), 4593. doi:10.3748/wjg.v18.i33.4593

5. Dukowicz, A. C., Lacy, B. E., & Levine, G. M. (2007). Small intestinal bacterial overgrowth: a comprehensive review. *Gastroenterology & hepatology, 3*(2), 112–122.

6. Tursi, A. (2015). Diverticulosis today: unfashionable and still under-researched. *Therapeutic Advances in Gastroenterology, 9*(2), 213-228. doi:10.1177/1756283x15621228

7. Painter, N. S., & Burkitt, D. P. (1971). Diverticular disease of the colon: a deficiency disease of Western civilization. *BMJ, 2*(5759), 450-454. doi:10.1136/bmj.2.5759.450

8. Lin, O. S., Soon, M., Wu, S., Chen, Y., Hwang, K., & Triadafilopoulos, G. (2000). Dietary habits and right-sided colonic diverticulosis. *Diseases of the Colon & Rectum, 43*(10), 1412-1418. doi:10.1007/bf02236638

9. Song, J. H., Kim, Y. S., Lee, J. H., Ok, K. S., Ryu, S. H., Lee, J. H., & Moon, J. S. (2010). Clinical characteristics of colonic diverticulosis in Korea: A prospective study. *The Korean Journal of Internal Medicine, 25*(2), 140. doi:10.3904/kjim.2010.25.2.140

10. Peery, A. F., Barrett, P. R., Park, D., Rogers, A. J., Galanko, J. A., Martin, C. F., & Sandler, R. S. (2012). A High-fiber diet does not protect against asymptomatic diverticulosis. *Gastroenterology, 142*(2), 266-272.e1. doi:10.1053/j.gastro.2011.10.035

11. Peery, A. F., Sandler, R. S., Ahnen, D. J., Galanko, J. A., Holm, A. N., Shaukat, A., … Baron, J. A. (2013). Constipation and a low-fiber diet are not associated with diverticulosis. *Clinical Gastroenterology and Hepatology, 11*(12), 1622-1627. doi:10.1016/j.cgh.2013.06.033

12. Floch, M. H. (2006). A hypothesis: Is diverticulitis a type of inflammatory bowel disease? *Journal of Clinical Gastroenterology, 40*(Supplement 3), S121-S125. doi:10.1097/01.mcg.0000225502.29498.ba

13. Ünlü, C., Daniels, L., Vrouenraets, B. C., & Boermeester, M. A. (2011). A systematic review of high-fibre dietary therapy in diverticular disease. *International Journal of Colorectal Disease, 27*(4), 419-427. doi:10.1007/s00384-011-1308-3

14. Schatzkin, A., Lanza, E., Corle, D., Lance, P., Iber, F., Caan, B., … Slattery, M. (2000). Lack of effect of a low-fat, high-fiber diet on the recurrence of colorectal adenomas. *New England Journal of Medicine, 342*(16), 1149-1155. doi:10.1056/nejm200004203421601

15. Alberts, D. S., Martínez, M. E., Roe, D. J., Guillén-Rodríguez, J. M., Marshall, J. R., Van Leeuwen, J. B., … Sampliner, R. E. (2000). Lack of effect of a high-fiber cereal supplement on the recurrence of colorectal adenomas. *New England Journal of Medicine, 342*(16), 1156-1162. doi:10.1056/nejm200004203421602

16. Lanza, E., Yu, B., Murphy, G., Albert, P. S., Caan, B., & Marshall, J. R. (2007). The polyp prevention trial continued follow-up study: No effect of a low-fat, high-fiber, high-fruit, and -vegetable diet on adenoma recurrence eight years after randomization. *Cancer Epidemiology Biomarkers & Prevention, 16*(9), 1745-1752. doi:10.1158/1055-9965.epi-07-0127

17. Bonithon-Kopp, C., Kronborg, O., Giacosa, A., Räth, U., & Faivre, J. (2000). Calcium and fibre supplementation in prevention of colorectal adenoma recurrence: a randomised intervention trial. *The Lancet, 356*(9238), 1300-1306. doi:10.1016/s0140-6736(00)02813-0

18. Honsek, C., Kabisch, S., Kemper, M., Gerbracht, C., Arafat, A. M., Birkenfeld, A. L., … Pfeiffer, A. F. (2018). Fibre supplementation for the prevention of type 2 diabetes and improvement of glucose metabolism: The randomised controlled optimal fibre trial (OptiFiT). *Diabetologia, 61*(6), 1295-1305. doi:10.1007/s00125-018-4582-6

19. Torre, M., Rodriguez, A. R., & Saura-Calixto, F. (1991). Effects of dietary fiber and phytic acid on mineral availability. *Critical Reviews in Food Science and Nutrition, 30*(1), 1-22. doi:10.1080/10408399109527539

20. Southgate, D. A. (1987). Minerals, trace elements, and potential hazards. *The American Journal of Clinical Nutrition, 45*(5), 1256-1266. doi:10.1093/ajcn/45.5.1256

21. Toma, R. B. and Curtis, D. 1986. Dietary fiber: effect on mineral bioavailability. *Food Technol.,* 40: 111 [Web of Science ®] [Google Scholar]

22. N.T. Davies (1978) The effects of dietary fibre on mineral availability, Journal of Plant Foods, 3:1-2, 113-123, DOI: 10.1080/0142968X.1978.11904209

23. Bertin, C., Rouau, X. and Thibault, J. F. 1988. Structure and properties of sugar beet fibres. *J. Sci. Food Agric.,* 44: 15, DOI: 10.1002/jsfa.2740440104

24. Kelsay, J. L. (1987). Effects of fiber, phytic acid, and oxalic acid in the diet on mineral bioavailability. *American Journal of Gastroenterology, 82*(10), 983-986. Retrieved from https://www.ncbi.nlm.nih.gov/pubmed/2821800

25. Laszlo, J. A. (1987). Mineral binding properties of soy hull. Modeling mineral interactions with an insoluble dietary fiber source. *Journal of Agricultural and Food Chemistry, 35*(4), 593-600. doi:10.1021/jf00076a037

26. Foster, M., Karra, M., Picone, T., Chu, A., Hancock, D. P., Petocz, P., & Samman, S. (2012). Dietary fiber intake increases the risk of zinc deficiency in healthy and diabetic women. *Biological Trace Element Research, 149*(2), 135-142. doi:10.1007/s12011-012-9408-7

27. Gaskins, A. J., Mumford, S. L., Zhang, C., Wactawski-Wende, J., Hovey, K. M., & Schisterman, E. F. (2009). Effect of daily fiber intake on reproductive function: the BioCycle Study. *The American Journal of Clinical Nutrition, 90*(4), 1061-1069. doi:10.3945/ajcn.2009.27990

28. Shultz, T. D., & Howie, B. J. (1986). In vitro binding of steroid hormones by natural and purified fibers. *Nutrition and Cancer, 8*(2), 141-147. doi:10.1080/01635588609513887

29. Lewis, S., Heaton, K., Oakey, R., & McGarrigle, H. (1997). Lower serum oestrogen concentrations associated with faster intestinal transit. *British Journal of Cancer, 76*(3), 395-400. doi:10.1038/bjc.1997.397

30. Howarth, N. C., Saltzman, E., McCrory, M. A., Greenberg, A. S., Dwyer, J., Ausman, L., ... Roberts, S. B. (2003). Fermentable and nonfermentable fiber supplements Did Not Alter Hunger, Satiety or Body Weight in a Pilot Study of Men and Women Consuming Self-Selected Diets. *The Journal of Nutrition, 133*(10), 3141-3144. doi:10.1093/jn/133.10.3141

31. Poutanen, K. S., Dussort, P., Erkner, A., Fiszman, S., Karnik, K., Kristensen, M., ... Mela, D. J. (2017). A review of the characteristics of dietary fibers relevant to appetite and energy intake outcomes in human intervention trials. *The American Journal of Clinical Nutrition*, ajcn157172. doi:10.3945/ajcn.117.157172

32. Aydin, Ö., Nieuwdorp, M., & Gerdes, V. (2018). The gut microbiome as a target for the treatment of type 2 diabetes. *Current Diabetes Reports, 18*(8). doi:10.1007/s11892-018-1020-6

33. Kieler, I. N., Osto, M., Hugentobler, L., Puetz, L., Gilbert, M. T., Hansen, T., ... Bjørnvad, C. R. (2019). Diabetic cats have decreased gut microbial diversity and a lack of butyrate producing bacteria. *Scientific Reports, 9*(1). doi:10.1038/s41598-019-41195-0

34. Davis, S. C., Yadav, J. S., Barrow, S. D., & Robertson, B. K. (2017). Gut microbiome diversity influenced more by the Westernized dietary regime than the body mass index as assessed using effect size statistic. *MicrobiologyOpen, 6*(4), e00476. doi:10.1002/mbo3.476

35. Do, M., Lee, E., Oh, M., Kim, Y., & Park, H. (2018). High-glucose or -fructose diet cause changes of the gut microbiota and metabolic disorders in mice without body weight change. *Nutrients, 10*(6), 761. doi:10.3390/nu10060761

36. So, D., Whelan, K., Rossi, M., Morrison, M., Holtmann, G., Kelly, J. T., ... Campbell, K. L. (2018). Dietary fiber intervention on gut microbiota composition in healthy adults: and meta-analysis. *The American Journal of Clinical Nutrition, 107*(6), 965-983. doi:10.1093/ajcn/nqy041

37. David, L. A., Maurice, C. F., Carmody, R. N., Gootenberg, D. B., Button, J. E., Wolfe, B. E., ... Turnbaugh, P. J. (2013). Diet rapidly and reproducibly alters the human gut microbiome. *Nature, 505*(7484), 559-563. doi:10.1038/nature12820

38. Lindefeldt, M., Eng, A., Darban, H., Bjerkner, A., Zetterström, C. K., Allander, T., ... Prast-Nielsen, S. (2019). The ketogenic diet influences taxonomic and functional composition of the gut microbiota in children with severe epilepsy. *npj Biofilms and Microbiomes, 5*(1). doi:10.1038/s41522-018-0073-2

39. Swidsinski, A., Dörffel, Y., Loening-Baucke, V., Gille, C., Göktas, Ö., Reißhauer, A., ... Bock, M. (2017). Reduced mass and diversity of the colonic microbiome in patients with multiple sclerosis and their improvement with ketogenic diet. *Frontiers in Microbiology, 8*. doi:10.3389/fmicb.2017.01141

40. Bosman, E. S., Albert, A. Y., Lui, H., Dutz, J. P., & Vallance, B. A. (2019). Skin exposure to narrow band ultraviolet (UVB) light modulates the human intestinal microbiome. *Frontiers in Microbiology, 10*. doi:10.3389/fmicb.2019.02410

41. Scheppach, W. (1994). Effects of short chain fatty acids on gut morphology and function. *Gut, 35*(1 Suppl), S35-S38. doi:10.1136/gut.35.1_suppl.s35

42. Goverse, G., Molenaar, R., Macia, L., Tan, J., Erkelens, M. N., Konijn, T., ... Mebius, R. E. (2017). Diet-derived short chain fatty acids stimulate intestinal epithelial cells to induce mucosal tolerogenic dendritic cells. *The Journal of Immunology, 198*(5), 2172-2181. doi:10.4049/jimmunol.1600165

43. Den Besten, G., Van Eunen, K., Groen, A. K., Venema, K., Reijngoud, D., & Bakker, B. M. (2013). The role of short-chain fatty acids in the interplay between diet, gut microbiota, and host energy metabolism. *Journal of Lipid Research, 54*(9), 2325-2340. doi:10.1194/jlr.r036012

44. Roediger, W., Moore, J. & Babidge, W. (1997). Colonic sulfide in pathogenesis and treatment of ulcerative colitis. *Dig Dis Sci 42*, 1571–1579. doi:10.1023/A:1018851723920

45. Lowery RP, Wilson JM, Sharp MH, et al (2017). The effects of exogenous ketones on biomarkers of Crohn's disease: A case report. *J Gastroenterol Dig Dis., 2(3):8-11*

46. Paoli, A., Mancin, L., Bianco, A., Thomas, E., Mota, J. F., & Piccini, F. (2019). Ketogenic diet and microbiota: Friends or enemies? *Genes, 10*(7), 534. doi:10.3390/genes10070534

47. Le Poul, E., Loison, C., Struyf, S., Springael, J., Lannoy, V., Decobecq, M., ... Detheux, M. (2003). Functional characterization of human receptors for short chain fatty acids and their role in polymorphonuclear cell activation. *Journal of Biological Chemistry, 278*(28), 25481-25489. doi:10.1074/jbc.m301403200

48. Mohd Badrin Hanizam Bin, A. (2016). *Gut microbial metabolome: regulation of host metabolism by SCFAs* (Doctoral dissertation, Imperial College London, London, England). Retrieved from http://hdl.handle.net/10044/1/42223

49. Depauw, S., Bosch, G., Hesta, M., Whitehouse-Tedd, K., Hendriks, W. H., Kaandorp, J., & Janssens, G. P. (2012). Fermentation of animal components in strict carnivores: A comparative study with cheetah fecal inoculum1,2. *Journal of Animal Science, 90*(8), 2540-2548. doi:10.2527/jas.2011-4377

50. Johansson, M. E., Gustafsson, J. K., Holmén-Larsson, J., Jabbar, K. S., Xia, L., Xu, H., ... Hansson, G. C. (2013). Bacteria penetrate the normally impenetrable inner colon mucus layer in both murine colitis models and patients with ulcerative colitis. *Gut, 63*(2), 281-291. doi:10.1136/gutjnl-2012-303207

51. Chassaing, B., Raja, S. M., Lewis, J. D., Srinivasan, S., & Gewirtz, A. T. (2017). Colonic microbiota encroachment correlates with dysglycemia in humans. *Cellular and Molecular Gastroenterology and Hepatology, 4*(2), 205-221. doi:10.1016/j.jcmgh.2017.04.001

52. Martinez-Medina, M., Denizot, J., Dreux, N., Robin, F., Billard, E., Bonnet, R., ... Barnich, N. (2013). Western diet induces dysbiosis with increased E coli in CEABAC10 mice, alters host barrier function favouring AIEC colonisation. *Gut, 63*(1), 116-124. doi:10.1136/gutjnl-2012-304119

53. Swidsinski, A., Loening-Baucke, V., Theissig, F., Engelhardt, H., Bengmark, S., Koch, S., ... Dorffel, Y. (2007). Comparative study of the intestinal mucus barrier in normal and inflamed colon. *Gut, 56*(3), 343-350. doi:10.1136/gut.2006.098160

54. Banwell, J. G., Howard, R., Kabir, I., & Costerton, J. W. (1988). Bacterial overgrowth by indigenous microflora in the phytohemagglutinin-fed rat. *Canadian Journal of Microbiology, 34*(8), 1009-1013. doi:10.1139/m88-177

Chapter 10

1. Singh, P. N., & Fraser, G. E. (1998). Dietary risk factors for colon cancer in a low-risk population. *American Journal of Epidemiology, 148*(8), 761-774. doi:10.1093/oxfordjournals.aje.a009697

2. Basen-Engquist, K., & Chang, M. (2010). Obesity and cancer risk: Recent review and evidence. *Current Oncology Reports, 13*(1), 71-76. doi:10.1007/s11912-010-0139-7

3. Giovannucci, E., Harlan, D. M., Archer, M. C., Bergenstal, R. M., Gapstur, S. M., Habel, L. A., ... Yee, D. (2010). Diabetes and cancer: A consensus report. *Diabetes Care, 33*(7), 1674-1685. doi:10.2337/dc10-0666

4. Lee, J. E., McLerran, D. F., Rolland, B., Chen, Y., Grant, E. J., Vedanthan, R., ... Sinha, R. (2013). Meat intake and cause-specific mortality: a pooled analysis of Asian prospective cohort studies. *The American Journal of Clinical Nutrition, 98*(4), 1032-1041. doi:10.3945/ajcn.113.062638

5. Key, T. J., Appleby, P. N., Spencer, E. A., Travis, R. C., Roddam, A. W., & Allen, N. E. (2009). Cancer incidence in vegetarians: Results from the European prospective investigation into cancer and nutrition (EPIC-Oxford). *The American Journal of Clinical Nutrition, 89*(5), 1620S-1626S. doi:10.3945/ajcn.2009.26736m

6. Parnaud, G., Peiffer, G., Taché, S., & Corpet, D. E. (1998). Effect of meat (beef, chicken, and bacon) on rat colon carcinogenesis. *Nutrition and Cancer, 32*(3), 165-173. doi:10.1080/01635589809514736

7. Markova, M., Koelman, L., Hornemann, S., Pivovarova, O., Sucher, S., Machann, J., ... Aleksandrova, K. (2019). Effects of plant and animal high protein diets on immune-inflammatory biomarkers: A 6-week intervention trial. *Clinical Nutrition*. doi:10.1016/j.clnu.2019.03.019

8. Hodgson, J. M., Ward, N. C., Burke, V., Beilin, L. J., & Puddey, I. B. (2007). Increased lean red meat intake does not elevate markers of oxidative stress and inflammation in humans. *The Journal of Nutrition, 137*(2), 363-367. doi:10.1093/jn/137.2.363

9. Johnston, B. C., Zeraatkar, D., Han, M. A., Vernooij, R. W., Valli, C., El Dib, R., ... Guyatt, G. H. (2019). Unprocessed red meat and processed meat consumption: Dietary guideline recommendations from the nutritional recommendations (NutriRECS) consortium. *Annals of Internal Medicine, 171*(10), 756. doi:10.7326/m19-1621

10. Bastide, N. M., Pierre, F. H., & Corpet, D. E. (2011). Heme iron from meat and risk of colorectal cancer: A meta-analysis and a review of the mechanisms involved. *Cancer Prevention Research, 4*(2), 177-184. doi:10.1158/1940-6207.capr-10-0113

11. Turner, N. D., & Lloyd, S. K. (2017). Association between red meat consumption and colon cancer: A systematic review of experimental results. *Experimental Biology and Medicine, 242*(8), 813-839. doi:10.1177/1535370217693117

12. Kruger, C., & Zhou, Y. (2018). Red meat and colon cancer: A review of mechanistic evidence for heme in the context of risk assessment methodology. *Food and Chemical Toxicology, 118*, 131-153. doi:10.1016/j.fct.2018.04.048

13. Carvalho, A. M., Miranda, A. M., Santos, F. A., Loureiro, A. P., Fisberg, R. M., & Marchioni, D. M. (2015). High intake of heterocyclic amines from meat is associated with oxidative stress. *British Journal of Nutrition, 113*(8), 1301-1307. doi:10.1017/s0007114515000628

14. Turesky, R. J. (2007). Formation and biochemistry of carcinogenic heterocyclic aromatic amines in cooked meats. *Toxicology Letters, 168*(3), 219-227. doi:10.1016/j.toxlet.2006.10.018

15. Rohrmann, S., Hermann, S., & Linseisen, J. (2009). Heterocyclic aromatic amine intake increases colorectal adenoma risk: findings from a prospective European cohort study. *The American Journal of Clinical Nutrition, 89*(5), 1418-1424. doi:10.3945/ajcn.2008.26658

16. Soulillou, J., Süsal, C., Döhler, B., & Opelz, G. (2018). No increase in colon cancer risk following induction with Neu5Gc-bearing rabbit anti-t cell IgG (ATG) in recipients of kidney transplants. *Cancers, 10*(9), 324. doi:10.3390/cancers10090324

17. Altman, M. O., & Gagneux, P. (2019). Absence of Neu5Gc and presence of anti-Neu5Gc antibodies in humans—An evolutionary perspective. *Frontiers in Immunology, 10*. doi:10.3389/fimmu.2019.00789

18. Watson, K., & Baar, K. (2014). mTOR and the health benefits of exercise. *Seminars in Cell & Developmental Biology, 36*, 130-139. doi:10.1016/j.semcdb.2014.08.013

19. Floyd, S., Favre, C., Lasorsa, F. M., Leahy, M., Trigiante, G., Stroebel, P., … O'Connor, R. (2007). The insulin-like growth factor-I–mTOR signaling pathway induces the mitochondrial pyrimidine nucleotide carrier to promote cell growth. *Molecular Biology of the Cell, 18*(9), 3545-3555. doi:10.1091/mbc.e06-12-1109

20. Mossmann, D., Park, S., & Hall, M. N. (2018). mTOR signalling and cellular metabolism are mutual determinants in cancer. *Nature Reviews Cancer, 18*(12), 744-757. doi:10.1038/s41568-018-0074-8

21. Paquette, M., El-Houjeiri, L., & Pause, A. (2018). mTOR pathways in cancer and autophagy. *Cancers, 10*(1), 18. doi:10.3390/cancers10010018

22. Levine, M., Suarez, J., Brandhorst, S., Balasubramanian, P., Cheng, C., Madia, F., … Longo, V. (2014). Low protein intake is associated with a major reduction in IGF-1, cancer, and overall mortality in the 65 and younger but not older population. *Cell Metabolism, 19*(3), 407-417. doi:10.1016/j.cmet.2014.02.006

23. Strasser, B., Volaklis, K., Fuchs, D., & Burtscher, M. (2018). Role of dietary protein and muscular fitness on longevity and aging. *Aging and Disease, 9*(1), 119. doi:10.14336/ad.2017.0202

24. Zhang, X., Wang, C., Dou, Q., Zhang, W., Yang, Y., & Xie, X. (2018). Sarcopenia as a predictor of all-cause mortality among older nursing home residents: a systematic review and meta-analysis. *BMJ Open, 8*(11), e021252. doi:10.1136/bmjopen-2017-021252

25. Gran, P., & Cameron-Smith, D. (2011). The actions of exogenous leucine on mTOR signalling and amino acid transporters in human myotubes. *BMC Physiology, 11*(1), 10. doi:10.1186/1472-6793-11-10

26. Friedman, A. N., Ogden, L. G., Foster, G. D., Klein, S., Stein, R., Miller, B., … Wyatt, H. R. (2012). Comparative effects of low-carbohydrate high-protein versus low-fat diets on the kidney. *Clinical Journal of the American Society of Nephrology, 7*(7), 1103-1111. doi:10.2215/cjn.11741111

27. Devries, M. C., Sithamparapillai, A., Brimble, K. S., Banfield, L., Morton, R. W., & Phillips, S. M. (2018). Changes in kidney function do not differ between healthy adults consuming higher- compared with lower- or normal-protein diets: A systematic review and meta-analysis. *The Journal of Nutrition, 148*(11), 1760-1775. doi:10.1093/jn/nxy197

28. Remer, T., & Manz, F. (1995). Potential renal acid load of foods and its influence on urine pH. *Journal of the American Dietetic Association, 95*(7), 791-797. doi:10.1016/s0002-8223(95)00219-7

29. Macdonald, H. M., New, S. A., Fraser, W. D., Campbell, M. K., & Reid, D. M. (2005). Low dietary potassium intakes and high dietary estimates of net endogenous acid production are associated with low bone mineral density in premenopausal women and increased markers of bone resorption in postmenopausal women. *The American Journal of Clinical Nutrition, 81*(4), 923-933. doi:10.1093/ajcn/81.4.923

30. Cuenca-Sánchez, M., Navas-Carrillo, D., & Orenes-Piñero, E. (2015). Controversies surrounding high-protein diet intake: Satiating effect and kidney and bone health. *Advances in Nutrition, 6*(3), 260-266. doi:10.3945/an.114.007716

31. Bonjour, J., Chevalley, T., Amman, P., & Rizzoli, R. (2014). Protein intake and bone health. *Nutrition and Bone Health*, 301-317. doi:10.1007/978-1-4939-2001-3_20

32. Calvez, J., Poupin, N., Chesneau, C., Lassale, C., & Tomé, D. (2011). Protein intake, calcium balance and health consequences. *European Journal of Clinical Nutrition, 66*(3), 281-295. doi:10.1038/ejcn.2011.196

33. Fam AG (2002). Gout, diet and the insulin resistance syndrome. *The Journal of Rheumatology*, 29:1350-1355.

34. Collier, A., Stirling, A., Cameron, L., Hair, M., & Crosbie, D. (2016). Gout and diabetes: A common combination. *Postgraduate Medical Journal, 92*(1089), 372-378. doi:10.1136/postgradmedj-2015-133691

35. Maiuolo J., Oppedisano F., Gratteri S., Muscoli C., Mollace V. (2016). Regulation of uric acid metabolism and excretion. *International Journal of Cardiology*, 213:8–14. doi: 10.1016/j.ijcard.2015.08.109

36. Jamnik, J., Rehman, S., Blanco Mejia, S., De Souza, R. J., Khan, T. A., Leiter, L. A., … Sievenpiper, J. L. (2016). Fructose intake and risk of gout and hyperuricemia: a systematic review and meta-analysis of prospective cohort studies. *BMJ Open, 6*(10), e013191. doi:10.1136/bmjopen-2016-013191

37. Grasgruber, P., Sebera, M., Hrazdíra, E., Cacek, J., & Kalina, T. (2016). Major correlates of male height: A study of 105 countries. *Economics & Human Biology, 21*, 172-195. doi:10.1016/j.ehb.2016.01.005

38. Kappeler, R., Eichholzer, M., & Rohrmann, S. (2013). Meat consumption and diet quality and mortality in NHANES III. *European Journal of Clinical Nutrition, 67*(6), 598-606. doi:10.1038/ejcn.2013.59

39. Mihrshahi, S., Ding, D., Gale, J., Allman-Farinelli, M., Banks, E., & Bauman, A. E. (2017). Vegetarian diet and all-cause mortality: Evidence from a large population-based Australian cohort - the 45 and up study. *Preventive Medicine, 97*, 1-7. doi:10.1016/j.ypmed.2016.12.044

40. Appleby, P. N., Crowe, F. L., Bradbury, K. E., Travis, R. C., & Key, T. J. (2015). Mortality in vegetarians and comparable nonvegetarians in the United Kingdom. *The American Journal of Clinical Nutrition, 103*(1), 218-230. doi:10.3945/ajcn.115.119461

41. Balan, E., Decottignies, A., & Deldicque, L. (2018). Physical activity and nutrition: Two promising strategies for telomere maintenance? *Nutrients, 10*(12), 1942. doi:10.3390/nu10121942

42. Kasielski, M., Eusebio, M., Pietruczuk, M., & Nowak, D. (2015). The relationship between peripheral blood mononuclear cells telomere length and diet - unexpected effect of red meat. *Nutrition Journal, 15*(1). doi:10.1186/s12937-016-0189-2

43. Rosero-Bixby, L., Dow, W. H., & Rehkopf, D. H. (2014). The Nicoya region of Costa Rica: A high longevity island for elderly males. *Vienna Yearbook of Population Research, Volume 11*, 109-136. doi:10.1553/populationyearbook2013s109

44. Pes, G. M., Tolu, F., Dore, M. P., Sechi, G. P., Errigo, A., Canelada, A., & Poulain, M. (2014). Male longevity in Sardinia, a review of historical sources supporting a causal link with dietary factors. *European Journal of Clinical Nutrition, 69*(4), 411-418. doi:10.1038/ejcn.2014.230

45. Shibata, H., Nagai, H., Haga, H., Yasumura, S., Suzuki, T., & Suyama, Y. (1992). Nutrition for the Japanese elderly. *Nutrition and Health, 8*(2–3), 165–175. https://doi.org/10.1177/026010609200800312

46. Chrysohoou, C., Pitsavos, C., Lazaros, G., Skoumas, J., Tousoulis, D., & Stefanadis, C. (2015). Determinants of all-cause mortality and incidence of cardiovascular disease (2009 to 2013) in older adults: The Ikaria study of the Blue Zones, *Angiology, 67*(6), 541-548. doi:10.1177/0003319715603185

47. Orlich, M. J., Singh, P. N., Sabaté, J., Jaceldo-Siegl, K., Fan, J., Knutsen, S., … Fraser, G. E. (2013). Vegetarian dietary patterns and mortality in adventist health study 2. *JAMA Internal Medicine, 173*(13), 1230. doi:10.1001/jamainternmed.2013.6473

48. Enstrom, J. E., & Breslow, L. (2008). Lifestyle and reduced mortality among active California Mormons, 1980–2004. *Preventive Medicine, 46*(2), 133-136. doi:10.1016/j.ypmed.2007.07.030

49. Appleby, P. N., Key, T. J., Thorogood, M., Burr, M. L., & Mann, J. (2002). Mortality in British vegetarians. *Public Health Nutrition, 5*(1), 29-36. doi:10.1079/phn2001248

50. Messerlian, C., Williams, P. L., Ford, J. B., Chavarro, J. E., Mínguez-Alarcón, L., & Dadd, R. (2018). The environment and reproductive health (EARTH) study: A prospective preconception cohort. *Human Reproduction Open, 2018*(2). doi:10.1093/hropen/hoy001

51. Orzylowska, E. M., Jacobson, J. D., Bareh, G. M., Ko, E. Y., Corselli, J. U., & Chan, P. J. (2016). Food intake diet and sperm characteristics in a blue zone: a Loma Linda study. *European Journal of Obstetrics & Gynecology and Reproductive Biology, 203*, 112-115. doi:10.1016/j.ejogrb.2016.05.043

52. Willcox, D. C., Willcox, B. J., Hsueh, W., & Suzuki, M. (2006). Genetic determinants of exceptional human longevity: insights from the Okinawa centenarian study. *AGE, 28*(4), 313-332. doi:10.1007/s11357-006-9020-x

53. Sebastiani, P., & Perls, T. T. (2012). The genetics of extreme longevity: Lessons from the New England centenarian study. *Frontiers in Genetics, 3.* doi:10.3389/fgene.2012.00277

54. Kucharski. H., & Zajac, J. (2009). *Handbook of vitamin C research. Daily requirements, dietary sources and adverse effects.* New York: Nova Biomedical Books.

55. Johnson, R. J., & Andrews, P. (2010). Fructose, uricase, and the back-to-Africa hypothesis. *Evolutionary Anthropology: Issues, News, and Reviews, 19*(6), 250-257. doi:10.1002/evan.20266

56. Ames, B. N., Cathcart, R., Schwiers, E., & Hochstein, P. (1981). Uric acid provides an antioxidant defense in humans against oxidant- and radical-caused aging and cancer: A hypothesis. *Proceedings of the National Academy of Sciences, 78*(11), 6858-6862. doi:10.1073/pnas.78.11.6858

57. Clemens, Z., & Tóth, C. (2016). Vitamin C and Disease: Insights from the evolutionary perspective. *Journal of Evolution and Health, 1*(1). doi:10.15310/2334-3591.1030

58. Bjelakovic, G., Nikolova, D., Gluud, L. L., Simonetti, R. G., & Gluud, C. (2012). Antioxidant supplements for prevention of mortality in healthy participants and patients with various diseases. *Cochrane Database of Systematic Reviews.* doi:10.1002/14651858.cd007176.pub2

59. Sesso, H. D., Buring, J. E., Christen, W. G., Kurth, T., Belanger, C., MacFadyen, J., … Bubes, V. (2008). vitamins E and C in the prevention of cardiovascular disease in Men. *JAMA, 300*(18), 2123. doi:10.1001/jama.2008.600

60. Padayatty, S. J., Katz, A., Wang, Y., Eck, P., Kwon, O., Lee, J., … Levine, M. (2003). Vitamin C as an antioxidant: Evaluation of its role in disease prevention. *Journal of the American College of Nutrition, 22*(1), 18-35. doi:10.1080/07315724.2003.10719272

61. Levine, M., Wang, Y., Padayatty, S. J., & Morrow, J. (2001). A new recommended dietary allowance of vitamin C for healthy young women. *Proceedings of the National Academy of Sciences, 98*(17), 9842-9846. doi:10.1073/pnas.171318198

62. Halliwell, B. (2000). Why and how should we measure oxidative DNA damage in nutritional studies? How far have we come? *The American Journal of Clinical Nutrition, 72*(5), 1082-1087. doi:10.1093/ajcn/72.5.1082

63. Zhang, S. M., Hunter, D. J., Rosner, B. A., Giovannucci, E. L., Colditz, G. A., Speizer, F. E., & Willett, W. C. (2000). Intakes of fruits, vegetables, and related nutrients and the risk of non-hodgkin's lymphoma among women. *Cancer Epidemiol Biomarkers, 9*(5), 477-485.

64. Duthie, S. J., Duthie, G. G., Russell, W. R., Kyle, J. A., Macdiarmid, J. I., Rungapamestry, V., ... Bestwick, C. S. (2017). Effect of increasing fruit and vegetable intake by dietary intervention on nutritional biomarkers and attitudes to dietary change: A randomised trial. *European Journal of Nutrition, 57*(5), 1855-1872. doi:10.1007/s00394-017-1469-0

65. Assimos D. G. (2004). Vitamin C supplementation and urinary oxalate excretion. *Reviews in urology, 6*(3), 167.

66. Nobile, S., & Woodhill, J. (2012). *Vitamin C: The mysterious redox-system a trigger of life?* Berlin, Germany: Springer Science & Business Media.

67. Thomas, L. D., Elinder, C., Tiselius, H., Wolk, A., & Åkesson, A. (2013). Ascorbic acid supplements and kidney stone incidence among men: A prospective study. *JAMA Internal Medicine, 173*(5), 386. doi:10.1001/jamainternmed.2013.2296

68. Cunningham, J. J., Ellis, S. L., McVeigh, K. L., Levine, R. E., & Calles-Escandon, J. (1991). Reduced mononuclear leukocyte ascorbic acid content in adults with insulin-dependent diabetes mellitus consuming adequate dietary vitamin C. *Metabolism, 40*(2), 146-149. doi:10.1016/0026-0495(91)90165-s

69. Song, J., Kwon, O., Chen, S., Daruwala, R., Eck, P., Park, J. B., & Levine, M. (2002). Flavonoid inhibition of sodium-dependent vitamin C transporter 1 (SVCT1) and glucose transporter isoform 2 (GLUT2), intestinal transporters for vitamin C and glucose. *Journal of Biological Chemistry, 277*(18), 15252-15260. doi:10.1074/jbc.m110496200

CHAPTER 11

1. Seneff, S., Davidson, R. M., Lauritzen, A., Samsel, A., & Wainwright, G. (2015). A novel hypothesis for atherosclerosis as a cholesterol sulfate deficiency syndrome. *Theoretical Biology and Medical Modelling, 12*(1). doi:10.1186/s12976-015-0006-1

2. Strott, C. A., & Higashi, Y. (2003). Cholesterol sulfate in human physiology. *Journal of Lipid Research, 44*(7), 1268-1278. doi:10.1194/jlr.r300005-jlr200

3. Manifold-Wheeler, B. C., Elmore, B. O., Triplett, K. D., Castleman, M. J., Otto, M., & Hall, P. R. (2015). Serum lipoproteins are critical for pulmonary innate defense against Staphylococcus aureus quorum sensing. *The Journal of Immunology, 196*(1), 328-335. doi:10.4049/jimmunol.1501835

4. Peterson, M. M., Mack, J. L., Hall, P. R., Alsup, A. A., Alexander, S. M., Sully, E. K., ... Gresham, H. D. (2008). Apolipoprotein B is an innate barrier against invasive Staphylococcus aureus infection. *Cell Host & Microbe, 4*(6), 555-566. doi:10.1016/j.chom.2008.10.001

5. Bhakdi, Sucharit & Tranum-Jensen, J & Utermann, G & Füssle, R. (1983). Binding and partial inactivation of Staphylococcus aureus α-toxin by human plasma low density lipoprotein. The Journal of biological chemistry. 258. 5899-904.

6. Miller M. B., Bassler B. L. (2001). Quorum sensing in bacteria. *Annu. Rev. Microbiol.* 55 165–199.

7. Feingold, K. R., Funk, J. L., Moser, A. H., Shigenaga, J. K., Rapp, J. H. & Grunfeld, C. (1995). Role for circulating lipoproteins in protection from endotoxin toxicity. *Infection and immunity, 63*(5), 2041-2046

8. Elias, E. R., Irons, M. B., Hurley, A. D., Tint, G. S., & Salen, G. (1997). Clinical effects of cholesterol supplementation in six patients with the Smith-Lemli-Opitz syndrome (SLOS). *American Journal of Medical Genetics, 68*(3), 305-310. doi:10.1002/(sici)1096-8628(19970131)68:3<305::aid-ajmg11>3.0.co;2-x

9. Ravnskov, U. (2003). High cholesterol may protect against infections and atherosclerosis. *QJM: An International Journal of Medicine, 96*(12), 927-934. doi:10.1093/qjmed/hcg150

10. Räihä, I., Marniemi, J., Puukka, P., Toikka, T., Ehnholm, C., & Sourander, L. (1997). Effect of serum lipids, lipoproteins, and apolipoproteins on vascular and nonvascular mortality in the elderly. *Arteriosclerosis, Thrombosis, and Vascular Biology, 17*(7), 1224-1232. doi:10.1161/01.atv.17.7.1224

11. Forette, F., De la Fuente, X., Golmard, J., Henry, J., & Hervy, M. (1982). The prognostic significance of isolated systolic hypertension in the elderly. Results of a ten year longitudinal survey. *Clinical and Experimental Hypertension. Part A: Theory and Practice, 4*(7), 1177-1191. doi:10.3109/10641968209060782

12. Forette, B., Tortrat, D., & Wolmark, Y. (1989). Cholesterol as risk factor for mortality in elderly women. *The Lancet, 333*(8643), 868-870. doi:10.1016/s0140-6736(89)92865-1

13. Risk of fatal coronary heart disease in familial hypercholesterolaemia. Scientific Steering Committee on behalf of the Simon Broome Register Group. (1991). *BMJ, 303*(6807), 893-896. doi:10.1136/bmj.303.6807.893

14. Weijenberg, M. P., Feskens, E. J., & Kromhout, D. (1996). Total and high density lipoprotein cholesterol as risk factors for coronary heart disease in elderly men during 5 years of follow-up: The Zutphen elderly study. *American Journal of Epidemiology, 143*(2), 151-158. doi:10.1093/oxfordjournals.aje.a008724

15. Weuenberg, M. P., Feskens, E. J., Bowles, C. H., & Kromhout, D. (1994). Serum total cholesterol and systolic blood pressure as risk factors for mortality from ischemic heart disease among elderly men and women. *Journal of Clinical Epidemiology, 47*(2), 197-205. doi:10.1016/0895-4356(94)90025-6

16. Zimetbaum, P., Frishman, W. H., Ooi, W. L., Derman, M. P., Aronson, M., Gidez, L. I., & Eder, H. A. (1992). Plasma lipids and lipoproteins and the incidence of cardiovascular disease in the very elderly.

The Bronx Aging Study. *Arteriosclerosis and Thrombosis: A Journal of Vascular Biology, 12*(4), 416-423. doi:10.1161/01.atv.12.4.416

17. Abbott, R. D., Curb, J., Rodriguez, B. L., Masaki, K. H., Yano, K., Schatz, I. J., ... Petrovitch, H. (2002). Age-related changes in risk factor effects on the incidence of coronary heart disease. *Annals of Epidemiology, 12*(3), 173-181. doi:10.1016/s1047-2797(01)00309-x

18. Chyou, P., & Eaker, E. D. (2000). Serum cholesterol concentrations and all-cause mortality in older people. *Age and Ageing, 29*(1), 69-74. doi:10.1093/ageing/29.1.69

19. Menotti, A., Mulder, I., Nissinen, A., Feskens, E., Giampaoli, S., Tervahauta, M., & Kromhaut, D. (2001). Cardiovascular risk factors and 10-year all-cause mortality in elderly European male populations. The FINE study. *European Heart Journal, 22*(7), 573-579. doi:10.1053/euhj.2000.2402

20. Krumholz, H. M. (1994). Lack of association between cholesterol and coronary heart disease mortality and morbidity and all-cause mortality in persons older than 70 years. *JAMA: The Journal of the American Medical Association, 272*(17), 1335-1340. doi:10.1001/jama.272.17.1335

21. Jónsson, Á., Sigvaldason, H., & Sigfússon, N. (1997). Total cholesterol and mortality after age 80 years. *The Lancet, 350*(9093), 1778-1779. doi:10.1016/s0140-6736(05)63609-4

22. Weverling-Rijnsburger, A. W., Blauw, G. J., Lagaay, A. M., Knock, D. L., Meinders, A. E., & Westendorp, R. G. (1997). Total cholesterol and risk of mortality in the oldest old. *The Lancet, 350*(9085), 1119-1123. doi:10.1016/s0140-6736(97)04430-9

23. Jacobs, D., Blackburn, H., Higgins, M., Reed, D., Iso, H., McMillan, G., ... Rifkind, B. (1992). Report on the conference on low blood cholesterol: Mortality associations. *Circulation, 86*(3), 1046-1060. doi:10.1161/01.cir.86.3.1046

24. Iribarren, C., Jacobs, D. R., Sidney, S., Claxton, A. J., & Feingold, K. R. (1998). Cohort study of serum total cholesterol and in-hospital incidence of infectious diseases. *Epidemiology and Infection, 121*(2), 335-347. doi:10.1017/s0950268898001435

25. Iribarren, C. (1997). Serum total cholesterol and risk of hospitalization, and death from respiratory disease. *International Journal of Epidemiology, 26*(6), 1191-1202. doi:10.1093/ije/26.6.1191

26. Neaton, J. D., & Wentworth, D. N. (1997). Low serum cholesterol and risk of death from aids. *AIDS, 11*(7), 929-930. Retrieved from https://journals.lww.com/aidsonline/Fulltext/1997/07000/Low_serum_cholesterol_and_risk_of_death_from_AIDS.14.aspx

27. Castelli W.P. Epidemiology of coronary heart disease: The Framingham study. Am J Med 1984;76:4–12. 10.1016/0002-9343(84)90952-5

28. Gofman, J., Lindgren, F., Elliott, H., Mantz, W., Hewitt, J., Strisower, B., . . . Lyon, T. (1950). The role of lipids and lipoproteins in atherosclerosis. *Science, 111*(2877), 166-186. Retrieved from http://www.jstor.org/stable/1676938

29. Camejo G, Fager G, Rosengren B, Hurt-Camejo E, Bondjers G. (1993). Binding of low density lipoproteins by proteoglycans synthesized by proliferating and quiescent human arterial smooth muscle cells. J Biol Chem.;268:14131–14137

30. Lundstam, U., Hurt-Camejo, E., Olsson, G., Sartipy, P., Camejo, G., & Wiklund, O. (1999). Proteoglycans contribution to association of Lp(a) and LDL with smooth muscle cell extracellular matrix. *Arteriosclerosis, Thrombosis, and Vascular Biology, 19*(5), 1162-1167. doi:10.1161/01.atv.19.5.1162

31. Flood, C., Gustafsson, M., Richardson, P. E., Harvey, S. C., Segrest, J. P., & Borén, J. (2002). Identification of the proteoglycan binding site in apolipoprotein B48. *Journal of Biological Chemistry, 277*(35), 32228-32233. doi:10.1074/jbc.m204053200

32. Nakashima, Y., Fujii, H., Sumiyoshi, S., Wight, T. N., & Sueishi, K. (2007). Early human atherosclerosis: Accumulation of lipid and proteoglycans in intimal thickenings followed by macrophage infiltration. *Arteriosclerosis, Thrombosis, and Vascular Biology, 27*(5), 1159-1165. doi:10.1161/atvbaha.106.134080

33. Fukuchi, M., Watanabe, J., Kumagai, K., Baba, S., Shinozaki, T., Miura, M., ... Shirato, K. (2002). Normal and oxidized low density lipoproteins accumulate deep in physiologically thickened intima of human coronary arteries. *Laboratory Investigation, 82*(10), 1437-1447. doi:10.1097/01.lab.0000032546.01658.5d

34. Goldstein, J. L., Ho, Y. K., Basu, S. K., & Brown, M. S. (1979). Binding site on macrophages that mediates uptake and degradation of acetylated low density lipoprotein, producing massive cholesterol deposition. *Proceedings of the National Academy of Sciences, 76*(1), 333-337. doi:10.1073/pnas.76.1.333

35. Lemieux, I., Lamarche, B., Couillard, C., Pascot, A., Cantin, B., Bergeron, J., ... Després, J. (2001). Total Cholesterol/HDL cholesterol ratio vs LDL cholesterol/HDL cholesterol ratio as indices of ischemic heart disease risk in men. *Archives of Internal Medicine, 161*(22), 2685. doi:10.1001/archinte.161.22.2685

36. Shestov, D. B., Deev, A. D., Klimov, A. N., Davis, C. E., & Tyroler, H. A. (1993). Increased risk of coronary heart disease death in men with low total and low-density lipoprotein cholesterol in the Russian Lipid Research Clinics Prevalence Follow-up Study. *Circulation, 88*(3), 846-853. doi:10.1161/01.cir.88.3.846

37. Beaglehole, R., Foulkes, M. A., Prior, I. A., & Eyles, E. F. (1980). Cholesterol and mortality in New Zealand Maoris. *BMJ, 280*(6210), 285-287. doi:10.1136/bmj.280.6210.285

38. Hamazaki, T., Okuyama, H., Ogushi, Y., & Hama, R. (2015). Towards a paradigm shift in cholesterol treatment. A re-examination of the cholesterol issue in Japan: Abstracts. *Annals of Nutrition and Metabolism, 66*(4), 1-116. doi:10.1159/000381654

39. Thorogood, M. D. (1994). Vegetarianism, coronary disease risk factors and coronary heart disease. *Current Opinion in Lipidology, 5*(1), 17-21. doi:10.1097/00041433-199402000-00004

40. Packard, J., Cobbe, S. M., Shepherd, J., Ford, I., Isles, C. G., McKillop, J. H., … Macfarlane, P. W. (1998). Influence of pravastatin and plasma lipids on clinical events in the west of Scotland coronary prevention study (WOSCOPS). *Circulation, 97*(15), 1440-1445. doi:10.1161/01.cir.97.15.1440

41. Sacks, F. M., Moyé, L. A., Davis, B. R., Cole, T. G., Rouleau, J. L., Nash, D. T., … Braunwald, E. (1998). Relationship between plasma LDL concentrations during treatment with pravastatin and recurrent coronary events in the cholesterol and recurrent events trial. *Circulation, 97*(15), 1446-1452. doi:10.1161/01.cir.97.15.1446

42. Schwartz, G., Olsson, A., & Ezekowitzet al, M. (2001). Effects of atorvastatin on early recurrent ischemic events in acute coronary syndromes. the miracl study: a randomized controlled trial. *ACC Current Journal Review, 10*(5), 23. doi:10.1016/s1062-1458(01)00368-3

43. Sabatine, M. S., Giugliano, R. P., Keech, A. C., Honarpour, N., Wiviott, S. D., Murphy, S. A., … Kuder, J. F. (2017). Evolocumab and clinical outcomes in patients with cardiovascular disease. *New England Journal of Medicine, 377*(8), 785-788. doi:10.1056/nejmc1708587

44. Castelli, W. P., Anderson, K., Wilson, P. W., & Levy, D. (1992). Lipids and risk of coronary heart disease. The Framingham study. *Annals of Epidemiology, 2*(1-2), 23-28. doi:10.1016/1047-2797(92)90033-m

45. Cordero, A., & Alegria-Ezquerra, E. (2009). TG/HDL ratio as surrogate marker for insulin resistance. *ESC Council for Cardiology Practice, 8*(16).

46. Karelis, A. D., Pasternyk, S. M., Messier, L., St-Pierre, D. H., Lavoie, J., Garrel, D., & Rabasa-Lhoret, R. (2007). Relationship between insulin sensitivity and the triglyceride–HDL-C ratio in overweight and obese postmenopausal women: a MONET study. *Applied Physiology, Nutrition, and Metabolism, 32*(6), 1089-1096. doi:10.1139/h07-095

47. Robins, S. J., Rubins, H. B., Faas, F. H., Schaefer, E. J., Elam, M. B., Anderson, J. W., & Collins, D. (2003). Insulin resistance and cardiovascular events with low HDL cholesterol: The veterans affairs HDL intervention trial (VA-HIT). *Diabetes Care, 26*(5), 1513-1517. doi:10.2337/diacare.26.5.1513

48. Semple, R. K., Sleigh, A., Murgatroyd, P. R., Adams, C. A., Bluck, L., Jackson, S., … Savage, D. B. (2009). Postreceptor insulin resistance contributes to human dyslipidemia and hepatic steatosis. *Journal of Clinical Investigation.* doi:10.1172/jci37432

49. Rashid, S., Watanabe, T., Sakaue, T., & Lewis, G. F. (2003). Mechanisms of HDL lowering in insulin resistant, hypertriglyceridemic states: The combined effect of HDL triglyceride enrichment and elevated hepatic lipase activity. *Clinical Biochemistry, 36*(6), 421-429. doi:10.1016/s0009-9120(03)00078-x

50. Karhapaa, P., Malkki, M., & Laakso, M. (1994). Isolated low HDL cholesterol. An insulin-resistant state. *Diabetes, 43*(3), 411-417. doi:10.2337/diabetes.43.3.411

51. Borén, J., & Williams, K. J. (2016). The central role of arterial retention of cholesterol-rich apolipoprotein-B-containing lipoproteins in the pathogenesis of atherosclerosis: a triumph of simplicity. *Current Opinion in Lipidology, 27*(5), 473-483. doi:10.1097/mol.0000000000000330

52. Linton MF, Yancey PG, Davies SS, Jerome WGJ, Linton EF, Vickers KC (2000). The role of lipids and lipoproteins in atherosclerosis [Updated 2015 Dec 24]In: De Groot LJ, Chrousos G, Dungan K, *et al.,* editors. Endotext [Internet]. South Dartmouth (MA): MDText.com, Inc.; 2000. Available from: https://www.ncbi.nlm.nih.gov/books/NBK343489/

53. Hurt-Camejo, E., & Camejo, G. (2018). ApoB-100 lipoprotein complex formation with intima proteoglycans as a cause of atherosclerosis and Its possible ex vivo evaluation as a disease biomarker. *Journal of Cardiovascular Development and Disease, 5*(3), 36. doi:10.3390/jcdd5030036

54. Hiukka, A., Stahlman, M., Pettersson, C., Levin, M., Adiels, M., Teneberg, S., … Boren, J. (2009). ApoCIII-enriched LDL in type 2 diabetes displays altered lipid composition, increased susceptibility for sphingomyelinase, and increased binding to biglycan. *Diabetes, 58*(9), 2018-2026. doi:10.2337/db09-0206

55. Olsson, U., Egnell, A., Lee, M. R., Lunden, G. O., Lorentzon, M., Salmivirta, M., … Camejo, G. (2001). Changes in matrix proteoglycans induced by insulin and fatty acids in hepatic cells may contribute to dyslipidemia of insulin resistance. *Diabetes, 50*(9), 2126-2132. doi:10.2337/diabetes.50.9.2126

56. Hulthe, J., Bokemark, L., Wikstrand, J., & Fagerberg, B. (2000). The metabolic syndrome, LDL particle size, and atherosclerosis. *Arteriosclerosis, Thrombosis, and Vascular Biology, 20*(9), 2140-2147. doi:10.1161/01.atv.20.9.2140

57. Wasty, F., Alavi, M. Z., & Moore, S. (1993). Distribution of glycosaminoglycans in the intima of human aortas: Changes in atherosclerosis and diabetes mellitus. *Diabetologia, 36*(4), 316-322. doi:10.1007/bf00400234

58. Rodriguéz-Lee, M., Bondjers, G., & Camejo, G. (2007). Fatty acid-induced atherogenic changes in extracellular matrix proteoglycans. *Current Opinion in Lipidology, 18*(5), 546-553. doi:10.1097/mol.0b013e3282ef534f

59. Srinivasan, S. R., Xu, J., Vijayagopal, P., Radhakrishnamurthy, B., & Berenson, G. S. (1993). Injury to the arterial wall of rabbits produces proteoglycan variants with enhanced low-density lipoprotein-binding property. *Biochimica et Biophysica Acta (BBA) - Lipids and Lipid Metabolism, 1168*(2), 158-166. doi:10.1016/0005-2760(93)90120-x

60. Howard, B. V., Robbins, D. C., Sievers, M. L., Lee, E. T., Rhoades, D., Devereux, R. B., … Howard, W. J. (2000). LDL cholesterol as a strong predictor of coronary heart disease in diabetic individuals with insulin resistance and low LDL. *Arteriosclerosis, Thrombosis, and Vascular Biology, 20*(3), 830-835. doi:10.1161/01. atv.20.3.830

61. Araújo, J., Cai, J., & Stevens, J. (2019). Prevalence of optimal metabolic health in american adults: National health and nutrition examination survey 2009–2016. *Metabolic Syndrome and Related Disorders, 17*(1), 46-52. doi:10.1089/met.2018.0105

62. Chiu, J., & Chien, S. (2011). Effects of disturbed flow on vascular endothelium: Pathophysiological basis and clinical perspectives. *Physiological Reviews, 91*(1), 327-387. doi:10.1152/physrev.00047.2009

63. Davies, P. F. (1995). Flow-mediated endothelial mechanotransduction. *Physiological Reviews, 75*(3), 519-560. doi:10.1152/physrev.1995.75.3.519

64. Gimbrone, M., Topper, J. N., Nagel, T., Anderson, K. R., & Garcia-Cardeña, G. (1999). Endothelial dysfunction, hemodynamic forces, and atherosclerosis. *Thrombosis and Haemostasis, 82*(08), 722-726. doi:10.1055/s-0037-1615903

65. Zhang, H., Sun, A., Shen, Y., Jia, J., Wang, S., Wang, K., & Ge, J. (2004). Artery interposed to vein did not develop atherosclerosis and underwent atrophic remodeling in cholesterol-fed rabbits. *Atherosclerosis, 177*(1), 37-41. doi:10.1016/j.atherosclerosis.2004.06.019

66. Finlayson, R., & Symons, C. (1961). Arteriosclerosis in wild animals in captivity [abstract]. *Proceedings of the Royal Society of Medicine, 54*(11), 973.

67. McCullagh, K. (1972). Arteriosclerosis in the african elephant Part 1. Intimal atherosclerosis and its possible causes. *Atherosclerosis, 16*(3), 307-335. doi:10.1016/0021-9150(72)90080-9

68. Finlayson, R., Symons, C., & Fiennes, R. N. (1962). Atherosclerosis: a comparative study. *British medical journal, 1*(5277), 501–507. doi:10.1136/bmj.1.5277.501

69. Bohorquez, F., & Stout, C. (1972). Arteriosclerosis in exotic mammals. *Atherosclerosis, 16*(2), 225-231. doi:10.1016/0021-9150(72)90056-1

70. Han, C. Y. (2016). Roles of reactive oxygen species on insulin resistance in adipose tissue. *Diabetes & Metabolism Journal, 40*(4), 272. doi:10.4093/dmj.2016.40.4.272

71. Kim, J., Wei, Y., & Sowers, J. R. (2008). Role of mitochondrial dysfunction in insulin resistance. *Circulation Research, 102*(4), 401-414. doi:10.1161/circresaha.107.165472

72. Gonzalez-Franquesa A., Patti ME. (2017) Insulin resistance and mitochondrial dysfunction. In: Santulli G. (eds) Mitochondrial Dynamics in Cardiovascular Medicine. Advances in Experimental Medicine and Biology, vol 982. Springer, Cham

73. Williams, K. J., & Wu, X. (2016). Imbalanced insulin action in chronic over nutrition: Clinical harm, molecular mechanisms, and a way forward. *Atherosclerosis, 247*, 225-282. doi:10.1016/j. atherosclerosis.2016.02.004

74. Gasior, M., Rogawski, M. A., & Hartman, A. L. (2006). Neuroprotective and disease-modifying effects of the ketogenic diet. *Behavioural Pharmacology, 17*(5-6), 431-439. doi:10.1097/00008877-200609000-00009

75. Basciano, H., Federico, L., & Adeli, K. (2005). Fructose, insulin resistance, and metabolic dyslipidemia. *Nutrition & metabolism, 2*(1), 5. doi:10.1186/1743-7075-2-5

76. Shapiro, A., Mu, W., Roncal, C., Cheng, K., Johnson, R. J., & Scarpace, P. J. (2008). Fructose-induced leptin resistance exacerbates weight gain in response to subsequent high-fat feeding. *American Journal of Physiology-Regulatory, Integrative and Comparative Physiology, 295*(5), R1370-R1375. doi:10.1152/ajpregu.00195.2008

77. Mehta, N. N., McGillicuddy, F. C., Anderson, P. D., Hinkle, C. C., Shah, R., Pruscino, L., … Reilly, M. P. (2009). Experimental endotoxemia induces adipose inflammation and insulin resistance in humans. *Diabetes*. doi:10.2337/db09-0729

78. Feingold KR, Grunfeld C (2019). The effect of inflammation and infection on lipids and lipoproteins. In Endotext. Edited by De Groot LJ, Chrousos G, Dungan K, Feingold KR, Grossman A, Hershman JM, Koch C, Korbonits M, McLachlan R, New M, et al. South Dartmouth (MA);

79. Straub, R. H. (2014). Insulin resistance, selfish brain, and selfish immune system: An evolutionarily positively selected program used in chronic inflammatory diseases. *Arthritis Research & Therapy, 16*(Suppl 2), S4. doi:10.1186/ar4688

80. Durante, A., & Bronzato, S. (2015). The increased cardiovascular risk in patients affected by autoimmune diseases: Review of the various manifestations. *Journal of Clinical Medicine Research, 7*(6), 379-384. doi:10.14740/jocmr2122w

81. De Kort, S., Keszthelyi, D., & Masclee, A. A. (2011). Leaky gut and diabetes mellitus: What is the link? *Obesity Reviews, 12*(6), 449-458. doi:10.1111/j.1467-789x.2010.00845.x

82. Joo, Myung & Yang, Jaemo & Youl, Jae & Cho, Ssang-Goo & Shim, Byung & Kim, Duk & Lee, Jaehwi. (2010). Bioavailability enhancing activities of natural compounds from medicinal plants. Journal of Medicinal Plants Research. 3. 1204-1211.

83. DeVries, J. H. (2013). Glucose variability: Where it is important and how to measure it. *Diabetes, 62*(5), 1405-1408. doi:10.2337/db12-1610

84. Service, F. J., Molnar, G. D., Rosevear, J. W., Ackerman, E., Gatewood, L. C., & Taylor, W. F. (1970). Mean amplitude of glycemic excursions, a measure of diabetic instability. *Diabetes, 19*(9), 644-655. doi:10.2337/ diab.19.9.644

85. Nieuwdorp, M., Van Haeften, T. W., Gouverneur, M. C., Mooij, H. L., Van Lieshout, M. H., Levi, M., … Stroes, E. S. (2006). Loss of endothelial glycocalyx during acute hyperglycemia coincides with endothelial dysfunction and coagulation activation in vivo. *Diabetes, 55*(2), 480-486. doi:10.2337/diabetes.55.02.06.db05-1103

86. Schött, U., Solomon, C., Fries, D., & Bentzer, P. (2016). The endothelial glycocalyx and its disruption, protection and regeneration: A narrative review. *Scandinavian Journal of Trauma, Resuscitation and Emergency Medicine, 24*(1). doi:10.1186/s13049-016-0239-y

87. Thaiss, C. A., Levy, M., Grosheva, I., Zheng, D., Soffer, E., Blacher, E., … Elinav, E. (2018). Hyperglycemia drives intestinal barrier dysfunction and risk for enteric infection. *Science, 359*(6382), 1376-1383. doi:10.1126/science.aar3318

88. Singh, A., Fridén, V., Dasgupta, I., Foster, R. R., Welsh, G. I., Tooke, J. E., … Satchell, S. C. (2011). High glucose causes dysfunction of the human glomerular endothelial glycocalyx. *American Journal of Physiology-Renal Physiology, 300*(1), F40-F48. doi:10.1152/ajprenal.00103.2010

89. Obrenovich, M. (2018). Leaky gut, leaky brain? *Microorganisms, 6*(4), 107. doi:10.3390/microorganisms6040107

90. Lindeberg, S., Eliasson, M., Lindahl, B., & Ahrén, B. (1999). Low serum insulin in traditional pacific islanders—The Kitava study. *Metabolism, 48*(10), 1216-1219. doi:10.1016/s0026-0495(99)90258-5

91. Lindberg, S., Nilsson-Ehle, P., Terént, A., Vessby, B., & Scherstén, B. (1994). Cardiovascular risk factors in a Melanesian population apparently free from stroke and ischaemic heart disease: the Kitava study. *Journal of Internal Medicine, 236*(3), 331-340. doi:10.1111/j.1365-2796.1994.tb00804.x

92. Schulz, L. O., & Chaudhari, L. S. (2015). High-risk populations: The Pimas of Arizona and Mexico. *Current Obesity Reports, 4*(1), 92-98. doi:10.1007/s13679-014-0132-9

93. Schulz, L. O., Bennett, P. H., Ravussin, E., Kidd, J. R., Kidd, K. K., Esparza, J., & Valencia, M. E. (2006). Effects of traditional and western environments on prevalence of type 2 diabetes in Pima Indians in Mexico and the U.S. *Diabetes Care, 29*(8), 1866-1871. doi:10.2337/dc06-0138

94. Creighton, B. C., Hyde, P. N., Maresh, C. M., Kraemer, W. J., Phinney, S. D., & Volek, J. S. (2018). Paradox of hypercholesterolaemia in highly trained, keto-adapted athletes. *BMJ Open Sport & Exercise Medicine, 4*(1), e000429. doi:10.1136/bmjsem-2018-000429

95. Wood, T., Stubbs, B., & Juul, S. (2018). Exogenous ketone bodies as promising neuroprotective agents for developmental brain injury. *Developmental Neuroscience, 40*(5-6), 451-462. doi:10.1159/000496564

96. Sävendahl, L., & Underwood, L. E. (1999). Fasting increases serum total cholesterol, LDL cholesterol and apolipoprotein B in healthy, nonobese humans. *The Journal of Nutrition, 129*(11), 2005-2008. doi:10.1093/jn/129.11.2005

97. Cohn, J. S., Wagner, D. A., Cohn, S. D., Millar, J. S., & Schaefer, E. J. (1990). Measurement of very low density and low density lipoprotein apolipoprotein (Apo) B-100 and high density lipoprotein Apo A-I production in human subjects using deuterated leucine. Effect of fasting and feeding. *Journal of Clinical Investigation, 85*(3), 804-811. doi:10.1172/jci114507

98. Hopkins, P. N., Stephenson, S., Wu, L. L., Riley, W. A., Xin, Y., & Hunt, S. C. (2001). Evaluation of coronary risk factors in patients with heterozygous familial hypercholesterolemia. *The American Journal of Cardiology, 87*(5), 547-553. doi:10.1016/s0002-9149(00)01429-6

99. Wiegman, A., Gidding, S. S., Watts, G. F., Chapman, M. J., Ginsberg, H. N., Cuchel, M., … European Atherosclerosis Society Consensus Panel (2015). Familial hypercholesterolaemia in children and adolescents: Gaining decades of life by optimizing detection and treatment. *European heart journal, 36*(36), 2425–2437. doi:10.1093/eurheartj/ehv157

100. Šebeštjen, M., Žegura, B., Gužič-Salobir, B., & Keber, I. (2001). Fibrinolytic parameters and insulin resistance in young survivors of myocardial infarction with heterozygous familial hypercholesterolemia. *Wien Klin Wochenschr, 113*(3-4), 113-118. Retrieved from https://www.ncbi.nlm.nih.gov/pubmed/11253736

101. Hill, J. S., Hayden, M. R., Frohlich, J., & Pritchard, P. H. (1991). Genetic and environmental factors affecting the incidence of coronary artery disease in heterozygous familial hypercholesterolemia. *Arteriosclerosis and Thrombosis: A Journal of Vascular Biology, 11*(2), 290-297. doi:10.1161/01.atv.11.2.290

102. Okuyama, H., Langsjoen, P. H., Hamazaki, T., Ogushi, Y., Hama, R., Kobayashi, T., & Uchino, H. (2015). Statins stimulate atherosclerosis and heart failure: Pharmacological mechanisms. *Expert Review of Clinical Pharmacology, 8*(2), 189-199. doi:10.1586/17512433.2015.1011125

103. Ahmadizar, F., Ochoa-Rosales, C., Glisic, M., Franco, O. H., Muka, T., & Stricker, B. H. (2019). Associations of statin use with glycaemic traits and incident type 2 diabetes. *British Journal of Clinical Pharmacology, 85*(5), 993-1002. doi:10.1111/bcp.13898

104. Schultz, B. G., Patten, D. K., & Berlau, D. J. (2018). The role of statins in both cognitive impairment and protection against dementia: a tale of two mechanisms. *Translational Neurodegeneration, 7*(1). doi:10.1186/s40035-018-0110-3

105. Enas, E. A., Kuruvila, A., Khanna, P., Pitchumoni, C. S., & Mohan, V. (2013). Benefits & risks of statin therapy for primary prevention of cardiovascular disease in Asian Indians - a population with the highest risk of premature coronary artery disease & diabetes. *The Indian journal of medical research, 138*(4), 461–491.

106. Golomb, B., Kane, T., & Dimsdale, J. (2004). Severe irritability associated with statin cholesterol-lowering drugs. *QJM*, *97*(4), 229-235. doi:10.1093/qjmed/hch035

107. Leppien, E., Mulcahy, K., Demler, T. L., Trigoboff, E., & Opler, L. (2018). Effects of statins and cholesterol on patient aggression: Is there a connection?. *Innovations in clinical neuroscience*, *15*(3-4), 24–27.

108. Cham, S., Koslik, H. J., & Golomb, B. A. (2015). Mood, personality, and behavior changes during treatment with statins: A case series. *Drug Safety - Case Reports*, *3*(1). doi:10.1007/s40800-015-0024-2

109. Ginter, E., Kajaba, I., & Sauša, M. (2012). Addition of statins into the public water supply? Risks of side effects and low cholesterol levels. *Cas Lek Cesk*, *151*(5), 243-247. Retrieved from https://www.ncbi.nlm.nih.gov/pubmed/22779765

110. Pedersen, T. R., Kjekshus, J., Berg, K., Haghfelt, T., Faergeman, O., Thorgeirsson, G., ... Pyörälä, K. (1994). Randomised trial of cholesterol lowering in 4444 patients with coronary heart disease: the Scandinavian Simvastatin Survival Study (4S). *The Lancet*, *344*(8934), 1383-1389. doi:10.1016/s0140-6736(94)90566-5

111. Sherriff, J. L., O'Sullivan, T. A., Properzi, C., Oddo, J., & Adams, L. A. (2016). Choline, its potential role in nonalcoholic fatty liver disease, and the case for human and bacterial genes. *Advances in Nutrition*, *7*(1), 5-13. doi:10.3945/an.114.007955

112. Koeth, R. A., Lam-Galvez, B. R., Kirsop, J., Wang, Z., Levison, B. S., Gu, X., ... Hazen, S. L. (2018). l-carnitine in omnivorous diets induces an atherogenic gut microbial pathway in humans. *Journal of Clinical Investigation*, *129*(1), 373-387. doi:10.1172/jci94601

113. Dambrova, M., Latkovskis, G., Kuka, J., Strele, I., Konrade, I., Grinberga, S., ... Liepinsh, E. (2016). Diabetes is associated with higher trimethylamine N-oxide plasma Levels. *Experimental and Clinical Endocrinology & Diabetes*, *124*(04), 251-256. doi:10.1055/s-0035-1569330

114. Valeur, J., Landfald, B., Berstad, A., & Raa, J. (2016). Trimethylamine N-oxide in seafood. *Journal of the American College of Cardiology*, *68*(25), 2916-2917. doi:10.1016/j.jacc.2016.08.077

115. Velasquez, M., Ramezani, A., Manal, A., & Raj, D. (2016). Trimethylamine N-oxide: The good, the bad and the unknown. *Toxins*, *8*(11), 326. doi:10.3390/toxins8110326

116. Janeiro, M., Ramírez, M., Milagro, F., Martínez, J., & Solas, M. (2018). Implication of trimethylamine N-oxide (TMAO) in disease: Potential biomarker or new therapeutic target. *Nutrients*, *10*(10), 1398. doi:10.3390/nu10101398

117. Cheung, W., Keski-Rahkonen, P., Assi, N., Ferrari, P., Freisling, H., Rinaldi, S., ... Slimani, N. (2017). A metabolomic study of biomarkers of meat and fish intake. *American Journal of Clinical Nutrition*, *105*(3), 600-608. doi:10.3945/ajcn.116.146639

118. Huc, T., Drapala, A., Gawrys, M., Konop, M., Bielinska, K., Zaorska, E., ... Ufnal, M. (2018). Chronic, low-dose TMAO treatment reduces diastolic dysfunction and heart fibrosis in hypertensive rats. *American Journal of Physiology-Heart and Circulatory Physiology*, *315*(6), H1805-H1820. doi:10.1152/ajpheart.00536.2018

119. Jia, J., Dou, P., Gao, M., Kong, X., Li, C., Liu, Z., & Huang, T. (2019). Assessment of causal direction between gut microbiota–dependent metabolites and cardiometabolic health: A bidirectional mendelian randomization analysis. *Diabetes*, *68*(9), 1747-1755. doi:10.2337/db19-0153

120. Lande, K. E., & Sperry, W. M. (1937). Human atherosclerosis in relation to the cholesterol content of the blood serum. *American Heart Journal*, *13*(1), 125. doi:10.1016/s0002-8703(37)90941-4

121. Paoli, A., Rubini, A., Volek, J. S., & Grimaldi, K. A. (2013). Beyond weight loss: A review of the therapeutic uses of very-low-carbohydrate (ketogenic) diets. *European Journal of Clinical Nutrition*, *67*(8), 789-796. doi:10.1038/ejcn.2013.116

122. Westman, E. C., Yancy, W. S., Mavropoulos, J. C., Marquart, M., & McDuffie, J. R. (2008). The effect of a low-carbohydrate, ketogenic diet versus a low-glycemic index diet on glycemic control in type 2 diabetes mellitus. *Nutrition & Metabolism*, *5*(1). doi:10.1186/1743-7075-5-36

123. Ebbeling, C. B., Feldman, H. A., Klein, G. L., Wong, J. M., Bielak, L., Steltz, S. K., ... Ludwig, D. S. (2018). Effects of a low carbohydrate diet on energy expenditure during weight loss maintenance: randomized trial. *BMJ*, k4583. doi:10.1136/bmj.k4583

124. Forsythe, C. E., Phinney, S. D., Fernandez, M. L., Quann, E. E., Wood, R. J., Bibus, D. M., ... Volek, J. S. (2007). Comparison of low fat and low carbohydrate diets on circulating fatty acid composition and markers of inflammation. *Lipids*, *43*(1), 65-77. doi:10.1007/s11745-007-3132-7

125. Pérez-Guisado, J., Muñoz-Serrano, A., & Alonso-Moraga, Á. (2008). Spanish ketogenic Mediterranean diet: A healthy cardiovascular diet for weight loss. *Nutrition Journal*, *7*(1). doi:10.1186/1475-2891-7-30

126. Pinto, A., Bonucci, A., Maggi, E., Corsi, M., & Businaro, R. (2018). Anti-oxidant and anti-inflammatory activity of ketogenic diet: New Perspectives for Neuroprotection in Alzheimer's Disease. *Antioxidants*, *7*(5), 63. doi:10.3390/antiox7050063

127. Van der Auwera, I., Wera, S., Van Leuven, F., & Henderson, S. T. (2005). A ketogenic diet reduces amyloid beta 40 and 42 in a mouse model of Alzheimer's disease. *Nutrition & metabolism*, *2*, 28. doi:10.1186/1743-7075-2-28

128. Gasior, M., Rogawski, M. A., & Hartman, A. L. (2006). Neuroprotective and disease-modifying effects of the ketogenic diet. *Behavioural Pharmacology*, *17*(5-6), 431-439. doi:10.1097/00008877-200609000-00009

129. Krikorian, R., Shidler, M. D., Dangelo, K., Couch, S. C., Benoit, S. C., & Clegg, D. J. (2012). Dietary ketosis enhances memory in mild cognitive impairment. *Neurobiology of Aging*, *33*(2), 425.e19-425.e27. doi:10.1016/j.neurobiolaging.2010.10.006

130. Włodarek, D. (2019). Role of ketogenic diets in neurodegenerative diseases (Alzheimer's disease and Parkinson's disease). *Nutrients*, *11*(1), 169. doi:10.3390/nu11010169

131. Mavropoulos, J. C., Yancy, W. S., Hepburn, J., & Westman, E. C. (2005). The effects of a low-carbohydrate, ketogenic diet on the polycystic ovary syndrome: a pilot study. *Nutrition & metabolism*, *2*, 35. doi:10.1186/1743-7075-2-35

132. Kirpich, I. A., Feng, W., Wang, Y., Liu, Y., Barker, D. F., Barve, S. S., & McClain, C. J. (2011). The type of dietary fat modulates intestinal tight junction integrity, gut permeability, and hepatic toll-like receptor expression in a mouse model of alcoholic liver disease. *Alcoholism: Clinical and Experimental Research*, *36*(5), 835-846. doi:10.1111/j.1530-0277.2011.01673.x

133. Silaste, M., Rantala, M., Alfthan, G., Aro, A., Witztum, J. L., Kesäniemi, Y. A., & Hörkkö, S. (2004). Changes in dietary fat intake alter plasma levels of oxidized low-density lipoprotein and lipoprotein(a). *Arteriosclerosis, Thrombosis, and Vascular Biology*, *24*(3), 498-503. doi:10.1161/01.atv.0000118012.64932.f4

134. Zhu, Y., Bo, Y., & Liu, Y. (2019). Dietary total fat, fatty acids intake, and risk of cardiovascular disease: A dose-response meta-analysis of cohort studies. *Lipids in Health and Disease*, *18*(1). doi:10.1186/s12944-019-1035-2

135. Grasgruber, P., Sebera, M., Hrazdira, E., Hrebickova, S., & Cacek, J. (2016). Food consumption and the actual statistics of cardiovascular diseases: An epidemiological comparison of 42 European countries. *Food & Nutrition Research*, *60*(1), 31694. doi:10.3402/fnr.v60.31694

CHAPTER 12

1. White Oak Pastures Team. (2019, June 4). White oak pastures beef reduces atmospheric carbon. Retrieved from http://blog.whiteoakpastures.com/blog/carbon-negative-grassfed-beef

2. Planas, G. M., & Kucacute, J. (1968). Contraceptive properties of Stevia rebaudiana. *Science*, *162*(3857), 1007-1007. doi:10.1126/science.162.3857.1007

3. Melis, M. (1999). Effects of chronic administration of Stevia rebaudiana on fertility in rats. *Journal of Ethnopharmacology*, *67*(2), 157-161. doi:10.1016/s0378-8741(99)00081-1

4. Kimata, H. (2007). Anaphylaxis by stevioside in infants with atopic eczema. *Allergy*, *62*(5), 565-566. doi:10.1111/j.1398-9995.2007.01317.x

5. Ruiz-Ojeda, F. J., Plaza-Díaz, J., Sáez-Lara, M. J., & Gil, A. (2019). Effects of sweeteners on the gut microbiota: A review of experimental studies and clinical trials. *Advances in Nutrition*, *10*(suppl_1), S31-S48. doi:10.1093/advances/nmy037

6. Suez, J., Korem, T., Zilberman-Schapira, G., Segal, E., & Elinav, E. (2015). Non-caloric artificial sweeteners and the microbiome: Findings and challenges. *Gut Microbes*, *6*(2), 149-155. doi:10.1080/19490976.2015.1017700

7. Payne, A. N., Chassard, C., & Lacroix, C. (2012). Gut microbial adaptation to dietary consumption of fructose, artificial sweeteners and sugar alcohols: Implications for host-microbe interactions contributing to obesity. *Obesity Reviews*, *13*(9), 799-809. doi:10.1111/j.1467-789x.2012.01009.x

8. Pearlman, M., Obert, J., & Casey, L. (2017). The association between artificial sweeteners and obesity. *Current Gastroenterology Reports*, *19*(12). doi:10.1007/s11894-017-0602-9

9. Dotson, C. D., Vigues, S., Steinle, N. I., & Munger, S. D. (2010). T1R and T2R receptors: The modulation of incretin hormones and potential targets for the treatment of type 2 diabetes mellitus. *Current opinion in investigational drugs (London, England : 2000)*, *11*(4), 447–454.

10. Joo, Myung & Yang, Jaemo & Youl, Jae & Cho, Ssang-Goo & Shim, Byung & Kim, Duk & Lee, Jaehwi. (2010). Bioavailability enhancing activities of natural compounds from medicinal plants. Journal of Medicinal Plants Research. 3. 1204-1211

11. Masterjohn, C., Park, Y., Lee, J., Noh, S., Koo, S., & Bruno, R. (2013). Dietary fructose feeding increases adipose methylglyoxal accumulation in rats in association with low expression and activity of glyoxalase-2. *Nutrients*, *5*(8), 3311-3328. doi:10.3390/nu5083311

12. Legeza, B., Marcolongo, P., Gamberucci, A., Varga, V., Bánhegyi, G., Benedetti, A., & Odermatt, A. (2017). Fructose, glucocorticoids and adipose tissue: Implications for the metabolic syndrome. *Nutrients*, *9*(5), 426. doi:10.3390/nu9050426

13. Basciano, H., Federico, L., & Adeli, K. (2005). Fructose, insulin resistance, and metabolic dyslipidemia. *Nutrition & metabolism*, *2*(1), 5. doi:10.1186/1743-7075-2-5

14. Elliott, S. S., Keim, N. L., Stern, J. S., Teff, K., & Havel, P. J. (2002). Fructose, weight gain, and the insulin resistance syndrome. *The American Journal of Clinical Nutrition*, *76*(5), 911-922. doi:10.1093/ajcn/76.5.911

15. Johnson, R. J., Sanchez-Lozada, L. G., & Nakagawa, T. (2010). The effect of fructose on renal biology and disease. *Journal of the American Society of Nephrology*, *21*(12), 2036-2039. doi:10.1681/asn.2010050506

16. DiNicolantonio, J. J., & Lucan, S. C. (2014). The wrong white crystals: Not salt but sugar as aetiological in hypertension and cardiometabolic disease. *Open Heart*, *1*(1), e000167. doi:10.1136/openhrt-2014-000167

17. Shapiro, A., Mu, W., Roncal, C., Cheng, K., Johnson, R. J., & Scarpace, P. J. (2008). Fructose-induced leptin resistance exacerbates weight gain in response to subsequent high-fat feeding. *American Journal of Physiology-Regulatory, Integrative and Comparative Physiology*, *295*(5), R1370-R1375. doi:10.1152/ajpregu.00195.2008

18. Vasselli, J. R. (2008). Fructose-induced leptin resistance: Discovery of an unsuspected form of the phenomenon and its significance. Focus on "Fructose-induced leptin resistance exacerbates weight gain in response to subsequent high-fat feeding," by Shapiro et al. *American Journal of Physiology-Regulatory, Integrative and Comparative Physiology, 295*(5), R1365-R1369. doi:10.1152/ajpregu.90674.2008

19. Softic, S., Meyer, J. G., Wang, G., Gupta, M. K., Batista, T. M., Lauritzen, H. P., … Kahn, C. R. (2019). Dietary sugars alter hepatic fatty acid oxidation via transcriptional and post-translational modifications of mitochondrial proteins. *Cell Metabolism, 30*(4), 735-753.e4. doi:10.1016/j.cmet.2019.09.003

20. DiNicolantonio, J. J., & Berger, A. (2016). Added sugars drive nutrient and energy deficit in obesity: A new paradigm. *Open Heart, 3*(2), e000469. doi:10.1136/openhrt-2016-000469

21. Do, M., Lee, E., Oh, M., Kim, Y., & Park, H. (2018). High-glucose or -fructose diet cause changes of the gut microbiota and metabolic disorders in mice without body weight change. *Nutrients, 10*(6), 761. doi:10.3390/nu10060761

22. Woelber, J. P., Bremer, K., Vach, K., König, D., Hellwig, E., Ratka-Krüger, P., … Tennert, C. (2016). An oral health optimized diet can reduce gingival and periodontal inflammation in humans - a randomized controlled pilot study. *BMC Oral Health, 17*(1). doi:10.1186/s12903-016-0257-1

23. Najeeb, S., Zafar, M., Khurshid, Z., Zohaib, S., & Almas, K. (2016). The role of nutrition in periodontal health: An update. *Nutrients, 8*(9), 530. doi:10.3390/nu8090530

24. Pritchard, A. B., Crean, S., Olsen, I., & Singhrao, S. K. (2017). Periodontitis, microbiomes and their role in Alzheimer's disease. *Frontiers in Aging Neuroscience, 9*. doi:10.3389/fnagi.2017.00336

25. Dominy, S. S., Lynch, C., Ermini, F., Benedyk, M., Marczyk, A., Konradi, A., … Potempa, J. (2019). Porphyromonas gingivalis in Alzheimer's disease brains: Evidence for disease causation and treatment with small-molecule inhibitors. *Science Advances, 5*(1), eaau3333. doi:10.1126/sciadv.aau3333

26. Crittenden, A. N., Sorrentino, J., Moonie, S. A., Peterson, M., Mabulla, A., & Ungar, P. S. (2017). Oral health in transition: The Hadza foragers of Tanzania. *PLOS ONE, 12*(3), e0172197. doi:10.1371/journal.pone.0172197

27. Butten, K., Johnson, N. W., Hall, K. K., Anderson, J., Toombs, M., King, N., & O'Grady, K. F. (2019). Risk factors for oral health in young, urban, Aboriginal and Torres Strait Islander children. *Australian dental journal, 64*(1), 72–81. doi:10.1111/adj.12662

28. Bhandari, M. R., & Kawabata, J. (2005). Bitterness and toxicity in wild yam (Dioscorea spp.) tubers of Nepal. *Plant Foods for Human Nutrition, 60*(3), 129-135. doi:10.1007/s11130-005-6841-1

29. Cordain, L., Miller, J. B., Eaton, S. B., Mann, N., Holt, S. H., & Speth, J. D. (2000). Plant-animal subsistence ratios and macronutrient energy estimations in worldwide hunter-gatherer diets. *The American Journal of Clinical Nutrition, 71*(3), 682-692. doi:10.1093/ajcn/71.3.682

30. Crittenden, A. N., & Schnorr, S. L. (2017). Current views on hunter□ gatherer nutrition and the evolution of the human diet. *American Journal of Physical Anthropology, 162*(S63), 84-109. doi:10.1002/ajpa.23148

31. Ben-Dor, M. (2015). Use of animal fat as a symbol of health in traditional societies suggests humans may be well adapted to its consumption. *Journal of Evolution and Health, 1*(1). doi:10.15310/2334-3591.1022

32. Hiernaux, J., & Hartono, D. B. (1980). Physical measurements of the adult Hadza of Tanzania. *Annals of Human Biology, 7*(4), 339-346. doi:10.1080/03014468000004411

33. Blackwell, A. D., Urlacher, S. S., Beheim, B., Von Rueden, C., Jaeggi, A., Stieglitz, J., … Kaplan, H. (2016). Growth references for Tsimane forager-horticulturalists of the Bolivian Amazon. *American Journal of Physical Anthropology, 162*(3), 441-461. doi:10.1002/ajpa.23128

34. Shephard, S., & Schlatter, C. (1998). Covalent binding of agaritine to DNA in vivo. *Food and Chemical Toxicology, 36*(11), 971-974. doi:10.1016/s0278-6915(98)00076-3

35. Toth, B., Nagel, D., Patil, K., Erickson, J., & Antonson, K. (1978). Tumor induction with the at-acetyl derivative of 4-hydroxymethyl- phenylhydrazine, a metabolite of agaritine of agaricus b/sporus1. *CANCER RESEARCH, 38*, 177-180. Retrieved from https://cancerres.aacrjournals.org/content/canres/38/1/177.full.pdf

36. I. Nor Hayati, A. Aminah, S. Mamot, I. Nor Aini & H.M. Noor Lida (2002) Physical characteristics of modified milkfat in high-melting fat preparation, International Journal of Food Sciences and Nutrition, 53:1, 43-54. doi:10.1080/09637480120057000

37. Xiong, Z., Cao, X., Wen, Q., Chen, Z., Cheng, Z., Huang, X., … Huang, Z. (2019). An overview of the bioactivity of monacolin K / lovastatin. *Food and Chemical Toxicology, 131*, 110585. doi:10.1016/j.fct.2019.110585

38. Friedman, M. (2015). Chemistry, nutrition, and health-promoting properties of Hericium erinaceus (lion's mane) mushroom fruiting bodies and mycelia and their bioactive compounds. *Journal of Agricultural and Food Chemistry, 63*(32), 7108-7123. doi:10.1021/acs.jafc.5b02914

39. Rucker, J. J., Iliff, J., & Nutt, D. J. (2018). Psychiatry & the psychedelic drugs. Past, present & future. *Neuropharmacology, 142*, 200-218. doi:10.1016/j.neuropharm.2017.12.040

40. Reiche, S., Hermle, L., Gutwinski, S., Jungaberle, H., Gasser, P., & Majić, T. (2018). Serotonergic hallucinogens in the treatment of anxiety and depression in patients suffering from a life-threatening disease: A systematic review. *Progress in Neuro-Psychopharmacology and Biological Psychiatry, 81*, 1-10. doi:10.1016/j.pnpbp.2017.09.012

41. Ross, S., Bossis, A., Guss, J., Agin-Liebes, G., Malone, T., Cohen, B., ... Schmidt, B. L. (2016). Rapid and sustained symptom reduction following psilocybin treatment for anxiety and depression in patients with life-threatening cancer: a randomized controlled trial. *Journal of Psychopharmacology, 30*(12), 1165-1180. doi:10.1177/0269881116675512

42. Griffiths, R. R., Johnson, M. W., Carducci, M. A., Umbricht, A., Richards, W. A., Richards, B. D., ... Klinedinst, M. A. (2016). Psilocybin produces substantial and sustained decreases in depression and anxiety in patients with life-threatening cancer: A randomized double-blind trial. *Journal of Psychopharmacology, 30*(12), 1181-1197. doi:10.1177/0269881116675513

43. Ames, B. N., Profet, M., & Gold, L. S. (1990). Dietary pesticides (99.99% all natural). *Proceedings of the National Academy of Sciences of the United States of America, 87*(19), 7777–7781. doi:10.1073/pnas.87.19.7777

44. Mennen, L. I., Walker, R., Bennetau-Pelissero, C., & Scalbert, A. (2005). Risks and safety of polyphenol consumption. *The American Journal of Clinical Nutrition, 81*(1), 326S-329S. doi:10.1093/ajcn/81.1.326s

45. Martini, D., Del Bo', C., Tassotti, M., Riso, P., Del Rio, D., Brighenti, F., & Porrini, M. (2016). Coffee consumption and oxidative stress: A review of human intervention studies. *Molecules, 21*(8), 979. doi:10.3390/molecules21080979

46. Vicente, S. J., Ishimoto, E. Y., & Torres, E. A. (2013). Coffee modulates transcription factor NRF2 and highly increases the activity of antioxidant enzymes in Rats. *Journal of Agricultural and Food Chemistry, 62*(1), 116-122. doi:10.1021/jf401777m

47. Tucker, J. D., Taylor, R. T., Christensen, M. L., Strout, C. L., & Hanna, M. (1989). Cytogenetic response to coffee in Chinese hamster ovary AUXB1 cells and human peripheral lymphocytes. *Mutagenesis, 4*(5), 343-348. doi:10.1093/mutage/4.5.343

48. Ishidate, M., Harnois, M., & Sofuni, T. (1988). A comparative analysis of data on the clastogenicity of 951 chemical substances tested in mammalian cell cultures. *Mutation Research/Reviews in Genetic Toxicology, 195*(2), 151-213. doi:10.1016/0165-1110(88)90023-1

49. Gilliland, K., & Bullock, W. (1984). Caffeine: A potential drug of abuse. *Advances in Alcohol & Substance Abuse, 3*(1-2), 53-73. doi:10.1300/j251v03n01_05

50. Jin, M., Yoon, C., Ko, H., Kim, H., Kim, A., Moon, H., & Jung, S. (2016). The relationship of caffeine intake with depression, anxiety, stress, and sleep in Korean adolescents. *Korean Journal of Family Medicine, 37*(2), 111. doi:10.4082/kjfm.2016.37.2.111

51. Richards, G., & Smith, A. (2015). Caffeine consumption and self-assessed stress, anxiety, and depression in secondary school children. *Journal of Psychopharmacology, 29*(12), 1236-1247. doi:10.1177/0269881115612404

52. Dearfield, K. L., Abernathy, C. O., Ottley, M. S., Brantner, J. H., & Hayes, P. F. (1988). Acrylamide: Its metabolism, developmental and reproductive effects, genotoxicity, and carcinogenicity. *Mutation Research/Reviews in Genetic Toxicology, 195*(1), 45-77. doi:10.1016/0165-1110(88)90015-2

53. Mucci, L. A., Sandin, S., & Magnusson, C. (2005). Acrylamide intake and breast cancer risk in Swedish women. *JAMA, 293*(11), 1322. doi:10.1001/jama.293.11.1326

54. Virk-Baker, M. K., Nagy, T. R., Barnes, S., & Groopman, J. (2014). Dietary acrylamide and human cancer: A systematic review of literature. *Nutrition and Cancer, 66*(5), 774-790. doi:10.1080/01635581.2014.916323

55. The effects of workplace hazards on male reproductive health. (1996). doi:10.26616/nioshpub96132

56. De Roos, A. J., Blair, A., Rusiecki, J. A., Hoppin, J. A., Svec, M., Dosemeci, M., ... Alavanja, M. C. (2005). Cancer incidence among glyphosate-exposed pesticide applicators in the agricultural health study. *Environmental Health Perspectives, 113*(1), 49-54. doi:10.1289/ehp.7340

57. Tarazona, J. V., Court-Marques, D., Tiramani, M., Reich, H., Pfeil, R., Istace, F., & Crivellente, F. (2017). Glyphosate toxicity and carcinogenicity: a review of the scientific basis of the European Union assessment and its differences with IARC. *Archives of Toxicology, 91*(8), 2723-2743. doi:10.1007/s00204-017-1962-5

58. Samanta, P., Pal, S., Mukherjee, A. K., & Ghosh, A. R. (2014). Biochemical effects of glyphosate based herbicide, Excel Mera 71 on enzyme activities of acetylcholinesterase (AChE), lipid peroxidation (LPO), catalase (CAT), glutathione-S-transferase (GST) and protein content on teleostean fishes. *Ecotoxicology and Environmental Safety, 107*, 120-125. doi:10.1016/j.ecoenv.2014.05.025

59. Hoagland, R. E., & Duke, S. O. (1982). Biochemical effects of glyphosate[N-(phosphonomethyl)glycine]. *ACS Symposium Series*, 175-205. doi:10.1021/bk-1982-0181.ch010

60. Micco, C., Grossi, M., Miraglia, M., & Brera, C. (1989). A study of the contamination by ochratoxin A of green and roasted coffee beans. *Food Additives and Contaminants, 6*(3), 333-339. doi:10.1080/02652038909373788

61. Soliman, K. M. (2002). Incidence, level, and behavior of aflatoxins during coffee bean roasting and decaffeination. *Journal of Agricultural and Food Chemistry, 50*(25), 7477-7481. doi:10.1021/jf011338v

62. Hussein, H., & Brasel, J. M. (2001). Toxicity, metabolism, and impact of mycotoxins on humans and animals. *Toxicology, 167*(2), 101-134. doi:10.1016/s0300-483x(01)00471-1

63. Randerath, K., Randerath, E., Agrawal, H. P., Gupta, R. C., Schurdak, M. E., & Reddy, M. V. (1985). Postlabeling methods for carcinogen-DNA adduct analysis. *Environmental Health Perspectives, 62*, 57. doi:10.2307/3430093

64. Pfohl-Leszkowicz, A., & Manderville, R. A. (2007). Ochratoxin A: An overview on toxicity and carcinogenicity in animals and humans. *Molecular Nutrition & Food Research, 51*(9), 1192-1192. doi:10.1002/mnfr.200790020

65. Doi, K., & Uetsuka, K. (2011). Mechanisms of mycotoxin-induced neurotoxicity through oxidative stress-associated pathways. *International Journal of Molecular Sciences, 12*(8), 5213-5237. doi:10.3390/ijms12085213

66. Hsieh, M., Chiu, H., Lin☐ Tan, D., & Lin, J. (2004). Does human ochratoxin A aggravate proteinuria in patients with chronic renal disease? *Renal Failure, 26*(3), 311-316. doi:10.1081/jdi-200026744

67. Reddy, K. R., Abbas, H. K., Abel, C. A., Shier, W. T., & Salleh, B. (2010). Mycotoxin Contamination of Beverages: Occurrence of Patulin in Apple Juice and Ochratoxin A in Coffee, Beer and Wine and Their Control Methods. *Toxins, 2*(2), 229-261. doi:10.3390/toxins2020229

68. Sugita-Konishi, Y., Nakajima, M., Tabata, S., Ishikuro, E., Tanaka, T., Norizuki, H., ... Kumagai, S. (2006). Occurrence of aflatoxins, ochratoxin A, and fumonisins in retail foods in Japan. *Journal of Food Protection, 69*(6), 1365-1370. doi:10.4315/0362-028x-69.6.1365

69. Kumagai, S., Nakajima, M., Tabata, S., Ishikuro, E., Tanaka, T., Norizuki, H., ... Sugita-Konishi, Y. (2008). Aflatoxin and ochratoxin A contamination of retail foods and intake of these mycotoxins in Japan. *Food Additives & Contaminants: Part A, 25*(9), 1101-1106. doi:10.1080/02652030802226187

70. Patel, S. S., Beer, S., Kearney, D. L., Phillips, G., & Carter, B. A. (2013). Green tea extract: A potential cause of acute liver failure. *World Journal of Gastroenterology, 19*(31), 5174. doi:10.3748/wjg.v19.i31.5174

71. Chandra, A. K., & De, N. (2012). Catechin induced modulation in the activities of thyroid hormone synthesizing enzymes leading to hypothyroidism. *Molecular and Cellular Biochemistry, 374*(1-2), 37-48. doi:10.1007/s11010-012-1503-8

72. Young, J., Dragsted L.O.*, Haraldsdóttir, J., Daneshvar, B., Kall, M., Loft, S., ... Sandström, B. (2002). Green tea extract only affects markers of oxidative status postprandially: lasting antioxidant effect of flavonoid-free diet. *British Journal of Nutrition, 87*(4), 343-355. doi:10.1079/bjnbjn2002523

73. Information sheet: Pharmaceuticals in drinking-water. Retrieved from https://www.who.int/water_sanitation_health/diseases-risks/risks/info_sheet_pharmaceuticals/en/

74. Jamshed, H., Beyl, R. A., Della Manna, D. L., Yang, E. S., Ravussin, E., & Peterson, C. M. (2019). Early time-restricted feeding improves 24-hour glucose levels and affects markers of the circadian clock, aging, and autophagy in Humans. *Nutrients, 11*(6), 1234. doi:10.3390/nu11061234

75. Ben-Dor, M. (2015). Use of animal fat as a symbol of health in traditional societies suggests humans may be well adapted to its consumption. *Journal of Evolution and Health, 1*(1). doi:10.15310/2334-3591.1022

76. Geleijnse, J. M., Vermeer, C., Grobbee, D. E., Schurgers, L. J., Knapen, M. H., Van der Meer, I. M., ... Hofman A, A. (2004). Dietary intake of menaquinone is associated with a reduced risk of coronary heart disease: The Rotterdam study. *The Journal of Nutrition, 134*(11), 3100-3105. doi:10.1093/jn/134.11.3100

77. Rodahl, K., & Moore, T. (1943). The vitamin A content and toxicity of bear and seal liver. *Biochemical Journal, 37*(2), 166-168. doi:10.1042/bj0370166

78. Rothman, K. J., Moore, L. L., Singer, M. R., Nguyen, U. D., Mannino, S., & Milunsky, A. (1996). Teratogenicity of high vitamin A intake. (1996). *New England Journal of Medicine, 334*(18), 1195-1197. doi:10.1056/nejm199605023341813

79. Arnhold, T., Nau, H., Meyer, S., Rothkoetter, H. J., & Lampen, A. D. (2002). Porcine intestinal metabolism of excess vitamin A differs following vitamin A supplementation and liver consumption. *The Journal of Nutrition, 132*(2), 197-203. doi:10.1093/jn/132.2.197

80. Meléndez-Hevia, E., De Paz-Lugo, P., Cornish-Bowden, A., & Cárdenas, M. L. (2009). A weak link in metabolism: The metabolic capacity for glycine biosynthesis does not satisfy the need for collagen synthesis. *Journal of Biosciences, 34*(6), 853-872. doi:10.1007/s12038-009-0100-9

81. López-Corcuera, B., Geerlings, A., & Aragón, C. (2001). Glycine neurotransmitter transporters: an update. *Molecular Membrane Biology, 18*(1), 13-20. doi:10.1080/09687680120521

82. Regina, M., Korhonen, V., Smith, T., Alakuijala, L., & Eloranta, T. (1993). Methionine toxicity in the rat in relation to hepatic accumulation of S-adenosylmethionine: Prevention by dietary stimulation of the hepatic transsulfuration pathway. *Archives of Biochemistry and Biophysics, 300*(2), 598-607. doi:10.1006/abbi.1993.1083

83. Sugiyama, K., Kushima, Y., & Muramatsu, K. (1987). Effect of dietary glycine on methionine metabolism in rats fed a high-methionine diet. *Journal of Nutritional Science and Vitaminology, 33*(3), 195-205. doi:10.3177/jnsv.33.195

84. Sanz, A., Caro, P., Ayala, V., Portero-Otin, M., Pamplona, R., & Barja, G. (2006). Methionine restriction decreases mitochondrial oxygen radical generation and leak as well as oxidative damage to mitochondrial DNA and proteins. *The FASEB Journal, 20*(8), 1064-1073. doi:10.1096/fj.05-5568com

85. Miller, R. A., Harrison, D. E., Astle, C. M., Bogue, M. A., Brind, J., Fernandez, E., ... Strong, R. (2019). Glycine supplementation extends lifespan of male and female mice. *Aging Cell, 18*(3), e12953. doi:10.1111/acel.12953

86. Schuchardt, J., Schneider, I., Meyer, H., Neubronner, J., Von Schacky, C., & Hahn, A. (2011). Incorporation of EPA and DHA into plasma phospholipids in response to different omega-3 fatty acid formula-

tions - a comparative bioavailability study of fish oil vs. krill oil. *Lipids in Health and Disease, 10*(1), 145. doi:10.1186/1476-511x-10-145

87. Stefánsson, V. (2018). The laboratory check. In *The Fat of the Land* (pp. 87)

88. Rockwell, D. (2003). *Giving voice to bear: North American Indian myths, rituals, and images of the bear.* Roberts Rinehart.

89. Bilsborough, S., & Mann, N. (2006). A review of issues of dietary protein intake in humans. *International Journal of Sport Nutrition and Exercise Metabolism, 16*(2), 129-152. doi:10.1123/ijsnem.16.2.129

90. Westman, E. C., Yancy, W. S., Mavropoulos, J. C., Marquart, M., & McDuffie, J. R. (2008). The effect of a low-carbohydrate, ketogenic diet versus a low-glycemic index diet on glycemic control in type 2 diabetes mellitus. *Nutrition & Metabolism, 5*(1). doi:10.1186/1743-7075-5-36

91. Fürst, S. N., Philipsen, T., & Joergensen, J. C. (2007). Ten-year follow-up of endometrial ablation. *Acta Obstetricia et Gynecologica Scandinavica, 86*(3), 334-338. doi:10.1080/00016340601089701

92. Bough, K. J., Wetherington, J., Hassel, B., Pare, J. F., Gawryluk, J. W., Greene, J. G., ... Dingledine, R. J. (2006). Mitochondrial biogenesis in the anticonvulsant mechanism of the ketogenic diet. *Annals of Neurology, 60*(2), 223-235. doi:10.1002/ana.20899

93. Yin, J., Nielsen, M., Li, S., & Shi, J. (2019). Ketones improves apolipoprotein E4-related memory deficiency via sirtuin 3. *Aging.* doi:10.18632/aging.102070

94. Elamin, M., Ruskin, D. N., Masino, S. A., & Sacchetti, P. (2018). Ketogenic diet modulates NAD+-dependent enzymes and reduces DNA damage in hippocampus. *Frontiers in Cellular Neuroscience, 12.* doi:10.3389/fncel.2018.00263

95. Milder, J., & Patel, M. (2012). Modulation of oxidative stress and mitochondrial function by the ketogenic diet. *Epilepsy Research, 100*(3), 295-303. doi:10.1016/j.eplepsyres.2011.09.021

96. Volek, J., Sharman, M., Gómez, A., Judelson, D., Rubin, M., Watson, G., ... Kraemer, W. (2004). Comparison of energy-restricted very low-carbohydrate and low-fat diets on weight loss and body composition in overweight men and women. *Nutrition & metabolism, 1*(1), 13. doi:10.1186/1743-7075-1-13

97. McClernon, F. J., Yancy, W. S., Eberstein, J. A., Atkins, R. C., & Westman, E. C. (2007). The effects of a low-carbohydrate ketogenic diet and a low-fat diet on mood, hunger, and other self-reported symptoms. *Obesity, 15*(1), 182-182. doi:10.1038/oby.2007.516

98. Bostock, E. C., Kirkby, K. C., & Taylor, B. V. (2017). The current status of the ketogenic diet in psychiatry. *Frontiers in Psychiatry, 8.* doi:10.3389/fpsyt.2017.00043

99. Gasior, M., Rogawski, M. A., & Hartman, A. L. (2006). Neuroprotective and disease-modifying effects of the ketogenic diet. *Behavioural Pharmacology, 17*(5-6), 431-439. doi:10.1097/00008877-200609000-00009

100. Wood, R. J., Volek, J. S., Liu, Y., Shachter, N. S., Contois, J. H., & Fernandez, M. L. (2006). Carbohydrate restriction alters lipoprotein metabolism by modifying VLDL, LDL, and HDL subfraction distribution and size in overweight men. *The Journal of Nutrition, 136*(2), 384-389. doi:10.1093/jn/136.2.384

101. Mensink, R. P., Zock, P. L., Kester, A. D., & Katan, M. B. (2003). Effects of dietary fatty acids and carbohydrates on the ratio of serum total to HDL cholesterol and on serum lipids and apolipoproteins: a meta-analysis of 60 controlled trials. *The American Journal of Clinical Nutrition, 77*(5), 1146-1155. doi:10.1093/ajcn/77.5.1146

102. Ginsberg, H., Olefsky, J. M., Kimmerling, G., Crapo, P., & Reaven, G. M. (1976). Induction of hypertriglyceridemia by a low-fat diet. *The Journal of Clinical Endocrinology & Metabolism, 42*(4), 729-735. doi:10.1210/jcem-42-4-729

103. Rovenský, J., Stancíková, M., Masaryk, P., Svík, K., & Istok, R. (2003). Eggshell calcium in the prevention and treatment of osteoporosis. *Int J Clin Pharmacol Res, 23*(2-3), 83-92. Retrieved from https://www.ncbi.nlm.nih.gov/pubmed/15018022

104. Schaafsma, A., Pakan, I., Hofstede, G., Muskiet, F., Veer, E. V. D., & Vries, P. D. (2000). Mineral, amino acid, and hormonal composition of chicken eggshell powder and the evaluation of its use in human nutrition. *Poultry Science, 79*(12), 1833–1838. doi: 10.1093/ps/79.12.1833

105. Nutraingredients-usa.com. (2010, April 23). Eggshell calcium tests safe for heavy metals, says ESM. Retrieved from https://www.nutraingredients-usa.com/Article/2010/04/23/Eggshell-calcium-tests-safe-for-heavy-metals-says-ESM

106. Hsu, D., Lee, C., Tsai, W., & Chien, Y. (2017). Essential and toxic metals in animal bone broths. *Food & Nutrition Research, 61*(1), 1347478. doi:10.1080/16546628.2017.1347478

107. Pal, S., Radavelli-Bagatini, S., Hagger, M., & Ellis, V. (2014). Comparative effects of whey and casein proteins on satiety in overweight and obese individuals: a randomized controlled trial. *European Journal of Clinical Nutrition, 68*(9), 980-986. doi:10.1038/ejcn.2014.84

108. De Vadder, F., Gautier-Stein, A., & Mithieux, G. (2013). Satiety and the role of µ-opioid receptors in the portal vein. *Current Opinion in Pharmacology, 13*(6), 959-963. doi:10.1016/j.coph.2013.09.003

109. Pal, S., Woodford, K., Kukuljan, S., & Ho, S. (2015). Milk intolerance, beta-casein and lactose. *Nutrients, 7*(9), 7285–7297. doi:10.3390/nu7095339

110. Elliott, R. B., Harris, D. P., Hill, J. P., Bibby, N. J., & Wasmuth, H. E. (1999). Type I (insulin-dependent) diabetes mellitus and cow milk: Casein variant consumption. *Diabetologia, 42*(3), 292-296. doi:10.1007/s001250051153

111. Tailford, K., Berry, C. L., Thomas, A. C., & Campbell JH, J. H. (2003). A casein variant in cow's milk is atherogenic. *Atherosclerosis, 170*(1), 13-19. doi:10.1016/s0021-9150(03)00131-x

112. Cade, R., Privette, M., Fregly, M., Rowland, N., Sun, Z., Zele, V., Wagemaker, H. & Edelstein, C. (2000) Autism and schizophrenia: Intestinal disorders, nutritional neuroscience, 3:1, 57-72, DOI: 10.1080/1028415X.2000.11747303

113. Pizzorno L. (2015). Nothing boring about boron. *Integrative medicine (Encinitas, Calif.), 14*(4), 35–48.

114. Ergul, A. B., Kara, M., Karakukcu, C., Tasdemir, A., Aslaner, H., Ergul, M. A., ... Torun, Y. A. (2018). High doses of boron have no protective effect against nephrolithiasis or oxidative stress in a rat model. *Biological Trace Element Research, 186*(1), 218-225. doi:10.1007/s12011-018-1294-1

115. Naghii, M. R., Einollahi, B., & Rostami, Z. (2012). Preliminary evidence hints at a protective role for boron in urolithiasis. *The Journal of Alternative and Complementary Medicine, 18*(3), 207-209. doi:10.1089/acm.2011.0865

116. Newnham, R. E. (1994). Essentiality of boron for healthy bones and joints. *Environmental Health Perspectives, 102*, 83. doi:10.2307/3431968

117. Mankarious, S., Lee, M., Fischer, S., Pyun, K. H., Ochs, H. D., Oxelius, V. A., & Wedgwood RJ, R. J. (1988). The half-lives of IgG subclasses and specific antibodies in patients with primary immunodeficiency who are receiving intravenously administered immunoglobulin. *J Lab Clin Med, 112*(5), 634-640. Retrieved from https://www.ncbi.nlm.nih.gov/pubmed/3183495

118. Tóth, C., Dabóczi, A., Howard, M., J. Miller, N., & Clemens, Z. (2016). Crohn's disease successfully treated with the paleolithic ketogenic diet. *International Journal of Case Reports and Images, 7*(9), 570. doi:10.5348/ijcri-2016102-cr-10690

119. Westman, E. C., Yancy, W. S., Mavropoulos, J. C., Marquart, M., & McDuffie, J. R. (2008). The effect of a low-carbohydrate, ketogenic diet versus a low-glycemic index diet on glycemic control in type 2 diabetes mellitus. *Nutrition & Metabolism, 5*(1). doi:10.1186/1743-7075-5-36

120. Yancy, W. S., Jr, Foy, M., Chalecki, A. M., Vernon, M. C., & Westman, E. C. (2005). A low-carbohydrate, ketogenic diet to treat type 2 diabetes. *Nutrition & metabolism, 2*, 34. doi:10.1186/1743-7075-2-34

121. Hussain, T. A., Mathew, T. C., Dashti, A. A., Asfar, S., Al-Zaid, N., & Dashti, H. M. (2012). Effect of low-calorie versus low-carbohydrate ketogenic diet in type 2 diabetes. *Nutrition, 28*(10), 1016-1021. doi:10.1016/j.nut.2012.01.016

122. Tóth, C., & Clemens, Z. (2015). Successful treatment of a patient with obesity, type 2 diabetes and hypertension with the paleolithic ketogenic diet. *International Journal of Case Reports and Images, 6*(3), 161. doi:10.5348/ijcri-201530-cr-10491

123. Tóth, C., & Clemens, Z. (2015). A child with type 1 diabetes mellitus (T1DM) successfully treated with the Paleolithic ketogenic diet: A 19-month insulin-freedom. *International Journal of Case Reports and Images, 6*(12), 752. doi:10.5348/ijcri-2015121-cr-10582

124. Tóth, C., & Clemens, Z. (2014). Type 1 diabetes mellitus successfully managed with the paleolithic ketogenic diet. *International Journal of Case Reports and Images, 5*(10), 699. doi:10.5348/ijcri-2014124-cr-10435

125. Clemens, Zsofia & Dabóczi, Andrea & Tóth, Csaba. (2019). Paleolithic ketogenic diet (PKD) as a standalone therapy in cancer: Case studies. 10.13140/RG.2.2.28600.19208.

126. Tóth, C., & Schimmer, Zsófia Clemens, M. (2018). Complete Cessation of Recurrent Cervical Intraepithelial Neoplasia (CIN) by the Paleolithic Ketogenic Diet: A Case Report. *Journal of Cancer Research and Treatment, 6*(1), 1-5. doi:10.12691/jcrt-6-1-1

127. Tóth, C., & Clemens, Z. (2017). Treatment of Rectal Cancer with the Paleolithic Ketogenic Diet: A 24-months Follow-up. *American Journal of Medical Case Reports, 5*(8), 205-216. doi:10.12691/ajmcr-5-8-3

128. Tóth, C., & Clemens, Z. (2015). Gilbert's syndrome successfully treated with the paleolithic ketogenic diet. *American Journal of Medical Case Reports, 3*(4), 117-120. doi:10.12691/ajmcr-3-4-9

129. Clemens, Z., Kelemen, A., Fogarasi, A., & Tóth, C. (2013). Childhood absence epilepsy successfully treated with the paleolithic ketogenic diet. *Neurology and Therapy, 2*(1-2), 71-76. doi:10.1007/s40120-013-0013-2

CHAPTER 13

1. Tóth, C., Dabóczi, A., Howard, M., J. Miller, N., & Clemens, Z. (2016). Crohn's disease successfully treated with the paleolithic ketogenic diet. *International Journal of Case Reports and Images, 7*(9), 570. doi:10.5348/ijcri-2016102-cr-10690

2. Wojtyniak, K., & Szajewska, H. (2017). Systematic review: Probiotics for functional constipation in children. *European Journal of Pediatrics, 176*(9), 1155-1162. doi:10.1007/s00431-017-2972-2

3. Koliaki, C., Kokkinos, A., Tentolouris, N., & Katsilambros, N. (2010). The effect of ingested macronutrients on postprandial ghrelin response: A critical review of existing literature data. *International Journal of Peptides, 2010*, 1-9. doi:10.1155/2010/710852

4. Palego, L., Betti, L., Rossi, A., & Giannaccini, G. (2016). Tryptophan biochemistry: Structural, nutritional, metabolic, and medical aspects in humans. *Journal of Amino Acids, 2016*, 1-13. doi:10.1155/2016/8952520

5. Daniel, P. M., Love, E. R., Moorhouse, S. R., & Pratt, O. E. (1981). The effect of insulin upon the in-flux of tryptophan into the brain of the rabbit. *The Journal of Physiology, 312*(1), 551-562. doi:10.1113/jphysiol.1981.sp013643

6. Gröber, U., Werner, T., Vormann, J., & Kisters, K. (2017). Myth or reality—Transdermal magnesium? *Nutrients, 9*(8), 813. doi:10.3390/nu9080813

7. Maintz, L., & Novak, N. (2007). Histamine and histamine intolerance. *The American Journal of Clinical Nutrition, 85*(5), 1185-1196. doi:10.1093/ajcn/85.5.1185

8. Cho, C., Fong, L., Ma, P., & Ogle, C. (1987). Zinc deficiency: Its role in gastric secretion and stress-induced gastric ulceration in rats. *Pharmacology Biochemistry and Behavior, 26*(2), 293-297. doi:10.1016/0091-3057(87)90121-3

9. Shafaghi, A., Hasanzadeh, J., Mansour-Ghanaei, F., Joukar, F., & Yaseri, M. (2016). The effect of zinc supplementation on the symptoms of gastroesophageal reflux disease: A randomized clinical trial. *Middle East Journal of Digestive Diseases, 8*(4), 289-296. doi:10.15171/mejdd.2016.38

10. Blumrich, M., Pack, R., Oesch, F., Petzinger, E., & Steinberg, P. (1994). Deficiency of bile acid transport and synthesis in oval cells from carcinogen-fed rats. *Hepatology, 19*(3), 722-727. doi:10.1002/hep.1840190326

11. LeBlanc, M., Gavino, V., Pérea, A., Yousef, I. M., Lévy, E., & Tuchweber, B. (1998). The role of dietary choline in the beneficial effects of lecithin on the secretion of biliary lipids in rats. *Biochimica et Biophysica Acta (BBA) - Lipids and Lipid Metabolism, 1393*(2-3), 223-234. doi:10.1016/s0005-2760(98)00072-1

12. Boyer, J. L. (2013). Bile formation and secretion. *Comprehensive Physiology.* doi:10.1002/cphy.c120027

13. Hofmann, A. F. (1989). Medical dissolution of gallstones by oral bile acid therapy. *The American Journal of Surgery, 158*(3), 198-204. doi:10.1016/0002-9610(89)90252-3

14. Kasbo, J., Tuchweber, B., Perwaiz, S., Bouchard, G., Lafont, H., Domingo, N., … Yousef, I. M. (2003). Phosphatidylcholine-enriched diet prevents gallstone formation in mice susceptible to cholelithiasis. *Journal of Lipid Research, 44*(12), 2297-2303. doi:10.1194/jlr.m300180-jlr200

15. Mahley, R. W. (2016). Apolipoprotein E: From cardiovascular disease to neurodegenerative disorders. *Journal of Molecular Medicine, 94*(7), 739-746. doi:10.1007/s00109-016-1427-y

16. Farrer, L. A., Cupples, A., Haines, J. L., Hyman, B., Kukull, W. A., Mayeux, R., … Myers, R. H. (1997). Effects of age, sex, and ethnicity on the association between apolipoprotein E genotype and Alzheimer disease. *JAMA, 278*(16), 1349. doi:10.1001/jama.1997.03550160069041

17. Trumble, B. C., Stieglitz, J., Blackwell, A. D., Allayee, H., Beheim, B., Finch, C. E., … Kaplan, H. (2017). Apolipoprotein E4 is associated with improved cognitive function in Amazonian forager-horticulturalists with a high parasite burden. *The FASEB Journal, 31*(4), 1508-1515. doi:10.1096/fj.201601084r

18. Vasunilashorn, S., Finch, C. E., Crimmins, E. M., Vikman, S. A., Stieglitz, J., Gurven, M., … Allayee, H. (2011). Inflammatory gene variants in the Tsimane, an indigenous Bolivian population with a high infectious load. *Biodemography and Social Biology, 57*(1), 33-52. doi:10.1080/19485565.2011.564475

19. Hall, K., Murrell, J., Ogunniyi, A., Deeg, M., Baiyewu, O., Gao, S., … Hendrie, H. (2006). Cholesterol, APOE genotype, and Alzheimer disease: An epidemiologic study of Nigerian Yoruba. *Neurology, 66*(2), 223-227. doi:10.1212/01.wnl.0000194507.39504.17

20. Huebbe, P., & Rimbach, G. (2017). Evolution of human apolipoprotein E (APOE) isoforms: Gene structure, protein function and interaction with dietary factors. *Ageing Research Reviews, 37*, 146-161. doi:10.1016/j.arr.2017.06.002

21. Finch, C., & Stanford, C. (2004). Meat-adaptive genes and the evolution of slower aging in humans. *The Quarterly Review of Biology, 79*(1), 3-50. doi:10.1086/381662

22. Talbot, K., Wang, H., Kazi, H., Han, L., Bakshi, K. P., Stucky, A., … Arnold, S. E. (2012). Demonstrated brain insulin resistance in Alzheimer's disease patients is associated with IGF-1 resistance, IRS-1 dysregulation, and cognitive decline. *Journal of Clinical Investigation, 122*(4), 1316-1338. doi:10.1172/jci59903

23. Zhao, N., Liu, C., Van Ingelgom, A. J., Martens, Y. A., Linares, C., Knight, J. A., … Bu, G. (2017). Apolipoprotein E4 impairs neuronal insulin signaling by trapping insulin receptor in the endosomes. *Neuron, 96*(1), 115-129.e5. doi:10.1016/j.neuron.2017.09.003

24. Fallaize, R., Carvalho-Wells, A. L., Tierney, A. C., Marin, C., Kieć-Wilk, B., Dembińska-Kieć, A., … Lovegrove, J. A. (2017). APOE genotype influences insulin resistance, apolipoprotein CII and CIII according to plasma fatty acid profile in the Metabolic Syndrome. *Scientific Reports, 7*(1). doi:10.1038/s41598-017-05802-2

25. Stoykovich, S., & Gibas, K. (2019). APOE ε4, the door to insulin-resistant dyslipidemia and brain fog? A case study. *Alzheimer's & Dementia: Diagnosis, Assessment & Disease Monitoring, 11*, 264-269. doi:10.1016/j.dadm.2019.01.009

26. Araújo, J., Cai, J., & Stevens, J. (2019). Prevalence of optimal metabolic health in american adults: National health and nutrition examination survey 2009–2016. *Metabolic Syndrome and Related Disorders, 17*(1), 46-52. doi:10.1089/met.2018.0105

27. Stoykovich, S., & Gibas, K. (2019). APOE ε4, the door to insulin-resistant dyslipidemia and brain fog? A case study. *Alzheimer's & Dementia: Diagnosis, Assessment & Disease Monitoring, 11*(1), 264-269. doi:10.1016/j.dadm.2019.01.009

28. Frayling, T. M., Timpson, N. J., Weedon, M. N., Zeggini, E., Freathy, R. M., Lindgren, C. M., ... McCarthy, M. I. (2007). A common variant in the FTO gene is associated with body mass index and predisposes to childhood and adult obesity. *Science (New York, N.Y.)*, *316*(5826), 889–894. doi:10.1126/science.1141634

29. Loos, R. J., & Yeo, G. S. (2013). The bigger picture of FTO—the first GWAS-identified obesity gene. *Nature Reviews Endocrinology*, *10*(1), 51-61. doi:10.1038/nrendo.2013.227

30. Phillips, C. M., Kesse-Guyot, E., McManus, R., Hercberg, S., Lairon, D., Planells, R., & Roche, H. M. (2012). High Dietary Saturated Fat Intake Accentuates Obesity Risk Associated with the Fat Mass and Obesity–Associated Gene in Adults. *The Journal of Nutrition*, *142*(5), 824-831. doi:10.3945/jn.111.153460

Chapter 14

1. White, R. R., & Hall, M. B. (2017). Nutritional and greenhouse gas impacts of removing animals from US agriculture. *Proceedings of the National Academy of Sciences*, *114*(48), E10301-E10308. doi:10.1073/pnas.1707322114

2. Rotz, C. A., Asem-Hiablie, S., Place, S., & Thoma, G. (2019). Environmental footprints of beef cattle production in the United States. *Agricultural Systems*, *169*, 1-13. doi:10.1016/j.agsy.2018.11.005

3. Qiancheng, M. (2018, April 9). NASA GISS: Science briefs: Greenhouse gases: Refining the role of carbon dioxide. Retrieved from https://www.giss.nasa.gov/research/briefs/ma_01/

4. The keeling curve. (2019, December). Retrieved from https://scripps.ucsd.edu/programs/keelingcurve/

5. Weil, Raymond & Brady, Nyle. (2016). The nature and properties of soils. 15th edition.

6. Swift, R. S. (2001). Sequestration of carbon by soil. *Soil Science*, *166*(11), 858-871.

7. Ontl, T. A. & Schulte, L. A. (2012) Soil carbon storage. *Nature Education Knowledge* 3(10):35

8. White Oak Pastures Team. (2019, June 4). White oak pastures beef reduces atmospheric carbon. Retrieved from http://blog.whiteoakpastures.com/blog/carbon-negative-grassfed-beef

Frequently Asked Questions

1. Descalzo, A., Rossetti, L., Grigioni, G., Irurueta, M., Sancho, A., Carrete, J., & Pensel, N. (2007). Antioxidant status and odour profile in fresh beef from pasture or grain-fed cattle. *Meat Science*, *75*(2), 299-307. doi:10.1016/j.meatsci.2006.07.015

2. Daley, C. A., Abbott, A., Doyle, P. S., Nader, G. A., & Larson, S. (2010). A review of fatty acid profiles and antioxidant content in grass-fed and grain-fed beef. *Nutrition Journal*, *9*(1). doi:10.1186/1475-2891-9-10

3. Charnley, G., & Doull, J. (2005). Human exposure to dioxins from food, 1999–2002. *Food and Chemical Toxicology*, *43*(5), 671-679. doi:10.1016/j.fct.2005.01.006

4. Mathews, K. H., & Johnson, R. (2013). *Alternative beef production systems: Issues and implications* (LDPM-218-01). Retrieved from Economic Research Service/USDA website: https://www.ers.usda.gov/webdocs/publications/37473/36491_ldpm-218-01.pdf?v=0

5. Albanito, L., Lappano, R., Madeo, A., Chimento, A., Prossnitz, E. R., Cappello, A. R., ... Maggiolini, M. (2015). Effects of atrazine on estrogen receptor α – and G protein–coupled receptor 30–mediated signaling and proliferation in cancer cells and cancer-associated fibroblasts. *Environmental Health Perspectives*, *123*(5), 493-499. doi:10.1289/ehp.1408586

6. Hayes, T. B., Khoury, V., Narayan, A., Nazir, M., Park, A., Brown, T., ... Gallipeau, S. (2010). Atrazine induces complete feminization and chemical castration in male African clawed frogs (Xenopus laevis). *Proceedings of the National Academy of Sciences*, *107*(10), 4612-4617. doi:10.1073/pnas.0909519107

7. Sydenham, E. W., Shephard, G. S., Thiel, P. G., Marasas, W. F., & Stockenstrom, S. (1991). Fumonisin contamination of commercial corn-based human foodstuffs. *Journal of Agricultural and Food Chemistry*, *39*(11), 2014-2018. doi:10.1021/jf00011a028

8. Yazar, S., & Omurtag, G. (2008). Fumonisins, trichothecenes and zearalenone in cereals. *International Journal of Molecular Sciences*, *9*(11), 2062-2090. doi:10.3390/ijms9112062

9. Wang, Z., Zheng, Y., Zhao, B., Zhang, Y., Liu, Z., Xu, J., ... Abliz, Z. (2015). Human metabolic responses to chronic environmental polycyclic aromatic hydrocarbon exposure by a metabolomic approach. *Journal of Proteome Research*, *14*(6), 2583-2593. doi:10.1021/acs.jproteome.5b00134

10. Russo, C., Ferk, F., Mišík, M., Ropek, N., Nersesyan, A., Mejri, D., ... Knasmüller, S. (2018). Low doses of widely consumed cannabinoids (cannabidiol and cannabidivarin) cause DNA damage and chromosomal aberrations in human-derived cells. *Archives of Toxicology*, *93*(1), 179-188. doi:10.1007/s00204-018-2322-9

11. O'Donnell,, M., Mente, A., Rangarajan, S., McQueen, M. J., Wang, X., Liu, L., ... Yan, H. (2014). Urinary sodium and potassium excretion, mortality, and cardiovascular events. *New England Journal of Medicine*, *371*(13), 1267-1267. doi:10.1056/nejmx140049

12. Azoulay, A., Garzon, P., & Eisenberg, M. J. (2001). Comparison of the mineral content of tap water and bottled waters. *Journal of General Internal Medicine*, *16*(3), 168-175. doi:10.1111/j.1525-1497.2001.04189.x

13. Huang, A. H. (2017). Plant lipid droplets and their associated proteins: Potential for rapid advances. *Plant Physiology*, *176*(3), 1894-1918. doi:10.1104/pp.17.01677

14. Leduc, V., Moneret-Vautrin, D. A., Tzen, J. T., Morisset, M., Guerin, L., & Kanny, G. (2006). Identification of oleosins as major allergens in sesame seed allergic patients. *Allergy, 61*(3), 349-356. doi:10.1111/j.1398-9995.2006.01013.x

15. Schwager, C., Kull, S., Behrends, J., Röckendorf, N., Schocker, F., Frey, A., ... Jappe, U. (2017). Peanut oleosins associated with severe peanut allergy—importance of lipophilic allergens for comprehensive allergy diagnostics. *Journal of Allergy and Clinical Immunology, 140*(5), 1331-1338.e8. doi:10.1016/j.jaci.2017.02.020

16. Li, D. D., & Fan, Y. M. (2009). Cloning, characterisation, and expression analysis of an oleosin gene in coconut (Cocos nuciferaL.) pulp. *The Journal of Horticultural Science and Biotechnology, 84*(5), 483-488. doi:10.1080/1 4620316.2009.11512552

17. Parthibane, V., Rajakumari, S., Venkateshwari, V., Iyappan, R., & Rajasekharan, R. (2011). Oleosin is bifunctional enzyme that has both monoacylglycerol acyltransferase and phospholipase activities. *Journal of Biological Chemistry, 287*(3), 1946-1954. doi:10.1074/jbc.m111.309955

18. Giannoulia, K., Banilas, G., & Hatzopoulos, P. (2007). Oleosin gene expression in olive. *Journal of Plant Physiology, 164*(1), 104-107. doi:10.1016/j.jplph.2006.03.016

19. McCarty, M. F., DiNicolantonio, J. J., & O'Keefe, J. H. (2015). Ketosis may promote brain macroautophagy by activating Sirt1 and hypoxia-inducible factor-1. *Medical Hypotheses, 85*(5), 631-639. doi:10.1016/j.mehy.2015.08.002

20. Jamshed, H., Beyl, R. A., Della Manna, D. L., Yang, E. S., Ravussin, E., & Peterson, C. M. (2019). Early Time-restricted feeding improves 24-hour glucose levels and affects markers of the circadian clock, aging, and autophagy in Humans. *Nutrients, 11*(6), 1234. doi:10.3390/nu11061234

21. Mandal, P. K. (2005). Dioxin: A review of its environmental effects and its aryl hydrocarbon receptor biology. *Journal of Comparative Physiology B, 175*(4), 221-230. doi:10.1007/s00360-005-0483-3

22. Kogevinas, M. (2001). Human health effects of dioxins: Cancer, reproductive and endocrine system effects. *APMIS, 109*(S103), S223-S232. doi:10.1111/j.1600-0463.2001.tb05771.x

23. Baars, A., Bakker, M., Baumann, R., Boon, P., Freijer, J., Hoogenboom, L., ... De Vries, J. (2004). Dioxins, dioxin-like PCBs and non-dioxin-like PCBs in foodstuffs: Occurrence and dietary intake in The Netherlands. *Toxicology Letters, 151*(1), 51-61. doi:10.1016/j.toxlet.2004.01.028

24. Kiviranta, H., Ovaskainen, M., & Vartiainen, T. (2004). Market basket study on dietary intake of PCDD/Fs, PCBs, and PBDEs in Finland. *Environment International, 30*(7), 923-932. doi:10.1016/j.envint.2004.03.002

25. Papadopoulos, A., Vassiliadou, I., Costopoulou, D., Papanicolaou, C., & Leondiadis, L. (2004). Levels of dioxins and dioxin-like PCBs in food samples on the Greek market. *Chemosphere, 57*(5), 413-419. doi:10.1016/j.chemosphere.2004.07.006

26. Elamin, M., Ruskin, D. N., Masino, S. A., & Sacchetti, P. (2018). Ketogenic diet modulates NAD+-dependent enzymes and reduces DNA damage in hippocampus. *Frontiers in Cellular Neuroscience, 12.* doi:10.3389/fncel.2018.00263

27. Milder, J., & Patel, M. (2012). Modulation of oxidative stress and mitochondrial function by the ketogenic diet. *Epilepsy Research, 100*(3), 295-303. doi:10.1016/j.eplepsyres.2011.09.021

28. Fürst, S. N., Philipsen, T., & Joergensen, J. C. (2007). Ten-year follow-up of endometrial ablation. *Acta Obstetricia et Gynecologica Scandinavica, 86*(3), 334-338. doi:10.1080/00016340601089701

29. Gasior, M., Rogawski, M. A., & Hartman, A. L. (2006). Neuroprotective and disease-modifying effects of the ketogenic diet. *Behavioural Pharmacology, 17*(5-6), 431-439. doi:10.1097/00008877-200609000-00009

30. Volek, J. S., Sharman, M. J., Love, D. M., Avery, N. G., G[oacute]mez, A. L., Scheett, T. P., & Kraemer, W. J. (2002). Body composition and hormonal responses to a carbohydrate-restricted diet. *Metabolism, 51*(7), 864-870. doi:10.1053/meta.2002.32037

31. Volek, J. S., & Sharman, M. J. (2004). Cardiovascular and Hormonal Aspects of Very-Low-Carbohydrate Ketogenic Diets. *Obesity Research, 12*(S11), 115S-123S. doi:10.1038/oby.2004.276

32. Gonzalez-Bono, E., Rohleder, N., Hellhammer, D. H., Salvador, A., & Kirschbaum, C. (2002). Glucose but not protein or fat load amplifies the cortisol response to psychosocial stress. *Hormones and Behavior, 41*(3), 328-333. doi:10.1006/hbeh.2002.1766

33. Dashti, H. M., Mathew, T. C., Hussein, T., Asfar, S. K., Behbahani, A., Khoursheed, M. A., ... Al-Zaid, N. S. (2004). Long-term effects of a ketogenic diet in obese patients. *Experimental and clinical cardiology, 9*(3), 200–205.

34. McGrice, M., & Porter, J. (2017). The effect of low carbohydrate diets on fertility hormones and outcomes in overweight and obese women: A systematic review. *Nutrients, 9*(3), 204. doi:10.3390/nu9030204

35. Mavropoulos, J. C., Yancy, W. S., Hepburn, J., & Westman, E. C. (2005). The effects of a low-carbohydrate, ketogenic diet on the polycystic ovary syndrome: A pilot study. *Nutrition & metabolism, 2,* 35. doi:10.1186/1743-7075-2-35

36. Kapetanakis, M., Liuba, P., Odermarsky, M., Lundgren, J., & Hallböök, T. (2014). Effects of ketogenic diet on vascular function. *European Journal of Paediatric Neurology, 18*(4), 489-494. doi:10.1016/j.ejpn.2014.03.006

37. Dostal, T., Plews, D. J., Hofmann, P., Laursen, P. B., & Cipryan, L. (2019). Effects of a 12-week very-low carbohydrate high-fat diet on maximal aerobic capacity, high-intensity intermittent exercise, and cardiac autonomic regulation: Non-randomized parallel-group study. *Frontiers in Physiology, 10.* doi:10.3389/fphys.2019.00912

38. Ebbeling, C. B., Feldman, H. A., Klein, G. L., Wong, J. M., Bielak, L., Steltz, S. K., ... Ludwig, D. S. (2018). Effects of a low carbohydrate diet on energy expenditure during weight loss maintenance: randomized trial. *BMJ*, k4583. doi:10.1136/bmj.k4583

39. Volek, J., Sharman, M., Gómez, A., Judelson, D., Rubin, M., Watson, G., ... Kraemer, W. (2004). Comparison of energy-restricted very low-carbohydrate and low-fat diets on weight loss and body composition in overweight men and women. *Nutrition & metabolism*, *1*(1), 13. doi:10.1186/1743-7075-1-13

40. Phinney, S., Bistrian, B., Wolfe, R., & Blackburn, G. (1983). The human metabolic response to chronic ketosis without caloric restriction: Physical and biochemical adaptation. *Metabolism*, *32*(8), 757-768. doi:10.1016/0026-0495(83)90105-1

41. Messina, G., Esposito, T., Lobaccaro, J., Esposito, M., Monda, V., Messina, A., ... Monda, M. (2016). Effects of low-carbohydrate diet therapy in overweight subject with autoimmune thyroiditis: possible synergism with ChREBP. *Drug Design, Development and Therapy, Volume 10*, 2939-2946. doi:10.2147/dddt.s106440

42. Cox, P., Kirk, T., Ashmore, T., Willerton, K., Evans, R., Smith, A., ... Clarke, K. (2016). Nutritional ketosis alters fuel preference and thereby endurance performance in athletes. *Cell Metabolism*, *24*(2), 256-268. doi:10.1016/j.cmet.2016.07.010

43. Volek, J. S., Freidenreich, D. J., Saenz, C., Kunces, L. J., Creighton, B. C., Bartley, J. M., ... Phinney, S. D. (2016). Metabolic characteristics of keto-adapted ultra-endurance runners. *Metabolism*, *65*(3), 100-110. doi:10.1016/j.metabol.2015.10.028

44. Holt, R., Roberts, G., & Scully, C. (2001). Dental damage, sequelae, and prevention. *Western Journal of Medicine*, *174*(4), 288-290. doi:10.1136/ewjm.174.4.288

45. McClellan, W. S., & Du Bois, E. F. (1930). Prolonged meat diets with a study of kidney function and ketosis. *Journal of Biological Chemistry*, *87*, 651-668. Retrieved from http://www.jbc.org/content/87/3/651.citation

46. Brehm, B. J., Seeley, R. J., Daniels, S. R., & D'Alessio, D. A. (2003). A randomized trial comparing a very low carbohydrate diet and a calorie-restricted low fat diet on body weight and cardiovascular risk factors in healthy women. *The Journal of Clinical Endocrinology & Metabolism*, *88*(4), 1617-1623. doi:10.1210/jc.2002-021480

47. Jabekk, P. T., Moe, I. A., Meen, H. D., Tomten, S. E., & Høstmark, A. T. (2010). Resistance training in overweight women on a ketogenic diet conserved lean body mass while reducing body fat. *Nutrition & Metabolism*, *7*(1), 17. doi:10.1186/1743-7075-7-17

48. Sidbury, J., & Dong, B. L. (1962). Ketosis in infants and children. *The Journal of Pediatrics*, *60*(2), 294-303. doi:10.1016/s0022-3476(62)80049-3

49. Wood, T., Stubbs, B., & Juul, S. (2018). Exogenous ketone bodies as promising neuroprotective agents for developmental brain injury. *Developmental Neuroscience*, *40*(5-6), 451-462. doi:10.1159/000499563

50. Rudolf, M. C., & Sherwin, R. S. (1983). Maternal ketosis and its effects on the fetus. *Clinics in Endocrinology and Metabolism*, *12*(2), 413-428. doi:10.1016/s0300-595x(83)80049-8

51. Lennerz, B. S., Barton, A., Bernstein, R. K., Dikeman, R. D., Diulus, C., Hallberg, S., ... Rhodes, E. T. (2018). Management of type 1 diabetes with a very low–carbohydrate diet. *Pediatrics*, *141*(6), e20173349. doi:10.1542/peds.2017-3349

ACKNOWLEDGEMENTS

There is nothing in my life that I have ever done like editing a book, and those who helped with this process will always have my profound gratitude. Dillon Randolph, you've been a champion throughout this process. Thank you so much for all of your help with edits, references, and lending an ear during times of feeling overwhelmed. Dad, what a joy it has been having you involved with this process. Thank you for all of your work helping me to craft this book into something that will positively affect the lives of others. I'd also like to thank Fairfax Hackley for the mentoring and suggestions regarding cover design. In addition, Joshua Fields Millburn and Ryan Nicodemus from The Minimalists for their support, and Jeff Sarris and Dave LaTulippe at SPYR for their additional design help.

I would also like to acknowledge others in the space who are fighting for the same things and helping others lead healthier lives. This tribe is too big to name every member, but it includes Dr. Shawn Baker, Dr. Ken Berry, Dr. Jaime Seeman, Dr. Gabrielle Lyon, Dr. Tommy Wood, Dr. Joe Mercola, Robb Wolf, Mikhaila Peterson, Anthony Gustin, Chris and Mark Bell, Kyle Kingsbury, Ben Greenfield, Danny Vega, Mark Sisson, Brian Sanders, Justin Nault, Ashley and Sarah Armstrong, Mike Mutzel, Judy Cho, Miki Ben-Dor, Bill von Hippel, and many others.

As a final acknowledgment, I would like to thank all of those in the health space who disagree with what I have written here and who have been willing to engage in conversations sharing their viewpoints. These individuals have been great teachers for me, and I look forward to many more conversations with them in the future. We must all seek truth, and the only way to do this is to challenge our ideas openly so that all may benefit from the discourse. I've got a feeling that after this book, there will be much more of this type of discussion in store!

Made in the USA
San Bernardino, CA
12 March 2020